Margaret Roberts

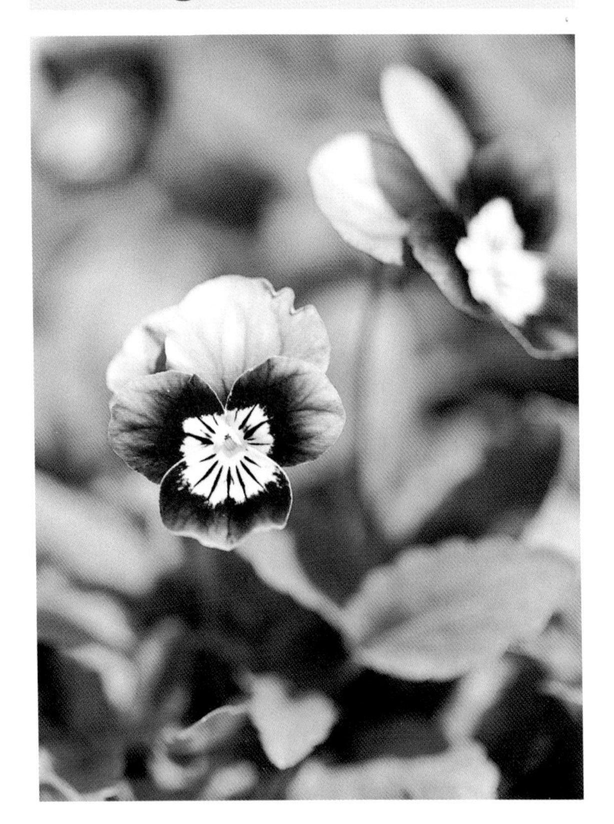

100 Edible & Healing Flowers

cultivating • cooking • restoring health

Text by **Margaret Roberts**

Photographs by **Phyllis Green**

Published by Struik Nature
(an imprint of Penguin Random House (Pty) Ltd)
Reg. No. 1953/000441/07
The Estuaries No 4, Oxbow Crescent,
Century Avenue, Century City 7441
PO Box 1144, Cape Town, 8000 South Africa

Visit **www.randomstruik.co.za** and join the Struik Nature Club
for updates, news, events, and special offers

First published in 2000 by Spearhead as *Edible & Medicinal Flowers*
New edition published in 2014 by Struik Nature

3 5 7 9 10 8 6 4 2

Publisher: Pippa Parker
Managing editor: Helen de Villiers
Editor: Julia Casciola
Project manager: Colette Alves
Design director: Janice Evans
Typesetting: Tessa Fortuin
Proofreader: Emsie du Plessis

Reproduction by Hirt & Carter Cape (Pty) Ltd
Printing and binding: Times Offset (M) Sdn Bhd, Malaysia

ISBN 978 1 77584 037 4 (Print)
ISBN 978 1 77584 152 4 (ePUB)
ISBN 978 1 77584 153 1 (ePDF)

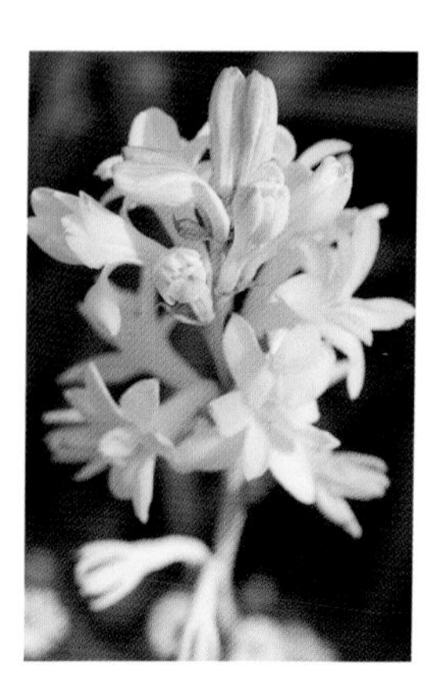

Sandy Roberts

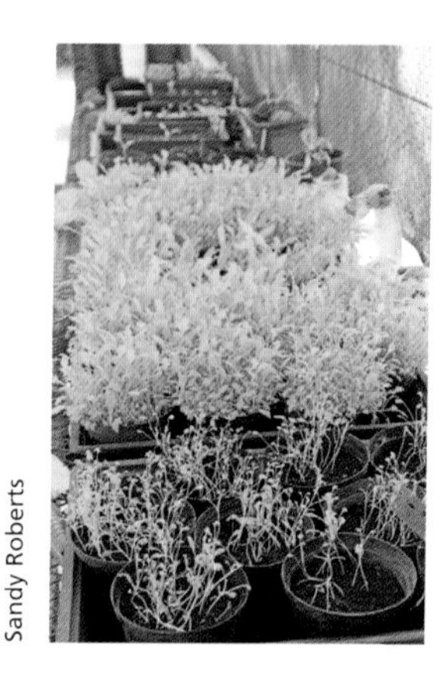

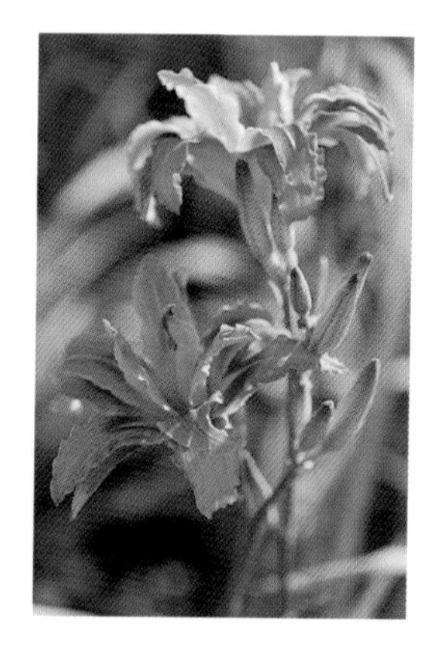

Sandy Roberts

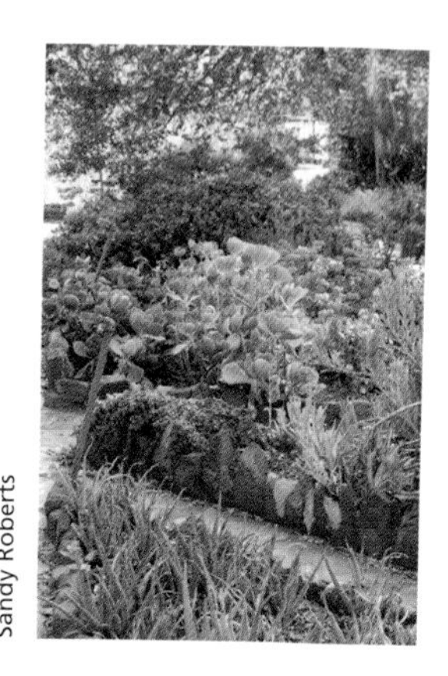

ALWAYS CONSULT YOUR DOCTOR BEFORE STARTING A HOME TREATMENT. THE INFORMATION IN THESE PAGES IS IN NO WAY INTENDED TO REPLACE YOUR DOCTOR'S ADVICE. ALWAYS BE 100% CERTAIN OF THE CORRECT IDENTIFICATION OF A PLANT BEFORE USING IT. WHEN IN DOUBT, DON'T USE!

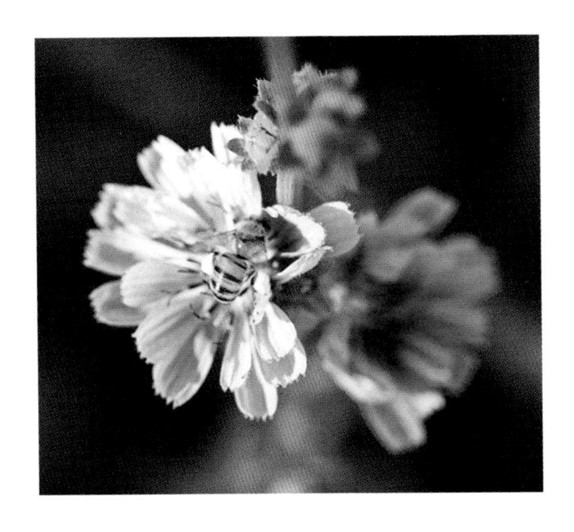

Contents

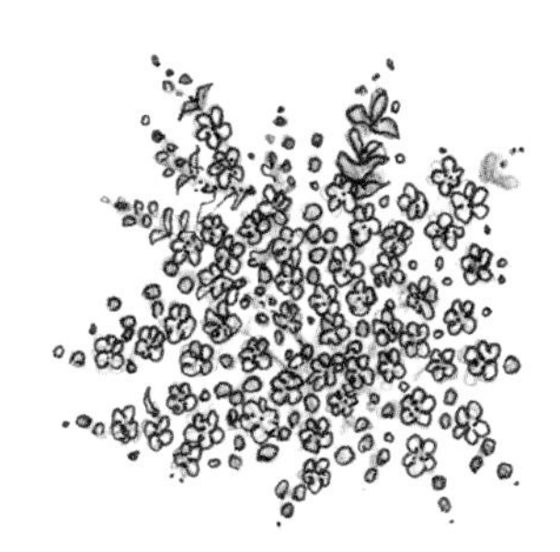

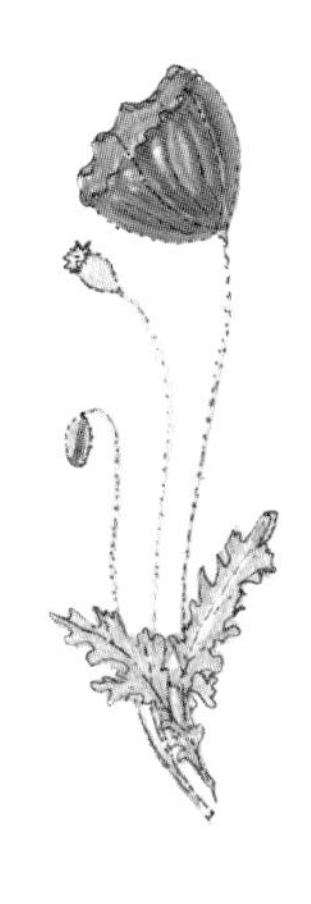

Acknowledgements

It is with great appreciation that I stand before a really amazing team of professional book creators. Thanks to Pippa Parker, who heads Struik Nature and whose unending and infectious ideas spark off so much I can hardly keep up! As a result of Janice Evans' incredible ability to create a visual feast, I look at this book in awe, and with the team of professional editors, layout designers, and competent and willing book creators like Colette Alves, I am thrilled to hand over my writings and recipes, knowing that they are putting in place a great and fascinating bouquet!

Once again, I thank my long-time friend, Annatjie van Wyk, who has played a part in so many of my books, for her patient typing of my many handwritten pages. Bless you for your ever willing assistance!

To Phyllis Green, for her numerous photographs of all the old familiar plants in the Herbal Centre gardens, and for the new beauties she has come to know and photograph, my most grateful thanks always.

To my daughter, Sandra, my endless gratitude for her new recipes and exciting food ideas, her endless support, her interest in all things edible that build health, and her kitchen garden that stretches further and further in front of her restaurant, which gives hotel school students and young chefs new ideas and inspiration.

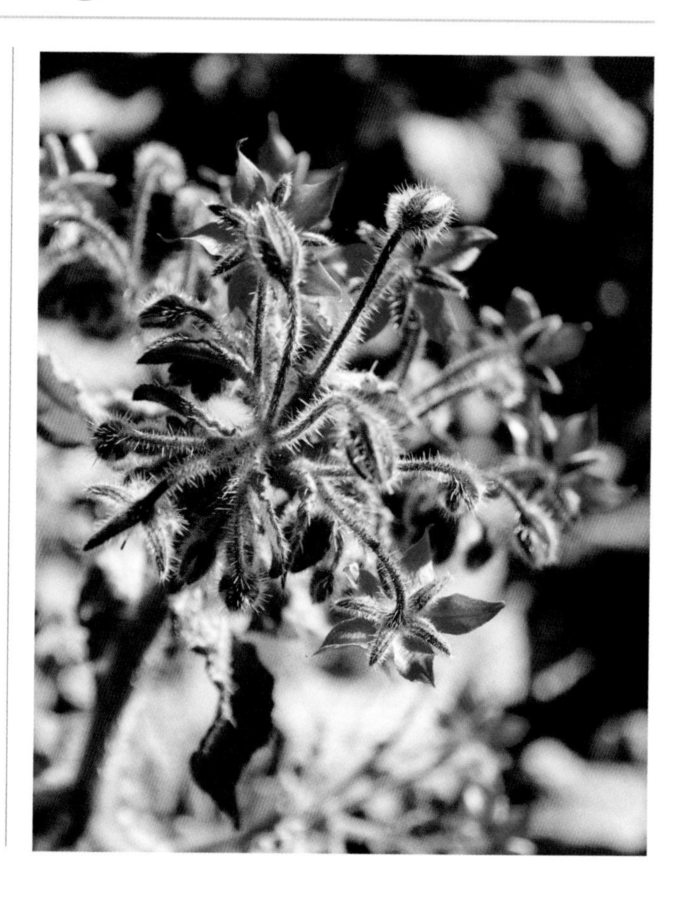

Flowers are surely the most beautiful of all God's creations. They say, 'I love you', 'I'm sorry', 'Please forgive me' and 'Thank you'. Flowers send blessings and good wishes. They are present in bouquets and posies at the beginning of our lives, throughout all the celebrations and great days, and also on the not-so-great days. And at the end of our lives, flowers speak of grief and mourning, of sympathy and compassion, of loss and the great change and challenge that death brings.

All the more precious is the role that flowers play in our day-to-day lives, where they can be incorporated into food, and used in bathing, washing, and healing of big and little wounds. Flowers are well loved, respected and appreciated. They thread their beauty into every aspect of our time here on Earth.

Is it any wonder, then, that they become our companions when all else becomes too much, too exhausting and too worrying? Just a breath of their fragrance, just a pause to look deep into the heart of a flower and experience that moment of upliftment, changes us for the better.

So here is a salute to flowers, a feeling of gratitude and wonder that nature gives us so much that betters, inspires and uplifts us. And here is to flower gardens everywhere!

Preface

In 2000 I wrote *Edible & Medicinal Flowers*, never dreaming that my gardens of flowers would reach into so many places, and so I was spurred on to rewrite it incorporating new recipes and the new flowers I have grown in the interim years.

Health, wellness and organic gardening go hand in hand, and with these easy-to-grow flowers and their vast edible and medicinal properties, I foresee an enjoyment of wellbeing, as people benefit from planting gardens of healing flowers.

And so I put into your hands my new recipes, thoughts, plantings – a garden of health and wealth – and I urge you to replan, rethink and replant your present garden into the paradise of food and natural medicine it was intended to be.

I dedicate this book to gardeners everywhere! May every page inspire you to grow your own edible and healing flowers close at hand for everyday use to build wellness and great positivity!

Margaret Roberts

Margaret Roberts
The Herbal Centre, De Wildt
North West Province, South Africa

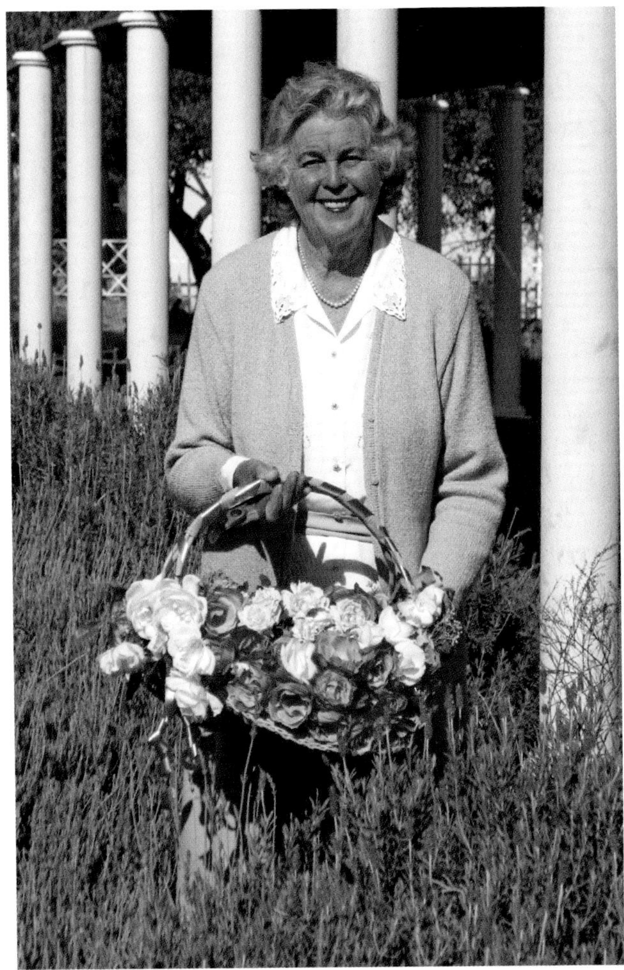

Sandy Roberts

The featured flowers

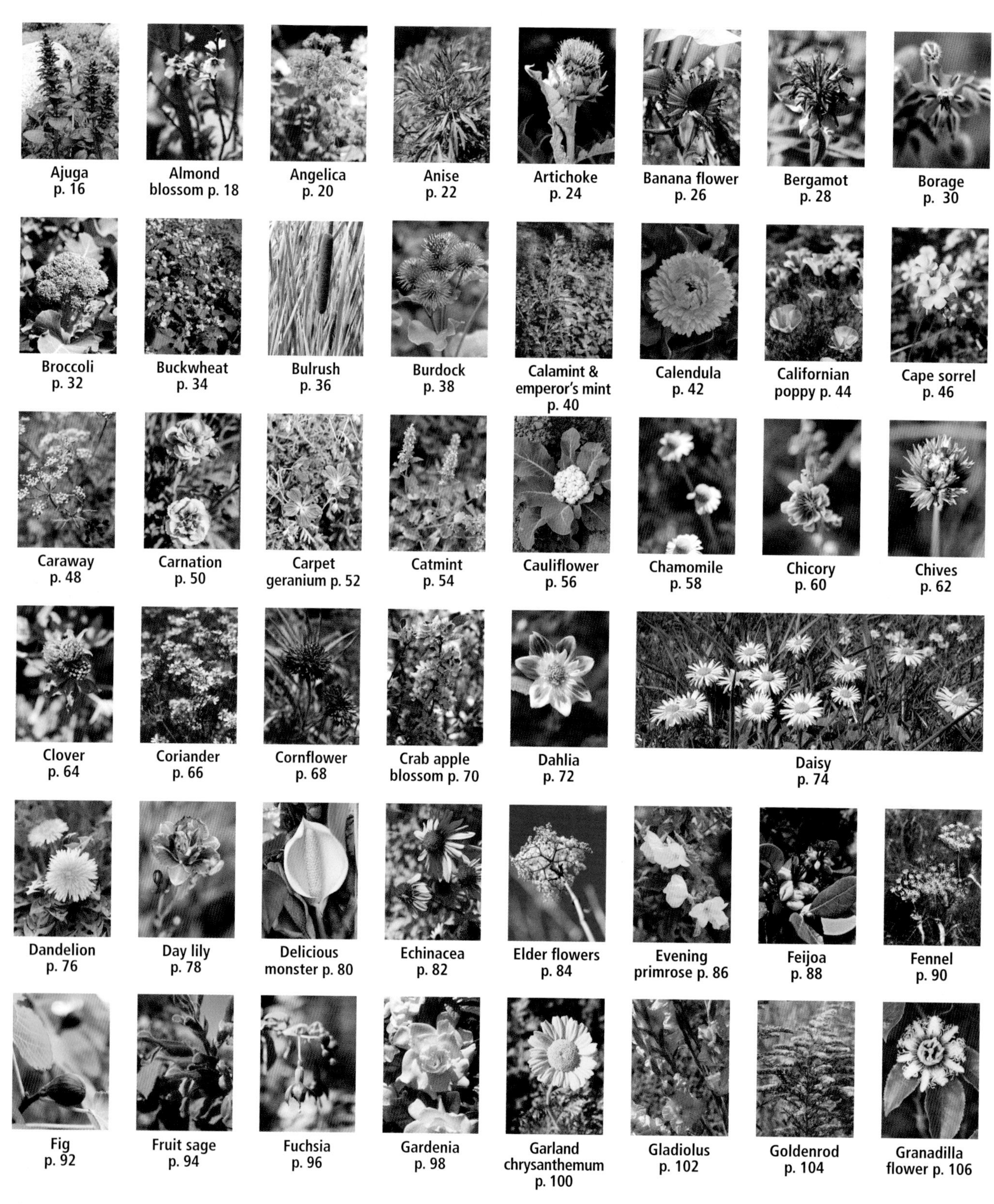

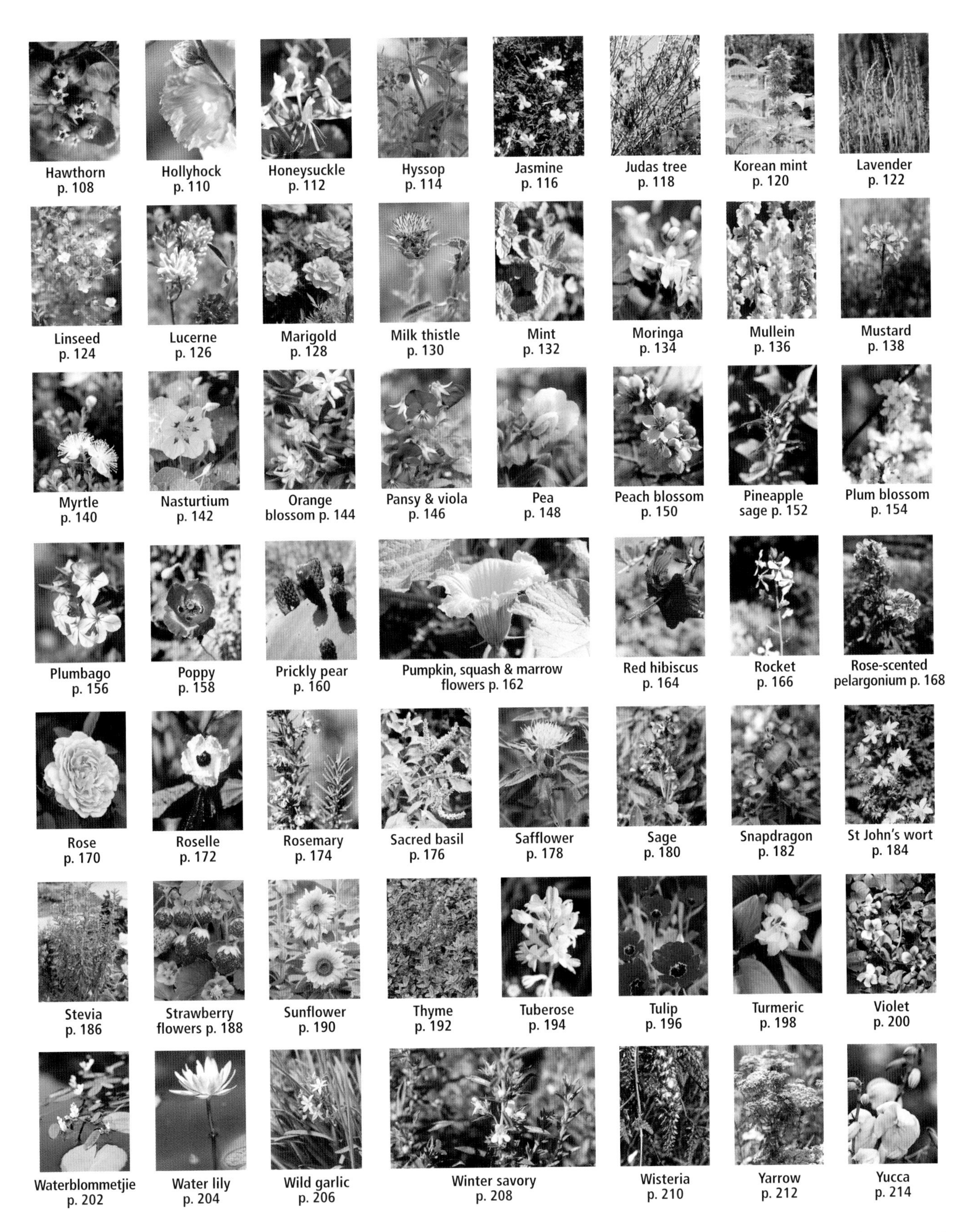

Introduction

There is nothing more appealing or exciting than creating a garden of flowers that can be eaten, incorporated in festivities, celebrations and feasts, and used as medicines or cosmetics.

Clever planting will ensure that the garden remains beautiful and fascinating throughout the seasons. Learning about the growth habits of every plant you bring into the garden will become an ongoing and rewarding interest. Find out about perennials (permanent plants), biennials (growing for about two years) and annuals (planted anew every year), which often bring the biggest colour splash to the garden. In this way, you can build a garden that is literally always rich in colour and interest. I set aside beds or edgings where I can grow perennials and annuals in quantity not only for cut flowers, but also to use in cosmetics, as well as for fragrance and medicinal purposes.

Food gardens interplanted with edible flowers become enchanting, and there is something uplifting about planting wheat, red poppies, chamomile and cornflowers together with rows of frilly lettuces and strawberries. No spring garden will ever be as varied and colourful as this one is – and you can make it happen!

Learn the value of the seemingly humble seed. I am passionate about these little gems; I save them, swop them, send them all over the country and the world. I continuously collect and store seeds in tins and glass jars that I have recycled, labelled and dated. My edible and medicinal gardens reflect this passion never-endingly.

I urge you to revitalise or re-invent your garden – it is like a small revolution that reawakens your interest. Cut out old trees and branches to let more sunshine in, replace old woody shrubs, creepers and perennials. Replace old hedges, repair or lift up old paving, and let light and sun into dark spaces. If tree roots hamper growth, create raised beds with new soil; new arches and fences for climbing plants can turn an uninteresting area into a fascinatingly beautiful garden, bright with sunshine and colour! If heavy trees overhang your only space, ask the neighbours if you could cut away the hanging branches. There are tree fellers who will do it expertly and reasonably quickly.

No matter how large or small our gardens – even if we only have a collection of pots and a sunny patch – it is vital for our health that we grow vegetables, fruits, healing herbs, shrubs and even a small lemon tree wherever we can.

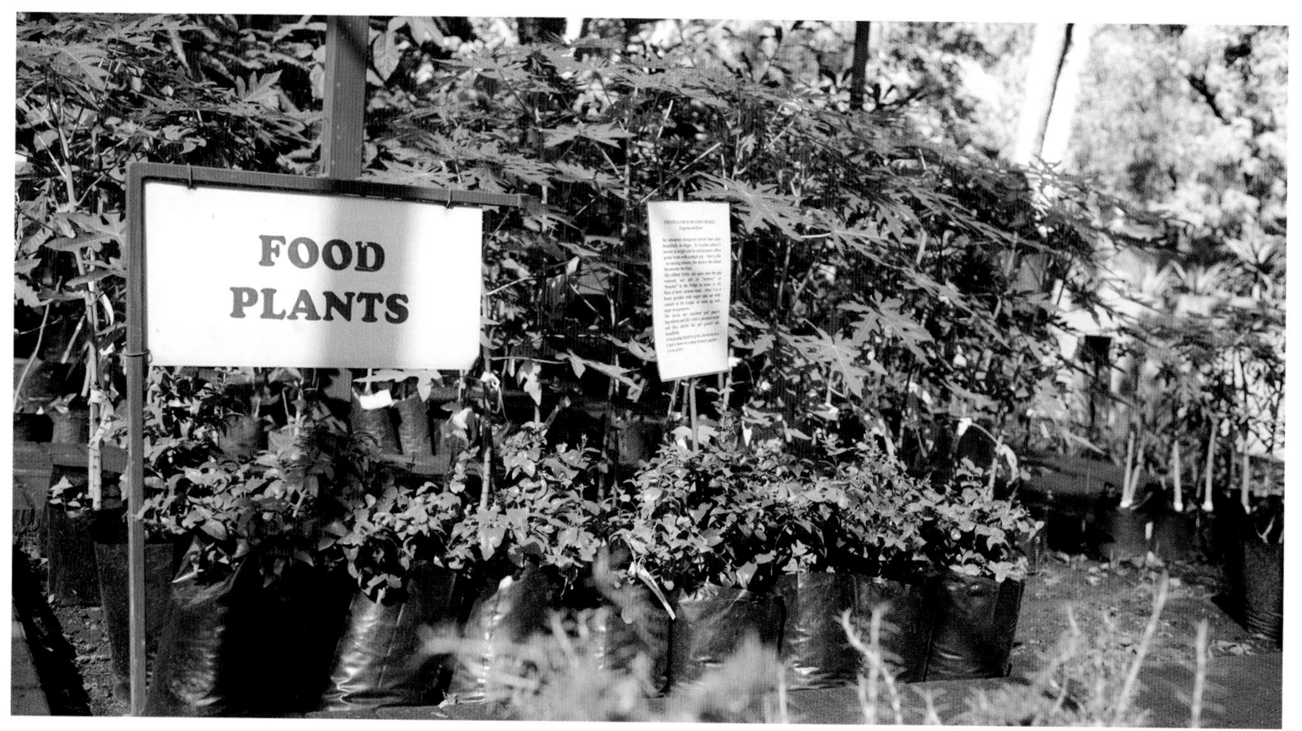

Food plants combine well wtih edible flowers, making for a beautiful and valuable garden. Here, in the nursery, food plants are ready for sale.

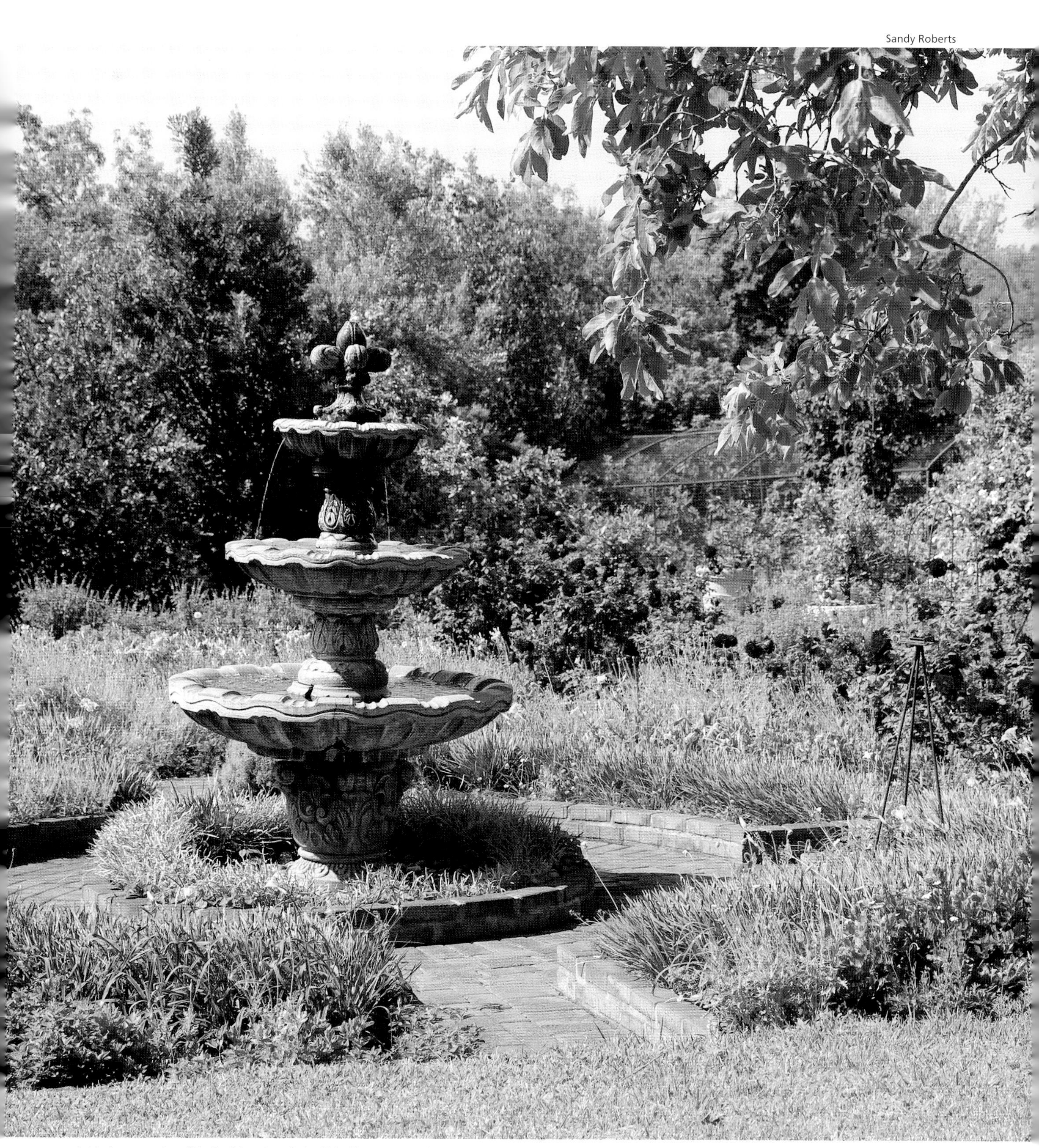

Sandy Roberts

A kitchen garden, filled with colourful edible flowers and fruit trees, planted around a beautiful ornamental fountain.

Planning your garden

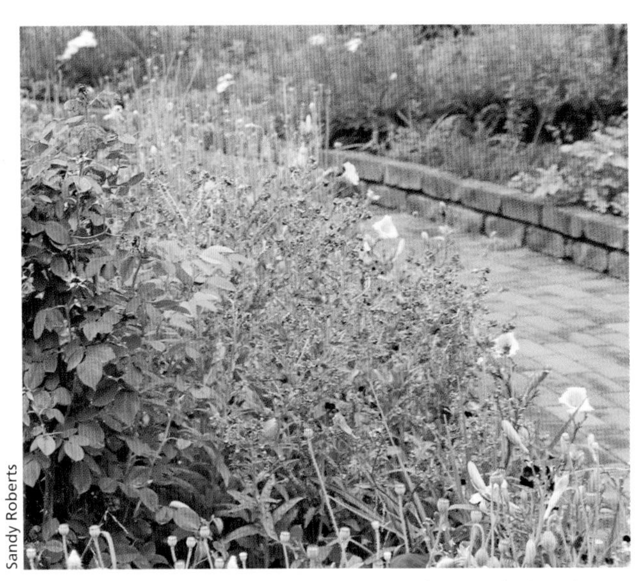
Sandy Roberts

Make sure your garden has easy-to-sweep paths to make it easier to manoeuvre wheelbarrows full of compost.

When planning a new flower garden, select the location very carefully. The best spot is usually one that gets full sun, as a minimum of six hours of sun daily will ensure a good harvest of flowers, fruit and vegetables throughout the year.

Once you have selected a spot, look out for invading trees, as well as old creepers that become woody and occupy too much light, and cut these back. Also, when planting new trees and shrubs, be mindful of how you plant them, considering the space they will require to grow into as the years pass. Before you know it, a once attractive garden can outgrow itself and need quite ruthless cutting back and chopping out.

The soil

Tired, depleted, really 'outgrown' soil needs to be replenished. This requires a lot of work and attention if you want your new garden to thrive. I have learned the hard way that new compost is essential – often several loads of it. Removing a 30–40-cm layer of old depleted soil is ideal, by the barrow load, especially when it's an old lawn. The old soil should be replaced by several loads of compost mixed with new top soil – this is the most vital part of the new garden and a budget for extra compost will be necessary. Just remember: the more compost you put in, the better. Soak each layer well and dig and dig again, turning it in well.

Making your own compost

It is really quite easy to make your own compost heap. Lawn mowings, raked leaves, weeds, prunings, kitchen vegetables and fruit peelings can all be thrown onto the compost heap.

First select a site for the heap, making sure it has easy access for a wheelbarrow. Clear the ground and spread an area as big as you can manage – 2 x 2 m is ideal – with twigs, prunings and rough clippings. This bottom layer will aerate the heap. Now add layers of leaves, raked up clippings, kitchen peelings and even grass mowings, veld grass and flower stalks, alternately with comfrey and yarrow leaves and flowers, and cattle or horse manure and grass from their stables and stalls.

Do this layer by layer, adding a little soil, and also layers of buckwheat as it matures. Buckwheat is an amazing soil improver and I grow it especially for this purpose. I also grow it over an empty flower or vegetable bed to dig back into the soil as it ripens – a practice known as green manuring.

Water the compost heap weekly to keep it moist and encourage decomposition. It will heat up steadily as the heap starts to decay. On top of the compost, sow a crop of amaranth, fenugreek, flax, oats or winter wheat and barley in winter. Once they mature to flowering stage, dig them in. This greatly invigorates the heap, adding excellent nutrients.

The greatest compost enemies are excessive moisture or excessive dryness! Should your heap become too wet or too dry, dismantle it and build it up again, layer by layer.

Remember, yarrow and comfrey are two of the most valuable compost makers. Grow them abundantly for continuous pickings for the compost heap – a heap that's worth its weight in gold!

Mulching

Mulching is very important – without it, weeds grow abundantly and the soil dries out rapidly. It is vital to prevent surface evaporation by covering beds with a 5-cm layer of mulch. Particularly in the summer heat, I have found mulching with dried leaves, straw, roughly chopped sprigs, prunings and twigs quite effective. These can all be mixed and sprinkled over the soil between plants. Water is able to run through the layer, but weeds are deterred, and the soil does not dry out so rapidly. Do not use green grass mowings as a mulch – it packs down, making a perfect nesting place for ants and crickets!

Plant options

Ground covers

Ajuga	perennial
Calamint	perennial
Cape sorrel	perennial
Catmint	perennial
Strawberry	perennial
Violet	perennial

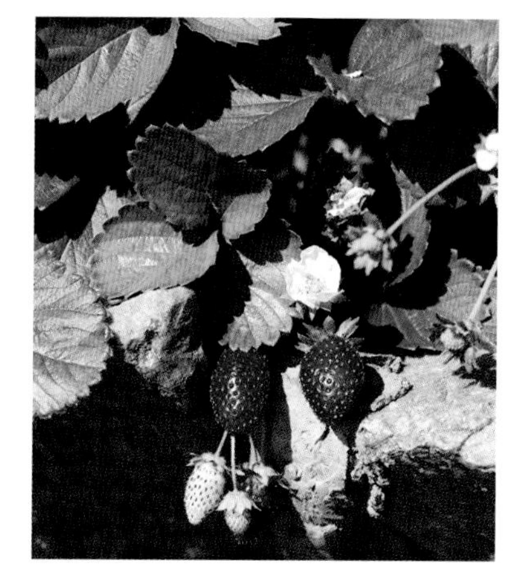

Low growing

Anise	annual
Calendula	annual
Caraway	annual
Carpet geranium	perennial
Chamomile	annual
Chives	perennial
Clover (Red)	short-lived perennial
Daisy	annual
Dandelion	perennial
Hyssop	perennial
Mint	perennial
Nasturtium	annual
Pansy and viola	annual
Sage	perennial
Wild garlic	perennial

Medium height

Bergamot	perennial
Broccoli	annual
Bulrush	perennial
Californian poppy	annual
Carnation	perennial
Cauliflower	annual
Coriander	annual
Cornflower	annual
Dahlia	perennial
Day lily	perennial
Echinacea	perennial
Evening primrose	perennial
Fuchsia	perennial
Gladiolus bulb	perennial
Korean mint	perennial
Linseed	annual
Lucern	perennial
Marigold	annual
Mustard	annual
Pineapple sage	perennial
Poppy	annual
Pumpkin and squash	annual
Rocket	annual
Safflower	annual
Snapdragon	annual
Stevia	perennial
Tuberose bulb	perennial
Tulip bulb	perennial
Turmeric bulb	perennial
Yarrow	perennial

Tall growing

Angelica	biennial
Artichoke	biennial
Borage	annual
Buckwheat	annual
Chicory	biennial
Fennel	perennial
Fruit sage	perennial
Garland chrysanthemum	winter annual
Golden rod	perennial
Hollyhock	biennial
Lavender	perennial
Milk thistle	annual
Mullein	biennial
Rose-scented pelargonium	perennial
Roselle	annual
Rosemary	perennial
Sacred basil	perennial
Sunflower	annual

Shrubs

Elder
Feijoa
Gardenia
Judas tree
Myrtle
Plumbago
Prickly pear
Rose
Yucca

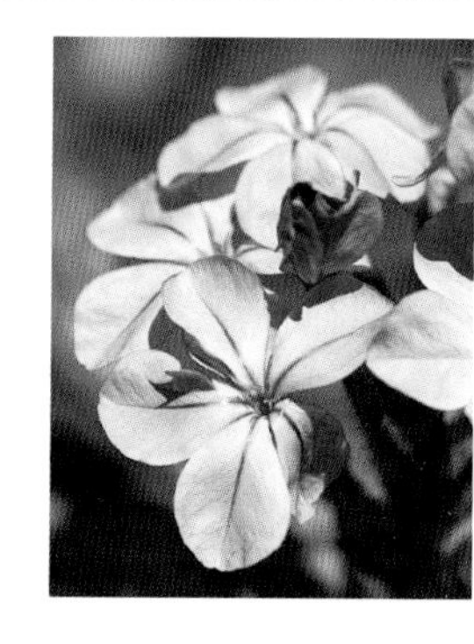

Trees

Almond
Banana
Crab apple
Fig
Hawthorn
Moringa
Orange
Peach
Plum

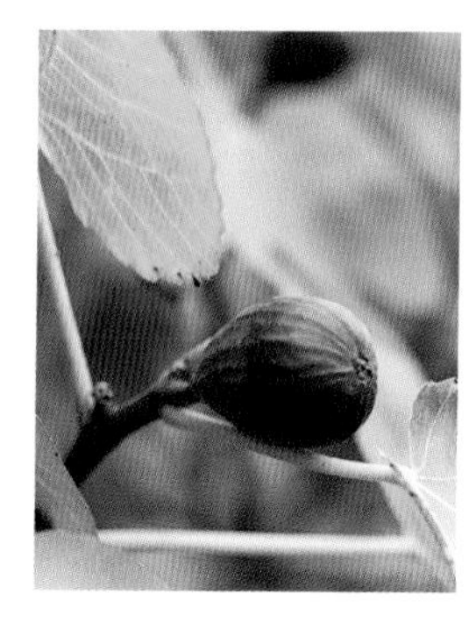

Vines

Delicious monster	perennial
Granadilla	short-lived perennial
Honeysuckle	perennial
Jasmine	perennial
Pea	annual
Wisteria	perennial

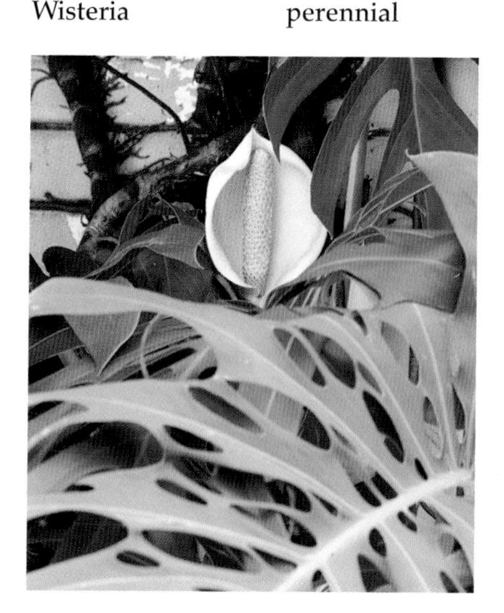

Propagating plants

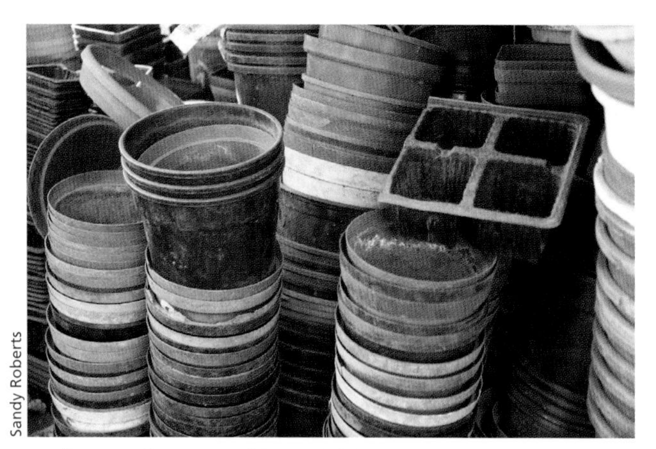
Sandy Roberts

A collection of pots is vital for establishing new plants and cuttings.

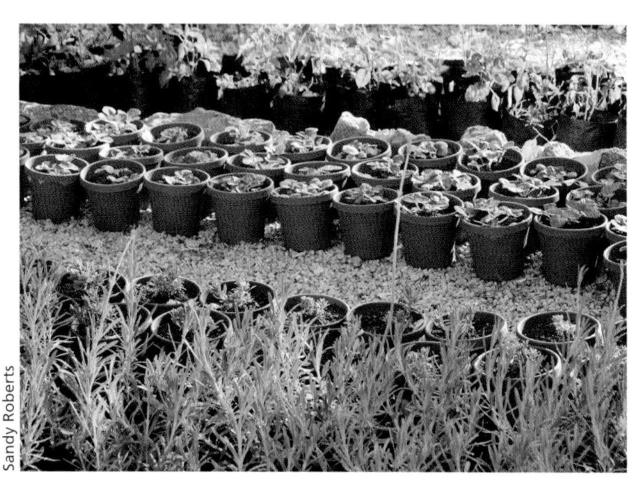
Sandy Roberts

Keep rooted cuttings in semi-shade to establish well before planting out.

Plants are propagated mainly by sowing seeds (in containers or directly in the garden), by cuttings, layering, root cuttings and root division. The most appropriate means of propagation for each plant is described in the individual flower entries, but as an easy reference the framework below is useful.

Sowing seeds in containers

It can be advantageous to start seeds in containers in sheltered positions. Perennial plants, which often take longer to germinate, can be started indoors in late winter and then moved outside to harden off in spring. The temperature and soil conditions can be controlled in the indoor environment, making it possible to produce superior seedlings and have more successful germination.

Commercially produced seed boxes are probably the easiest to handle and come ready with drainage holes. Any container can be used for his purpose, however. You can line strong cartons and tomato boxes with plastic and make a few drainage holes. Place a few small stones at the bottom of the container and then fill it with your soil mixture to within 15 mm of the top. The soil mixture should be loose, well-draining and yet able to hold water. Equal parts of sand, garden loam and a fine, well-matured compost make a good basic mixture. Sieve the mixture through a 6-mm mesh screen to remove clods and sticks, and press down well in the container. Soak with water.

The seeds should be sprinkled evenly over the surface and covered with a depth of soil approximately twice the diameter of the seed. Water carefully, using a fine spray to ensure the seeds are not washed out of the soil or exposed. Alternatively, soak the bottom of the seed tray in a pan of water so that the moisture is drawn up into the soil by capillary action. The secret of successful seed sowing is to ensure that the soil never dries out in those first critical weeks of germination.

Make sure you label the containers clearly so that you are sure which seeds you have sown, and cover them with hessian or a pane of glass to protect them from the drying effect of the wind. Seeds do not need light until they have sprouted but fresh air is needed to prevent fungus formation, so lift the cover for a couple of hours each day and check to see that the soil has not dried out. Water daily with a fine spray.

Once the seeds have germinated, the container can be moved to partial shade with good light but not full sun. Rotate the container daily so that the seeds receive equal exposure to light. Keep the soil moist but do not over-water as the seedlings are liable to damp off at this stage. Once two sets of true leaves have formed, the seedlings can be transplanted into bigger containers, or, if sturdy enough, they can be planted into prepared beds in the garden and shaded until stronger. To establish the seedlings well, plant them into the new containers in a richer mixture of soil: two parts garden loam, one part river sand and one part sifted peat moss or compost. Space the seedlings wider apart, at least 5 cm, and water carefully until they are well established.

When the plants are strong and big enough, place the seed box in the sun for increasing periods over the course of a few days in order to strengthen them before planting out. Plant them out in a prepared bed that is well-composted and has a good amount of leaf mould added to it. Use two spadefuls of compost and one spadeful of leaf mould or old manure to a square metre of soil.

Sowing seeds directly in the garden

Seeds can also be sown directly in the garden, providing there is no danger of frost and that the soil has begun to warm up. Some seeds that fare well sown directly into their site are aniseed, buckwheat, caraway, cornflower, field poppy, linseed, mustard and nasturtium.

Begin by choosing a spot that is suitable for the plant and then turn the soil to a depth of 30 cm, breaking up the clods. If the soil does not drain well, add organic compost, leaf mould, chopped hay or peat moss to lighten it. Fork and level well, then make shallow drills (draw the rake over the soil to indicate the lines) and sow the seeds into the drills, spacing them well. Cover with soil to the depth of roughly twice the diameter of the seed, press down well with the back of the rake and water with a fine spray, making sure you don't expose the seeds. As new seedlings look alike, label the row so that you know what is planted in that spot.

In our climate, it is usually necessary to make a low protective frame of sticks. The frame should be 20 cm above the soil; anything higher will need side flaps to counteract the slanting rays of the hot spring sunshine. Drive forked sticks into the soil at each of the four corners of the bed. Onto these, tie long sticks or reeds to form the frame, and also a few cross reeds tied at intervals. Place a hessian covering over the frame, tying it in place with string. Alternatively, you can use a thin layer of thatching grass over the frame. Secure it by tying sticks over it to weight it down against the wind. If it is difficult to create a shaded area, I make a small dam around each seed, or a long row of built-up earth, and put dried leaves and grass into it to create a little shade for the germinating seeds. Ensure that the seeds remain moist by watering at least twice a day.

Most annual seeds take 12–14 days to germinate, and perennials take a little longer – sometimes from three weeks up to a month. The soil must be kept moist throughout this period.

Broadcasting is another method you can use to plant seeds. This method is employed when you want to cover a certain area rather than plant rows. Prepare the soil as above, water well and scatter the seeds evenly over the area. Cover the area with sand, and water and shade it as you would rows of seeds.

Cuttings

Growing plants from cuttings is an easier method of propagation and is a much quicker process than growing from seed. Many herbs grow well from cuttings for example, bergamot, catmint, lavender, mint, pineapple sage, rosemary, sage, St John's wort, the thymes and wormwood.

You can take cuttings at any time during the growing season from healthy, well-established plants. Strong new tip growth makes the best cuttings. Using a sharp knife or clippers, make the cutting just below a leaf bud or node. The cutting should be between 8 cm and 15 cm long. The cuttings must be kept damp – place them between layers of wet newspaper or cloth and keep them out of the sun until you are ready to plant them.

Have seed boxes ready, about 10 cm in depth and filled with river sand. A pot or jam tin will suffice if you have just a few cuttings, as long as it has good drainage (place a few stones in the bottom of the container). Wet

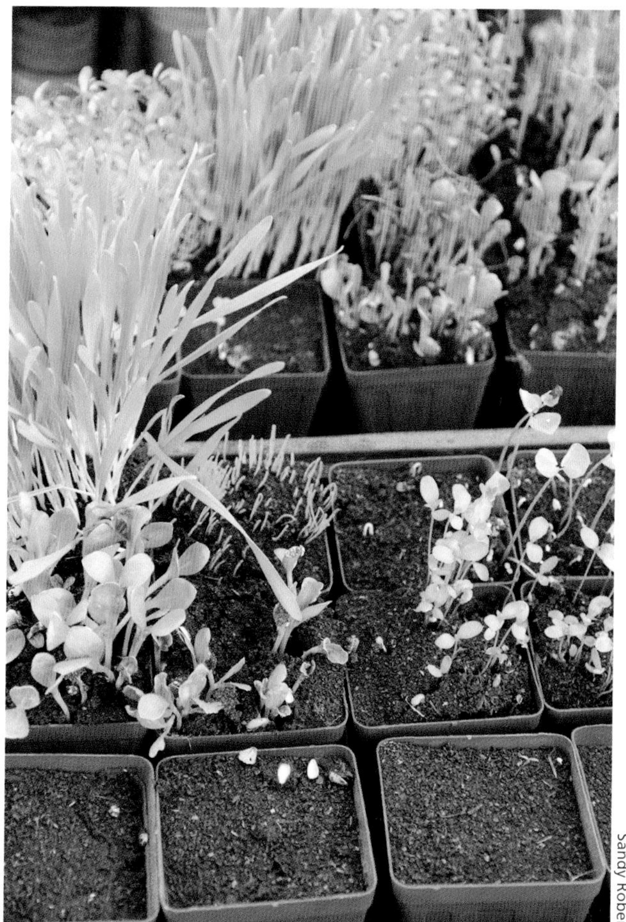
Sandy Roberts

Seed collections can be ongoing for continuous variety.

the sand well and use a stick to make a row of holes, about 5–8 cm deep. Strip the lower leaves from the cuttings and press each one into its prepared hole. You can dip the cut end into a hormone rooting powder first. Press down firmly and complete the rows. Water the cuttings again and place in a protected, warm place in the shade. If you take the cuttings before winter, create a miniature greenhouse by covering them with plastic, supported on a frame or wire arches, with the edges tucked under stones to keep out draughts.

It will take a month to seven weeks for the cuttings to take and form strong roots of their own and during this time they must not dry out. Allow them to harden off a little in the sun before transplanting, and take care when removing them from their seed tray – shake the box out gently on its side so as not to pull away the tender new roots.

The plants should be transplanted into prepared beds that have been well dug with compost and old manure (two spadefuls of compost and one spadeful of manure per square metre). Use extra compost if you do not have old manure. Prepare a hole, place the cutting into it, cover the roots with soil, press down firmly and water well. The cuttings must not dry out. Mulch with coarse compost. When the plants are established, water regularly once- or twice-weekly.

Layering

Creeping plants such as catmint, elder, honeysuckle, the mints, the thymes and winter savory will take root while still attached to the parent plant if they are brought into contact with soil. Many flowers, in fact, send down roots naturally from little tufts or branches that touch the ground, so this is a quick and easy way to make new plants.

Choose a strong, healthy tuft, twig or branch growing close to the ground. Prepare a shallow hole below it, and fill it with sand, soil and a little compost. First scratch a small raw place on the underside of the branch, then apply a little hormone powder and bend the branch down into the hole. Use a heavy wire arch to anchor it in place. Firm down with soil and give it a good watering. Place a stone over the area to keep the soil above the branch undisturbed.

After six weeks, check on the progress, gently scraping away a little of the soil. Once good roots are established, sever the stem from the parent plant and leave it undisturbed for three weeks. The new plant is now ready for transplanting to a different position. Prepare a hole with well-mixed soil and compost and fill it with water. Carefully dig out the plant, with a lot of soil around it, and place it in the hole, covering the roots with soil and pressing down firmly. Make a small dam around it and water well. Check twice a week to ensure it does not dry out completely.

Root cuttings

It is easy to propagate any plant that sends up suckers, for example bergamot, catmint, elder, goldenrod, the mints and yarrow. Choose strong suckers and chop them off with a spade, taking as much root as possible. Prepare a deep seed box, filling it with light garden soil with a little compost worked into it (four spadefuls of soil to one spadeful of compost).

The root cuttings must be placed horizontally in the box and covered with soil. Firm them down and water well. Put the box in the shade, making sure that it is not in a draught. It is important to keep the cuttings moist. When new growth and leaf buds appear, transplant into individual pots, where the cuttings can develop into strong plants. Keep them partially shaded, then place them in the sun for lengthening periods each day to harden off. Once they are established, plant out in the garden in well-prepared beds.

Root division

It is best to divide plants in autumn or early spring, when they are not forming new growth. Bergamot, chives, goldenrod, strawberries, violet and yarrow are among the plants that divide well.

Dig out a clump and place it on a firm surface. Then, using two forks back to back with their prongs firmly in the clump, pull them apart and split the clump open. Repeat this process if necessary, or simply pull apart the clumps until the sections are suitably small, and replant in newly prepared soil. Fairly rich soil is needed for these perennials, so dig in three spadefuls of compost and two spadefuls of old manure per square metre of garden soil. Make sure the soil remains moist until the newly planted pieces have adjusted.

The central portion or original mother plant often becomes woody and stunted and needs to be discarded. If you replant in the original position, where the soil will have become depleted, first dig in some compost and old manure.

Separate perennials every 2–3 years and give a yearly feed of compost and old manure. Perennials form the backbone of the flower garden so they deserve the best care in order to continue their good work.

Sandy Roberts

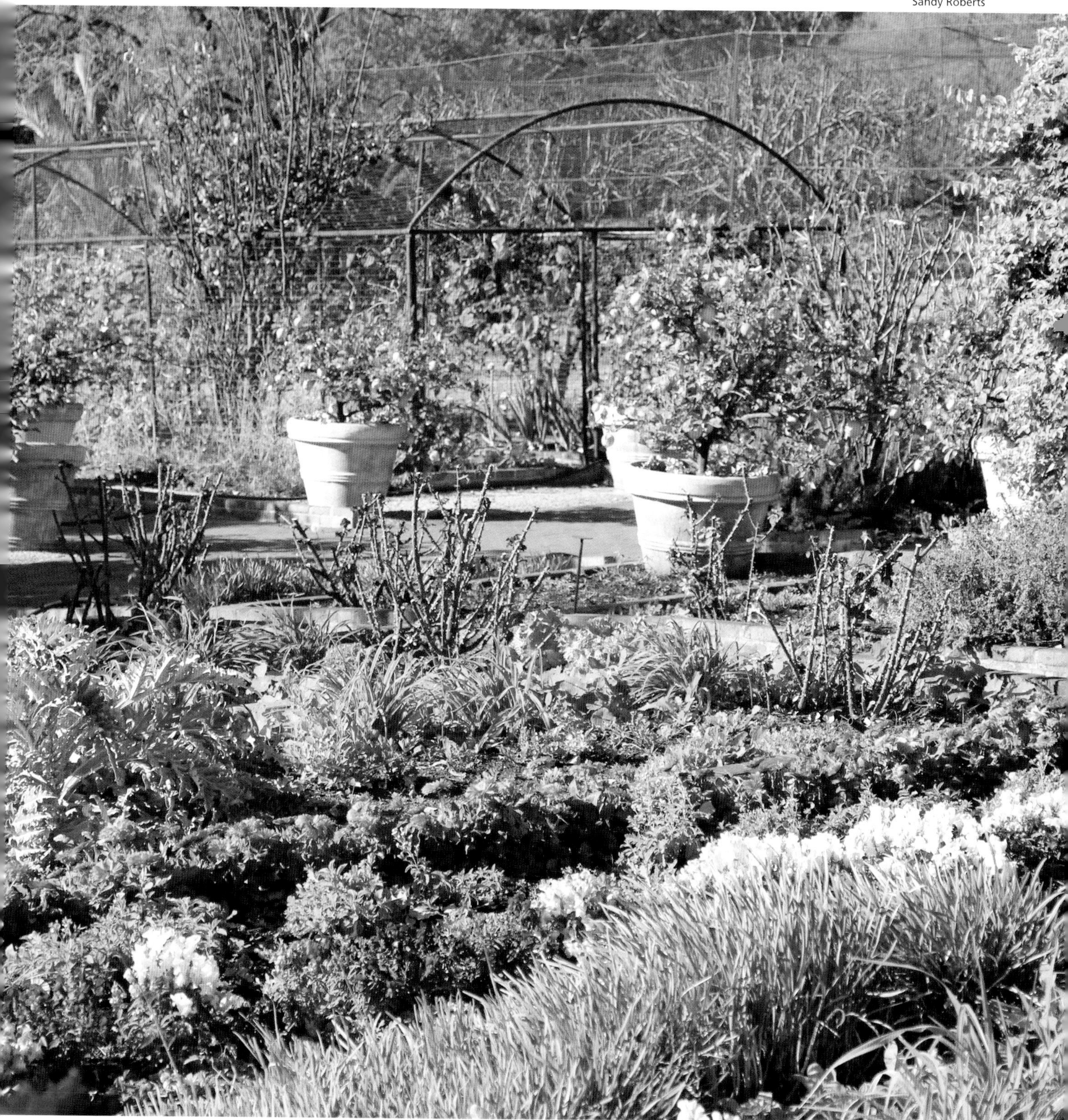

The Herbal Centre's kitchen garden is filled with a constant supply of edible flowers. The cage in the background protects tender radishes, cauliflowers, broccoli and newly sown spinach. Meyer lemons thrive in pots and make an attractive feature.

Ajuga

Ajuga reptans ● **Carpet bugle**

Ajuga is a favourite old-fashioned ground cover grown for centuries to cover moist ground as a neat and attractive path edging, while its pretty blue flowers have been used for food flavourings and medicines. No cottage garden was without it and it became a valuable ingredient in a popular medication kept in every household, known as 'traumatick decoction', which was registered in the London Dispensatory in 1694. This marvellous medication was used to treat injuries, falls, wounds, broken bones or 'miner's accident' and it was also used by carpenters and stoneworkers. Its common name was 'carpenter's herb', and it was made into ointments, lotions and even dried and powdered and spread over injuries of all descriptions.

Nicholas Culpeper, the famous English herbalist, encouraged all gardeners and farmers to grow it and wrote about it in *The English Physician Enlarged* in 1653: 'If the virtues of it (ajuga) make you fall in love with it (as they will if you be wise), keep a syrup of it to take inwardly, an ointment and a plaister to use outwardly, always by you.' Culpeper used it as a wound herb and considered it to be a cure for hangovers. It was grown around inns so that it could be picked and made into a strong tea to ease a hangover. Today it can still be found lining the paths to pubs in Europe and England, along with ivy, which was said to cure drunkenness!

Ajuga belongs to a genus of around 50 species native to Eurasia, with a few species native to tropical Africa and Australia.

CULTIVATION

Ajuga requires deeply dug, richly composted soil that is kept moist. It thrives in light shade in the midsummer heat and needs a light frost cover during the midwinter months. The flowering tips are edible and can be picked at any time of the year except during the coldest months, when it does not flower prolifically. Propagation is by division of the clump, with rooted tufts replanted in rich moist soil. Occasionally you will find ajuga seed.

MEDICINAL USES

Ajuga has been used as a home remedy through the centuries. Rubs, lotions and ointments made for rheumatic and arthritic pains became a valuable trade around the 1660s. The leaves and flowering heads were gathered in the summer, dried, and made into lotions to wash wounds, grazes and minor burns.

By the mid-17th century, monks in Britain and Europe had created a soothing oil as a panacea for many ailments, and old herbals had explicit and complicated methods of making the comforting and popular medication. Often combined with other herbs to give it scent, these ointments, oils or lards were sold as cure-alls.

When dried, the entire herb is a bitter astringent and was made into a tea for coughs, stomach ulcers, bronchitis and flu with a high temperature. In some herbals it was even used to treat heart ailments, all with excellent results.

To make ajuga tea, pour a cup of boiling water over ¼ cup fresh flowering tops, six crushed cloves and a thin sliver of lemon rind, the length of your little finger. Allow the tea to stand for five minutes, strain, sweeten with a touch of honey and sip slowly as a gentle laxative, or for tired, aching legs. The tea was also taken to lower high blood pressure, for excessive menstruation, to clear mouth ulcers and a sore throat, and for laryngitis and loss of voice. Monks in medieval England used the tea to wash wounds and for coughs, colds and varicose ulcers, with the honey included.

In the Mediterranean area, the flowers and flowering tips were warmed in olive oil on a slow fire and applied to bruises and sprains using a soft cloth, as hot as could be tolerated.

I began making ajuga oil and lotion early on in my herbal work when experimenting with herbs that could ease pain. What finally made me aware of its valuable pain-reducing effects was that I found the farm dogs constantly lying on my ajuga plantings. So I stuffed ajuga pillows for the dogs' baskets and made ajuga tea to add to their drinking water, and ajuga lotion for everyone's bath – dogs, children and the whole family!

Ajuga lotion to relieve pain and wash wounds

2 cups fresh ajuga flowering sprigs and leaves
½ cup whole cloves, lightly crushed
2 litres water

Simmer the ajuga, cloves and water in a heavy-bottomed stainless steel pot, with the lid on, for 30 minutes. Stir often. Set the lotion aside to cool, then strain. Add a cupful to the bathwater. In the case of a bad sprain or bruise, soak a facecloth in the warm brew and wrap it around the area, cover it with a warm towel, and relax for 10 minutes.

Ancient 'ajuga syrop' for aches and fatigue

1 cup ajuga flowering sprigs
1 litre water
1 cup honey
1 teaspoon aniseed, lightly crushed
1 teaspoon finely grated fresh ginger
1 pinch cayenne pepper
1 tablespoon brandy

Simmer the ingredients together for 20 minutes and stir well, then strain. Cool the syrup and keep in a glass bottle in the fridge. Warm half a cup at a time and sip slowly for great fatigue, aches and pains all over, and a feeling of not coping.

Ajuga orange and ginger syrup for pain relief

This Mediterranean recipe from near Sicily ideally needs an organically grown orange and organically grown ginger.

1 cup fresh ajuga flowering sprigs
¼ cup finely grated orange rind
½ cup finely grated ginger
¾ cup honey
¼ cup fresh flowering thyme sprigs
10 crushed cloves
1 litre water

Simmer all the ingredients together in the water for 20 minutes, with the lid on. Allow the syrup to cool, keeping it covered. Strain and pour into a glass bottle and take one tablespoonful in a little hot water for aches and pains, bruises, tumours, circulatory ailments, internal bleeding and excessive menstruation.

Ajuga massage cream for aches and pains

1 cup good aqueous cream
1 cup fresh flowering ajuga sprigs
1 teaspoon powdered cloves
1 teaspoon rose-geranium essential oil

Simmer the aqueous cream, ajuga and cloves together in a double boiler for 20 minutes. Stir often. Leave the cream to cool for 15 minutes, then strain and add the essential oil. Spoon the cream into a sterilised jar. Use warm as a gently soothing massage cream. It is wonderful for a stiff neck.

CULINARY USES

Ajuga and butter bean stir-fry

SERVES 4–6

This is a much-loved vegetarian dish served in many cultures.

500 g big white butter beans
2 onions, finely chopped
½ cup of olive oil
1 cup chopped green pepper
2 cups chopped fresh pineapple pieces
½ cup chopped parsley
1 cup chopped ajuga flowering tops
Sea salt and freshly ground black pepper
Juice of 1 lemon

Soak the butter beans overnight. In the morning, boil them in fresh water with no salt, simmering until tender. Strain the beans. In a deep, heavy-bottomed pan, fry the onions in olive oil until lightly brown. Add the butter beans and stir-fry. Add the green pepper, pineapple, parsley and ajuga flower tops and gently stir-fry. Finally, season with salt and pepper, add lemon juice and serve piping hot with rice or crusty brown bread.

> **COOK'S NOTE**
> **The pretty mauve-blue flowers can be pulled from their calyxes and added to salads and stir-fries, or sprinkled over cakes, desserts and drinks.**

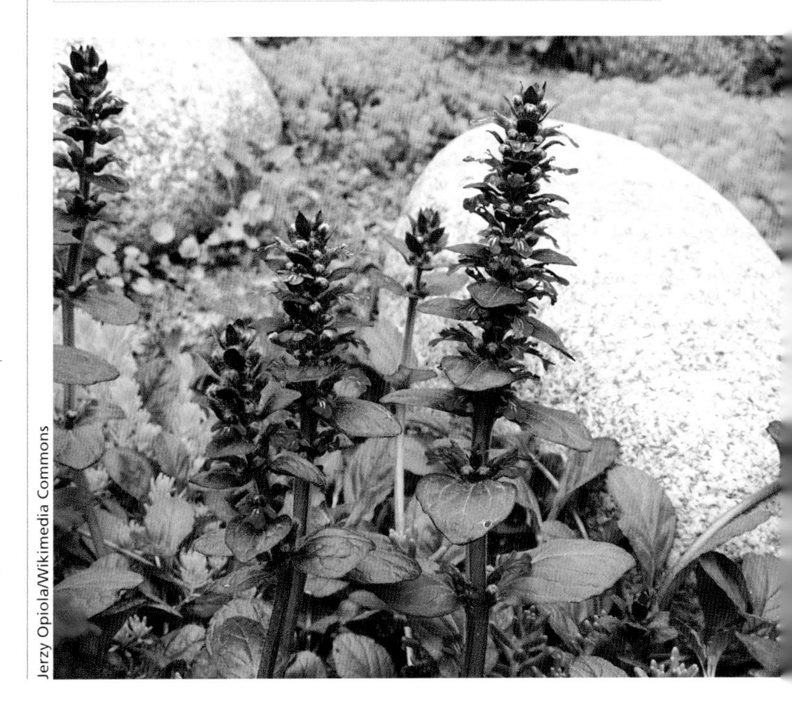
Jerzy Opiola/Wikimedia Commons

Almond blossom

Prunus dulcis ● *P. amygdalus*

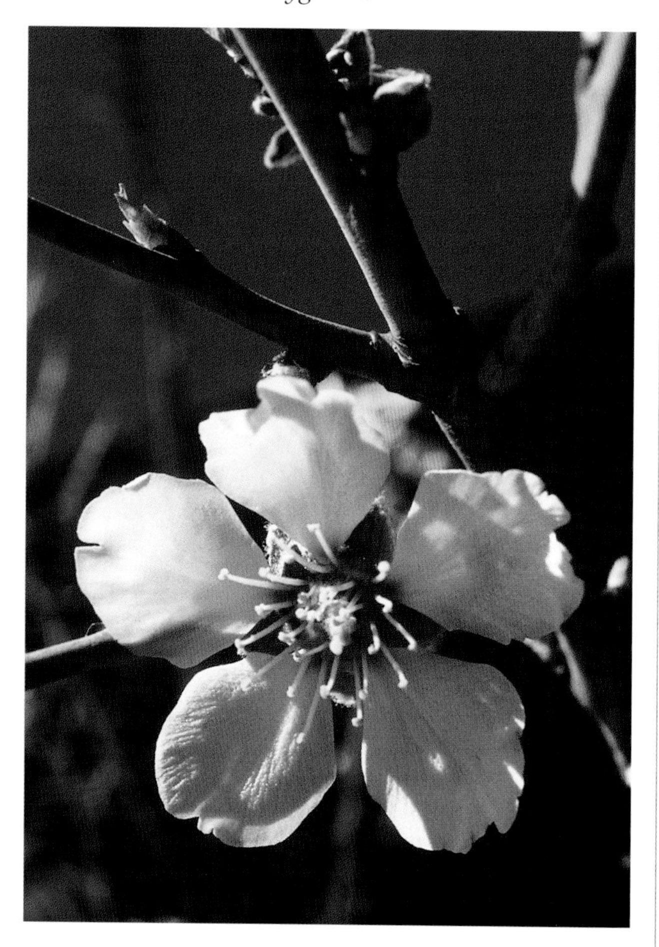

Almonds are rich in protein and are considered to be so nourishing and valuable that almond trade is still as brisk today as it was 3 000 years ago! And the dried flower petals are still gathered today in great calico sheets spread under the trees in spring, and used in cosmetics and soaps in Central and western Asia.

CULTIVATION

Almond trees grow up to 6 m in height and need full sun and deeply dug, richly composted soil. They need a deep weekly watering, increasing to twice-weekly in the hot dry months. Trees should be planted 4 m apart. They do not self-fertilise, so plant three or four varieties together, or ask a neighbour to plant one type and you plant the other to ensure fertilisation. Almond trees thrive with pruning in midwinter only to shape them and open out very tangled branches. I spray mine with a seaweed foliar feed throughout the year, and clip and train the supple branches to shape the trees, and am rewarded with masses of blossoms and a small collection of nuts for my efforts. Underplant almond trees with chives, garlic chives, lucerne and red clover, as this will increase the yield of fruit.

MEDICINAL USES

The delicate blossoms contain small amounts of B vitamins, particularly biotin and niacin, as well as vitamin E and traces of several amino acids. The petals and nuts contain calcium, magnesium, iron, phosphorus, potassium, sodium and zinc. Because the blossoms and nuts are so rich in these vitamins and minerals, they are a superb energy food. The ancient Phoenicians used the petals in honey as a tonic and sprinkled them into gruels and stews to boost muscular strength in soldiers. They used crushed petals as a poultice over skin spots, and mixed the crushed petals with oil in cases of dry skin and sunburn. Crushed petals are also soothing when applied to insect bites.

A tea made from the whole flower makes a refreshing mouthwash and gargle that clears up mouth ulcers and sore inflamed gums, and as a bonus, sweetens the breath. To make almond blossom tea, add ¼ cup almond blossoms and one sprig of peppermint or spearmint to a cup of boiling water. Allow the tea to stand for five minutes, then strain and drink.

Almonds have been cultivated for over 3 000 years and through the centuries 'almond milk' has been a much cherished and enjoyed energy drink.

Almond milk

This is excellent for recovery after an illness, during exam times or to help the elderly regain energy and vitality. Stir in a few almond petals for extra vitamins and minerals. Almond petals can be dried for use in winter-time drinks.

1 cup almonds
2 cups boiled water

Soak the almonds in the boiled water overnight. Next morning, blend in a liquidiser or food processor, adding a little more boiled water if needed to make the paste a little softer. Add 1–2 tablespoons of paste per glass and top up with milk, apple juice or grape juice.

CULINARY USES

Almond blossom milk energiser

SERVES 1

This drink is a quick pick-me-up at the end of a busy day, or a lunchtime energiser much loved by children.

1 glass full-cream milk
1–2 tablespoons roughly chopped almonds
1 banana, peeled
1 dessertspoon honey
1 dessertspoon almond blossom petals, stripped off their calyxes

Briefly liquidise half the milk and all the almonds until the almonds disintegrate. Add the banana, honey, almond blossom petals and the rest of the milk. Blend until well mixed. Pour immediately into a glass and drink it slowly.

> COOK'S NOTE
> **Use blossoms and seeds (nuts) from your own trees when cooking or making teas so that you know they are organically grown and not irradiated or sprayed.**

Almond blossom and strawberry ice-cream

SERVES 6–8

The first strawberries appear in spring just as the almond trees come into bloom. I make this special ice-cream at that time as a much-appreciated treat after the winter. It is one of the prettiest desserts, perfect for a spring birthday party or a wedding.

4–5 cups hulled and sliced strawberries
3 tablespoons white sugar
Juice of 1 lemon
1 tin condensed milk
3 cups thick cream
1 cup almond blossom petals

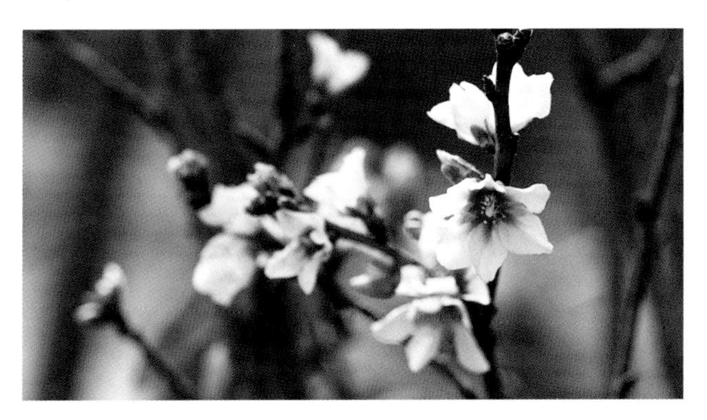

Liquidise the strawberries and sugar. Add the lemon juice. Pour into a bowl and whisk in the condensed milk until it starts to thicken. In another bowl, whisk the cream until it doubles in bulk, then add to the strawberry and condensed milk mixture. Fold in the almond blossom petals. Pour into two shallow ice-cream trays and freeze. Stir every now and then to break up the ice crystals. Serve sprinkled with more almond blossom petals and fresh strawberries in attractive glass bowls.

Almond blossom chocolate cake

SERVES 6–8

This is real angel food, wickedly rich, but so superb you will want to make it often for special occasions. Take care not to overcook it or it will dry out; I leave it slightly underdone and moist in the centre. Since it contains no flour it cannot upset the digestion. It is best made a day ahead as it matures beautifully. It can also be served as a dessert.

175 g milk or dark chocolate, broken into pieces
4 tablespoons butter
4 tablespoons castor sugar
3 large eggs, separated
6 tablespoons ground almonds
1 cup fresh fine brown breadcrumbs

Icing
175 ml thick cream
¾ cup icing sugar
2–4 tablespoons dark rum
1 cup almond blossom petals, stripped off their calyxes

Preheat the oven to 190°C. Warm the chocolate in a double boiler with the butter until both are melted and well mixed. Whisk the sugar and egg yolks together and add this to the chocolate and butter mixture. Stir in four tablespoons of the ground almonds (keep the other two tablespoons aside), and the breadcrumbs. Beat the egg whites and fold into the mixture very gently and evenly.

Grease a springform cake tin (20 cm in diameter) with a good layer of butter and sprinkle in the remaining ground almonds. Spoon in the cake mixture and bake in the centre of the oven for 25 minutes until almost done. Allow to cool in the tin on a wire rack. It will deflate slightly.

Gently remove the cake from the springform tin and place on a plate. To make the icing, whip the cream, sweeten to taste with the icing sugar and add the rum, and fold in about two tablespoons of the almond blossom petals. Pipe the cream or spread it decoratively over the cake and sprinkle the remaining almond blossom petals over it.

Angelica

Angelica archangelica • **Garden angelica**

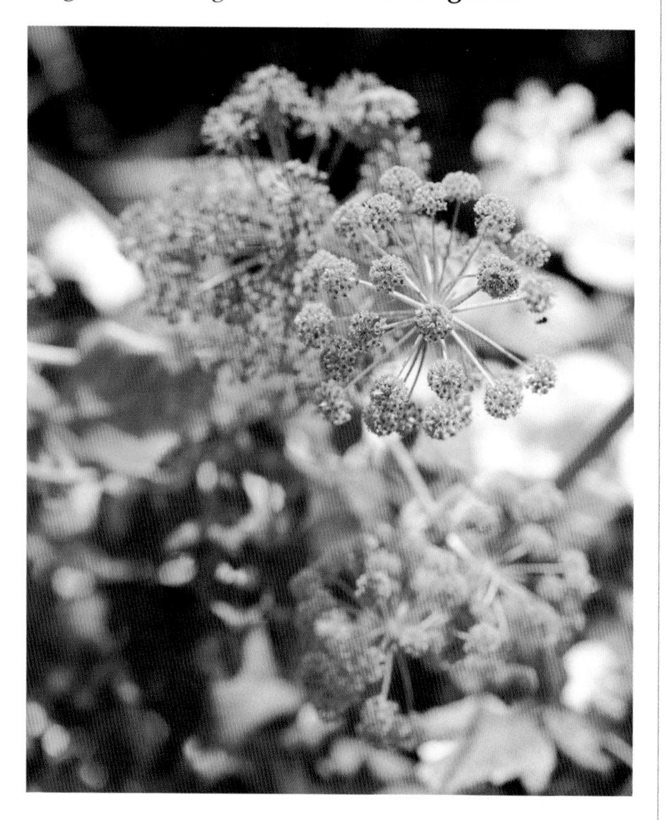

According to the medieval herbals, angelica is an ancient herb of the angels, 'praised for its virtues'. It originated in the cool moist meadows of Europe, and has remained a plant of great value. All parts of it are used, and it has been listed in the pharmacopoeias of Britain, Europe and China for centuries. In the present British pharmacopoeia it is listed as a urinary antiseptic for easing cystitis, and for inflammatory rheumatic conditions.

In addition to its medicinal properties, angelica is cultivated for its oils, fragrance and soothing constituents used in cosmetics, colognes, soaps and lotions. It is also used extensively in the food industry as a flavouring; in liqueurs and alcoholic drinks; and in a delicious soft drink with fruit sugars.

The main growers are Belgium, Germany and Hungary, and to a lesser extent Britain. The whole plant is utilised, from the roots to the flowers, and the seeds are used to produce an oil that has bactericidal and fungicidal properties.

CULTIVATION

Angelica is tricky to propagate only if the seed is not fresh – and by fresh I mean literally just matured, ripe and starting to fall off the umbels. So sure am I of my fresh organically grown seeds that I sow only two seeds per four-litre planting bag and both come up in the rich moist compost. Keep the seedlings moist, shaded and protected until they are 5 cm high, then gradually move them out into the sun for short periods each day, extending the time little by little until they are strong. Their final position in the garden should be in light shade or partial shade. They grow beautifully under 40% shade cloth for commercial plantings.

Angelica is a robust biennial and takes cold winters if protected. A light-as-a-feather covering of plant fleece bought at your nursery or hardware shop, draped over sturdy wire hoops and tucked down at root level with a stone or two, makes a protective tent. Lift up the northern side on a sunny winter day, and cover again at night. In a frost-free area there is no need to cover, and as angelica's homeland has bitter winters, the plants adjust easily.

Water once-weekly in winter and two or three times a week in summer; angelicas prefer a long slow stream to their roots rather than an overhead spray.

Deeply dug soil with a lot of compost is essential. Plant angelicas 1–1.5 m apart as the leaves are around 60 cm in length and often in width. Great umbels of beautiful 'lace flowers' appear in its second year. These have a branched habit so that a row of angelica looks spectacular in the garden. The flowers attract many beneficial insects that control and prey on aphids, whitefly, red spider and flies.

I partner angelica with *Salvia leucantha* 'Midnight' (the showy bright purple variety) and they thrive together in light shade but with late afternoon sun. Seed sown in autumn will ensure a mass of seedlings in spring and early summer. Angelica is cut once the flowers turn to seed.

MEDICINAL USES

Traditionally, angelica was regarded as a gift from the Archangel Michael and was used as a protection against evil and a cure for all ills. In the 15th century it was rated one of the most important medicinal plants by John Parkinson, an esteemed herbalist, in northern Europe and Asia, where it is found naturally. Angelica has remained a valuable and versatile herb that today still holds its place as a medicinal tea.

Angelica flower tea is still one of the favourite medicinal teas, and is available in specialist shops from China to Greenland to Central Asia. It has a bittersweet aromatic taste and remains a popular tea as an anti-inflammatory, for indigestion and digestive upsets, to relax muscle spasms, for bronchial coughs and tight chests and for the female reproductive system after giving birth. Angelica tea was often served in hospitals overseas.

To make angelica tea, fill half a cup with dried angelica flowers, or use fresh flowers with a piece of finely chopped stem and a piece of leaf. Top up and fill the cup with boiling water, and allow the tea to stand for five minutes, stirring continuously. The tea is a respected treatment for anorexia, menstrual and obstetric problems, poor circulation, chronic fatigue, flu, catarrh, urinary problems including cystitis, pleurisy, to increase perspiration and thus lower fevers, and as a strong expectorant.

Angelica is also used for migraines, taken in tablet or capsule form. Alternatively, take angelica tea at the first sign of a migraine, and sip frequently and consistently a little at a time.

WARNING: Do not take angelica in any form if you are pregnant or diabetic, even mildly diabetic.

Angelica poultice

Use this poultice for menstrual cramps, cystitis pains and colic.

4–6 angelica leaves and stems
(pick the whole compound leaf)
Boiling water
Towel
Pure cotton

Warm the leaves and stems in a large pot of boiling water. Lay them on a towel and cover with a piece of cotton. Place over the area of pain, cotton side against the body. Cover with another towel and a hot-water bottle. Rest for 15–20 minutes, keeping everything as hot as possible. Once the pain eases, rest for a further 10 minutes. Interestingly, angelica poultices were listed in ancient medical texts for treating aching feet and rheumatic joints – done exactly this way.

CULINARY USES

Sweet angelica spice for stir-fries and noodles

This sugary spice is still popular in the market places of Asia.

10–15 umbels of just-opened flowers, stalks attached
1 litre water
1 cup soft treacle sugar
1 teaspoon chopped fresh chilli
1 teaspoon crushed coriander seeds
1 teaspoon crushed cardamom pods

Cut the umbels with stalks attached, and set aside. Select a heavy-bottomed pot and simmer the water with the treacle sugar, chopped fresh chilli (if the chillies are not ripe use dried chilli a little at a time and taste for heat), coriander seeds and cardamom pods. Simmer for 20 minutes, stirring frequently.

Now dip each fresh flower head into the sugary mixture, gently submerging and turning it so that every part is covered. Shake off the excess syrup and tie a string to the stalk so that it can be suspended. Hang in an airy place to dry.

Once dry and brittle, discard the stalks, and crumble the flowers over fried fish, fried mushrooms, stir-fries, soups, noodles and rice. This flavoursome spice can also be served as a condiment in small bowls.

Angelica and orange marmalade

Try this marmalade with cheese and biscuits – it is delicious!

4 sweet oranges
2 rough-skinned lemons
1 cup finely chopped angelica leaves and stems
4 cups treacle sugar
4 cups water

Squeeze the juice from the oranges and lemons and mince the skins. Put the juice and minced skins into a bowl. Tie up the chopped angelica in a muslin square, push it into the fruit and leave it covered overnight. Next morning, boil the juice, skin and angelica for two hours. Remove the angelica bag and discard. Add the sugar and simmer, stirring constantly. Test for setting (a little will set on a cold saucer), then switch off the stove. Leave the jam to cool, stirring often to disperse the peel evenly. While still warm, pour the jam into sterilised jars, seal and label.

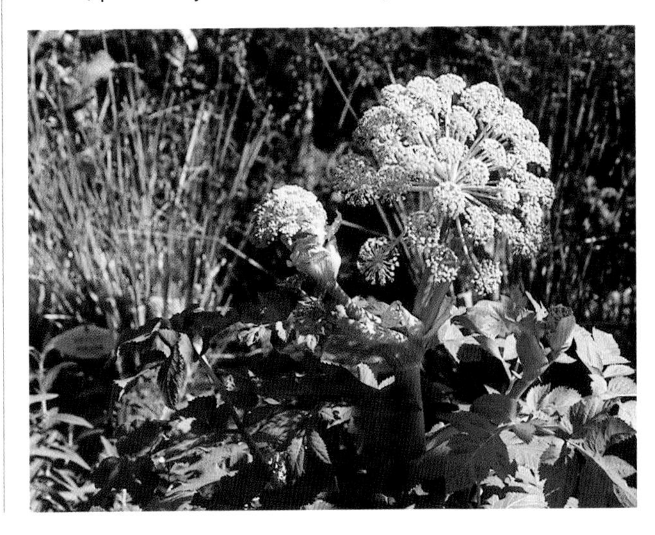

Anise

Pimpinella anisum

Anise is native to the eastern Mediterranean areas as well as western Asia and North Africa, where it still grows wild as a wayside weed. Because it is so short-lived, it often appears in spring and again in late summer, drawing bees and butterflies to it in droves with its sweet liquorice fragrance.

Remarkably, anise has been cultivated in Egypt for over 4 000 years. Pharaonic texts show that even then it was used as a digestive herb, diuretic and to help ease toothache. The Greeks used it too; Dioscorides wrote in the first century that aniseed 'warms, dries and dissolves, facilitates breathing, relieves pain, provokes urine and eases thirst'. Modern medical science has proved that these ancient uses of this marvellous herb were indeed correct.

CULTIVATION

Anise is an attractive, short-lived annual growing up to 50 cm in height with pretty, feathery flowers typical of the Umbelliferae, often mistakenly called lace flowers. It is a rewarding plant to grow as it demands nothing more than good, well-composted soil, full sun and a twice-weekly watering. It thrives on neglect, gives a swift return on its easily and quickly raised seeds, and is a delight to the eye and palate with its fragile beauty, tender buds and leaves, and pungent seeds. When growing anise in the garden I have found that the more one picks, the more flowers are produced.

MEDICINAL USES

Aniseed (and to some extent the leaves and flowers) helps with all digestive ailments, from colic and bloating to nausea, flatulence, heartburn and tummy rumblings, in all age groups, from infants through to the very elderly. Both the seeds and flowers are antispasmodic. Simply chewing a few seeds or flowers will ease period pain, asthma, bronchitis and coughing (it helps to dry up phlegm and is a known expectorant), and for whooping cough there is nothing better.

Doctors are now looking at anise flowers and seeds to help with irregular heartbeat and to ease anxiety. Stress is ever-increasing in our frenetic fast-paced lives, and anise's extraordinary antispasmodic effect can be relied on to ease tight chest pains and distressed breathing. Sit quietly, take several deep breaths, and slowly sip a cup of anise health tea. It is also excellent for children writing exams, especially with a sprig of peppermint in the tea to boost concentration and promote clear thinking. When there is a tension headache this tea often gives immediate results, and in the case of a chill, shock or severe agitation this remarkably soothing tea is definitely worth trying. Anise flowers in the diet and a tea made from the seeds helps breast-milk production in nursing mothers, and reduces acidity. All in all, anise really should be used more than it is!

Anise health tea

SERVES 1

I find this tea superb after a heavy meal or when I have dined out, or eaten rich or spicy food. It also helps with cramps and coughs and every other ailment mentioned above. I even travel with a little jar of aniseed and some dried flowers to ensure that I have a good night. Omit the honey if you prefer the tea unsweetened.

2 teaspoons aniseed
1 tablespoon fresh flowers and leaves
Honey

Pour a cup of boiling water over the seeds, flowers and leaves and allow the tea to stand for five minutes. Stir well, strain, sweeten with a touch of honey, and sip slowly.

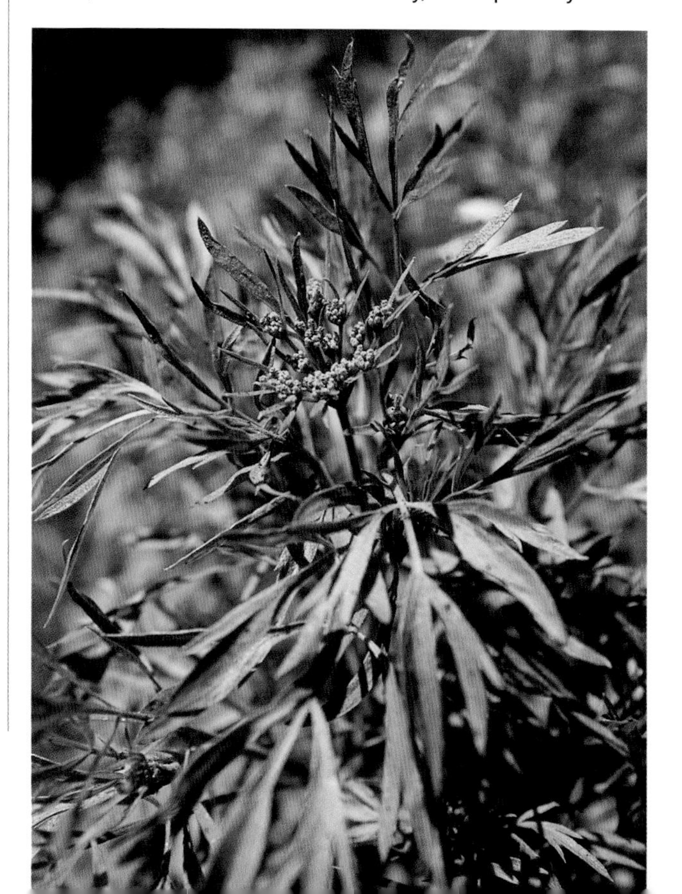

Anise de-stress vinegar

This excellent de-stressing vinegar can be used in two ways: mixed with water, it makes a delicious, soothing beverage at the end of a frantically busy day; used in the bath, it literally calms, untangles and eases you – lie back and enjoy its comforting presence. Be sure to make lots of this precious vinegar while your aniseed plants are in flower!

1 large bottle apple cider vinegar
Anise sprigs, flowers and leaves
1 tablespoon aniseeds

Press aniseeds, and as many sprigs, flowers and leaves as possible, into the vinegar. Keep in a warm place out of direct sunlight and shake up daily. After 10 days, strain out the flowers, leaves and seeds and replace with fresh ones. Keep it in a warm place for a further 10 days, shaking daily. Repeat the process if needed. Finally, strain, pour into a clean bottle and label. For easy identification, push in one fresh flowering sprig or a tablespoon of seeds.

To take orally, mix two teaspoons of vinegar in a glass of chilled water and sip slowly, especially on a hot afternoon. For a soothing bath, add a dash to the water and relax.

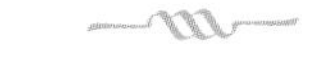

CULINARY USES

Anise apple dessert

SERVES 6

This dessert is quick, easy and delicious served either hot with cream and custard, or cold with ice-cream.

6 Golden Delicious apples
A few thin strips of fresh ginger
Sultanas
½ cup honey
1 cup sunflower seeds
1 cup anise flowers, stripped off their stems
½ cup soft butter

Core the unpeeled apples and place them in a steamer. Press some ginger and a few sultanas into the cores, and steam for 15 minutes. Mix the honey with the sunflower seeds, anise flowers and the butter, and spoon over the apples. Cover and steam for a further 15 minutes. Serve either hot or cold, with the fragrant sauce poured over the fruit.

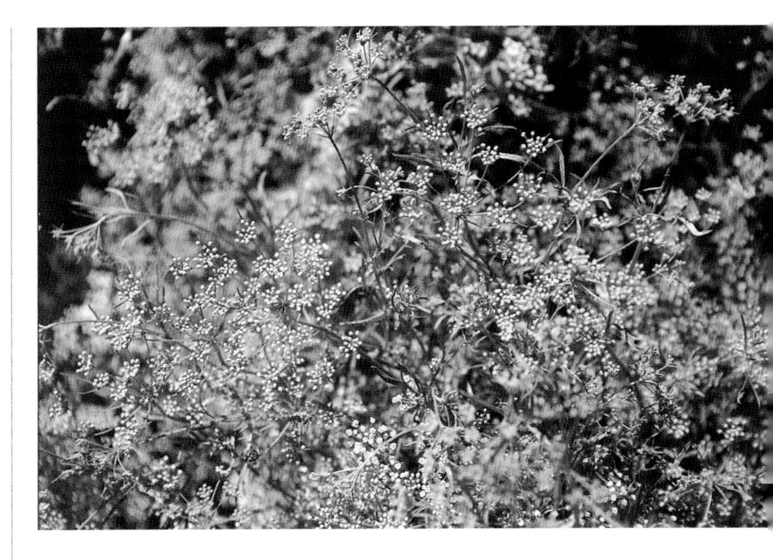

Anise pasta confetti salad

SERVES 4–6

I make this bright salad for summer picnics when the anise flowers are at their best. It keeps well in the fridge.

300 g pasta shells or any small pasta
2 carrots, peeled and finely grated
1 red pepper, finely chopped
2 sticks celery and their leaves, finely chopped
2 tablespoons parsley, finely chopped
6 radishes, finely chopped

Dressing
½ cup grape vinegar
¾ cup anise flowers, stripped off their stems
½ cup water
½ cup honey
2 teaspoons mustard powder
3 tablespoons olive oil

Cook the pasta in rapidly boiling water until *al dente*. Drain, rinse in cold water and leave to cool. Mix with the carrots, red pepper, celery, parsley and radishes, and refrigerate.

Place the dressing ingredients in a screw-top bottle and shake well. Leave to stand and infuse. Just before serving, shake the dressing, pour over the pasta salad and mix well.

COOK'S NOTE

Anise leaves give a refreshing taste when chopped into salads, soups and stews, and sprinkled on fritters, the freshly chopped leaves and flowers will aid digestion.

Artichoke

Cynara scolymus • **Globe artichoke**

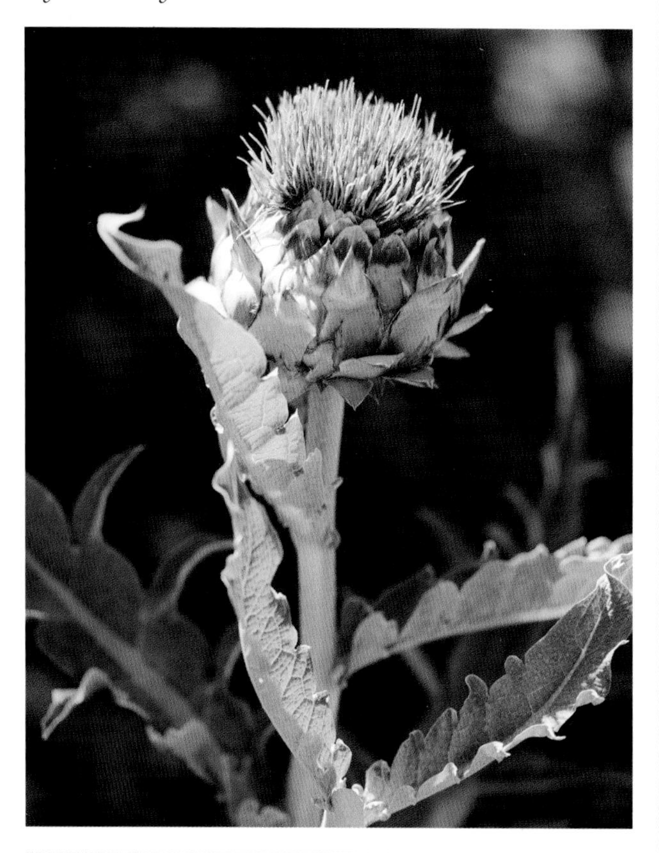

Greatly esteemed by the ancient Greeks and Romans, the artichoke was used as both a food and a medicine, and finds its place in the pharmacopoeias of the world from the earliest times. In the first century AD, Dioscorides recommended using mashed artichoke root as a deodorant, applying it as a scrub to the armpits and feet to fend off offensive odours!

The Italians are considered the best artichoke growers in the world and fields of the beautiful silvery-grey leaves, fat juicy buds and thistle-like purple flowers grace the Italian landscape. As a garden plant it is eye-catching, and a row in the vegetable garden will give three or four years of spring-flowering heads.

CULTIVATION

Native to the Mediterranean region, this much-loved plant thrives in warmth and sun, and needs richly composted, deeply dug, moist, loamy soil – the richer the soil the better. Artichokes are propagated by seed, with the seeds sown 1.5 m apart in rows. They grow over 1 m in height and produce beautiful flowers during spring and early summer. After flowering, new shoots will appear at the base, which in turn will mature the following season into new flower-bearing plants. Although the artichoke is considered to be a perennial, it is often planted as an annual or a biennial, or renewed every three or four years. Cut the flowering heads back after reaping the unopened flower buds, and mulch well. Leave some buds to mature and dry on the stems before cutting, and reap your own organic seed.

MEDICINAL USES

Although all parts of the globe artichoke are medicinal, the young flower buds and leaves have the highest levels of beneficial constituents for high cholesterol, gall bladder ailments, nausea, indigestion and abdominal bloating, distension and flatulence. All parts of the plant are bitter and stimulate digestive secretions, which in turn help to cleanse the liver and move toxins out of the system, protecting against infection. Current medical research is indicating that artichoke can boost the immune system, and simply adding globe artichokes to the diet will help to promote the flow of bile to the gall bladder, ensuring a healthy liver.

The globe artichoke is rich in vitamins A, C and all the B-vitamins, especially folic acid, biotin and niacin. The whole plant contains insulin, a polysaccharide that helps to control blood sugar, hence it is especially valuable for diabetics. It also contains cynarin, predominantly in the flower scales and leaves, which tones and improves the functioning of the arterial lining. In addition, artichokes are rich in natural and easily utilised iron, magnesium, phosphorus, potassium and manganese, and have been found to help with anaemia, glandular disorders, obesity, kidney ailments, diarrhoea and even chronic halitosis. They are also a good diuretic.

The seeds from the mature flowering head make an excellent tea. To make the tea, pour a cup of boiling water over 1–2 teaspoons of crushed seeds from your own organically grown plants. Allow the tea to stand for five minutes, stirring every now and then. Strain and sip slowly. Add a squeeze or two of fresh lemon juice for more flavour, if desired.

You can dry the flower heads after the flowers have matured by cutting them in half and drying them in a warm dry place. Turn them frequently. Once they are bone dry, store in airtight glass jars. In this way you will have this precious natural medicine year-round and not only in spring when artichokes begin their flowering cycle.

CAUTION: Women who are pregnant or breast-feeding should avoid the globe artichoke as it contains a substance that curdles milk.

Old Mediterranean liver tonic remedy

2 tablespoons fresh artichoke juice (1 cup artichoke leaves, 2–3 young flower buds and ½ cup hot water)
1 cup wine or hot water

To make the artichoke juice, liquefy the chopped artichoke leaves and flower buds with the hot water, and strain. Add the wine or hot water to the juice, and take one cupful daily as a liver cleanser and high cholesterol treatment.

CULINARY USES

Pickled artichokes

MAKES 1 LARGE JAR

Serve these delicious pickled artichokes with cheese and salads or finely chopped over mushroom dishes.

6 young tender artichoke buds
1 sprig origanum
2 bay leaves
2 sprigs parsley
2 cups brown grape vinegar
1½ cups brown sugar
½ cup mustard seeds

Select young tender buds, cut off the tough outer leaves and pare away the tops of the leaves, leaving the base. Scoop out any of the fluffy flower parts, the thistle's 'choke', and cut the heart into quarters. Pack into a glass jar, and add the origanum, bay leaves and parsley. Boil up the vinegar with brown sugar and mustard seeds for 10 minutes. Pour the hot mixture over the artichoke hearts, seal and label. Leave them to mature for at least a month before eating.

Artichokes with mint and yoghurt

SERVES 4

This recipe is delicious as a summer starter or even as a supper dish. The dressing is a healthy alternative to butter.

4 large artichokes, trimmed
1 sprig mint
Salt

Dressing
1 cup plain yoghurt
2 tablespoons finely chopped mint
4 spring onions, finely chopped
Juice of 1 lemon
2 tablespoons olive oil
Sea salt and black pepper to taste

Boil the artichokes in water with a sprig of mint and salt for about 45 minutes until they are tender. Drain. Remove the tough outer leaves and open out the centres. Pull away the tight tiny pale leaves, and using a teaspoon, scrape out the thistle-like fluff, the choke. Leave to cool. Mix the dressing ingredients together and pour into the centre of each artichoke. Dip each scale into the dressing and enjoy!

Artichoke dip

SERVES 6

This is the most delicious and nourishing dip I know. Serve it with savoury biscuits, chips, celery and carrot-sticks, or use it as a filling for baked potatoes. Use tinned artichoke hearts if it is not artichoke season.

250 g artichoke hearts, freshly cooked and finely chopped
2 tablespoons finely chopped parsley
1 medium onion, finely chopped
2 tablespoons parmesan cheese
½–¾ cup good mayonnaise
Juice of 1 lemon
Sea salt and black pepper to taste

Mix the ingredients together well. For a smoother dip, whirl everything together in a blender. I often ring the changes with one of the following: ½ cup chopped green pepper, ¾ cup chopped fresh brown mushrooms, or ¾ cup mashed avocado. Try spreading a little as a pizza topping.

COOK'S NOTE

Try sprouting your own organic artichoke seeds and see how delicious they are – the slight bitterness improves with a little lemon juice. Soak the seeds overnight, then spread on wet cotton wool in a shallow glass dish. Cover with another layer of cotton wool and keep moist. Check daily. Once they have sprouted, remove the top layer of cotton wool and keep the little sprouts moist with a frequent spritz spray of water. Eat with salads when 2–3 cm high.

Banana flower

Musa species

The banana tree or palm is a huge-leafed, exotic tropical plant that can grow up to 3–4 m in height, with a magnificent sheath of leaves at its crown. Each mature shoot produces an exquisite flowering stalk, which hangs under the protective canopy of giant leaves. Ideally it needs hot, moist, tropical air, but it will survive and even produce fruit against a sunny wall where it is protected against cold winds.

The banana is thought to have originated in Indo-Malaysia and eastern Asia. The ancient Egyptians are known to have eaten the Abyssinian banana, *Musa ensete*, and many varieties have been recorded in the tropical and subtropical regions of the world over the centuries.

CULTIVATION

Growing bananas is a fascinating hobby. Viable shoots can be cut away from the parent plant and propagated in full sun in moist, richly composted soil, and a stem will flower and fruit in about 15 months. Once the main shoot has fruited, it can be cut out to allow space for the next shoot to emerge. The clump or 'stool', as it is known botanically, can live for 60–70 years, sending up new fruit shoots continuously, but commercial growers keep the clump going for usually no more than 8–10 years, before replacing it with new stock.

Apply a fresh load of compost annually and dig it in carefully around the plant so as not to damage the emerging shoots. In January I dump a barrow load on top of the clump as well and give it a deep twice-weekly watering. The leaves really need moisture, so spray them with a hose often during hot dry periods. The best varieties to grow in South Africa, all of which have edible flowers, are *Musa* 'Cavendish', *Musa* 'Williams', *Musa* 'Grand Nain' selec American, and selec Israeli.

MEDICINAL USES

The ancient Egyptians used banana leaves, fruit and flowering sheaths as a wound dressing, often mashing the fruit and applying it as a poultice over rashes, infected scratches, grazes and burns, covered either with a banana skin or with a leaf warmed in hot water. Today many surfers worldwide use mashed banana pulp on sunburnt shoulders and noses. Hikers rub aching heels, corns and blisters with the inside of a banana skin and use the flowering bract, magenta in colour and spongy and crisp when young, as a heel guard, pressed into shoes to ease cracks in the heel.

COSMETIC USES

In Hawaii, flowering bracts are boiled in twice the volume of water, together with a few ripe banana skins, as a hair rinse for scalp problems, oily hair and hair that falls out. Boil for 20 minutes, cool, strain and use as a scalp massage and hair rinse. Sceptics wonder how this can possibly help, but just look at the Hawaiians' beautiful thick glossy hair!

Banana flower cream for cracked heels and dry skin

1½ cups good aqueous cream
1 cup finely sliced banana flower bracts
½ cup finely sliced skin of a partially ripe banana
2 teaspoons thinly pared skin of a lemon
2 teaspoons vitamin E oil
1 teaspoon lemon essential oil

Simmer the aqueous cream, banana bracts, banana skin and lemon rind in a double boiler, pressing down well and bruising the bracts. Simmer for 20 minutes. Cool for 10 minutes, and strain. Add the vitamin E and lemon essential oils and mix thoroughly. Store in a sterilised glass jar. Massage often into cracked heels and dry skin on the feet and legs.

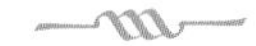

CULINARY USES

Banana blossom paella

SERVES 4–6

This is an easy-to-prepare Mauritian recipe that varies from village to village as the ingredients become available through the season.

4 medium onions, chopped
4 cups white fish, skinned, deboned and cubed
A few shrimps or langoustines, shelled and deveined
¼–½ cup olive oil
2 cups banana flowers, shredded and rinsed
2 green or red sweet peppers, cut into strips
½ cup desiccated coconut
½ cup sesame seeds
Juice of 1 lemon
Sea salt and cayenne pepper to taste
½ cup chopped mint

Brown the onions and seafood in the oil in a large wok. Add the banana flowers and stir-fry for about 10 minutes. Then add the green or red peppers and stir-fry, turning frequently. Add all the other ingredients except the mint and keep stir-frying. Finally, add the mint, and serve immediately on a bed of rice. Add a little water to the juices in the pan and pour over the paella.

COOK'S NOTE

In Sri Lanka, banana buds are a well-loved vegetable boiled and served with lemon juice, salt and fish, and in China they are pickled. Always prepare the flowers with salt and lemon juice before cooking with them, as described in the recipe above.

Banana flower kari-kari

SERVES 4

This quick and delicious dish was probably first enjoyed in the Philippines. It has many variants, but this is the plainest.

2 cups thinly shredded banana flowers, turned in salt and lemon juice
4 cups slivered topside beef
Sunflower oil
3 garlic cloves, thinly slivered
2 medium onions, thinly sliced
2 cups chopped green spring onions
1–2 tablespoons grated ginger root
2 tablespoons soy sauce
1 cup water
Sea salt and black pepper to taste

Prepare the banana flowers with salt and lemon juice as described in the cook's note. Meanwhile, gently sauté the beef in the oil until brown, then add the garlic and onions. When soft, add the banana flowers that have been drenched in fresh lemon juice. Add the spring onions and grated ginger root, soy sauce and water, and salt and pepper to taste. Simmer gently for about 10 minutes, adding more water if necessary. Serve with rice or pasta.

COOK'S NOTE

To prepare banana flowers for cooking, remove the tough, sheath-like covering from the flowers. Slice the flowers thinly crosswise, sprinkle with salt, and let them stand for an hour. Squeeze them with the salt, add lemon juice and squeeze again, then rinse. This removes any milky sap and astringency and makes the flowers more tender.

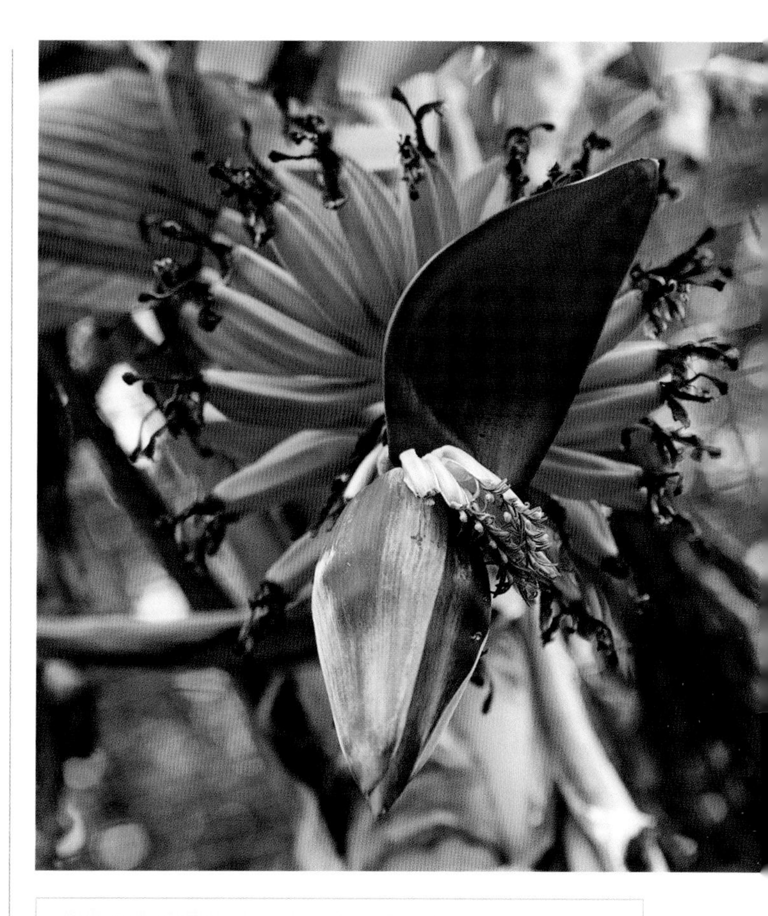

COOK'S NOTE

To ring the changes, add bacon, chopped green pepper or celery, peeled tomatoes, or thinly sliced aubergines to the banana flower kari-kari, or experiment with your own combinations.

Banana flower and mushroom sauce

SERVES 4

2 medium onions, minced
½–¾ cup olive oil
3 cups brown mushrooms, finely chopped
2 cups banana flowers, thinly sliced and prepared (see cook's note)
1–2 tablespoons rich soy sauce
½ tablespoon Worcestershire sauce
1 cup seedless raisins, soaked overnight and then finely chopped
1 cup minced celery
2 tablespoons lemon juice
Sea salt and cayenne pepper to taste
2 cups water

Brown the onions in the olive oil. Add the remaining ingredients and stir-fry until tender. Serve hot with rice.

Bergamot

Monarda didyma ● **Bee balm** ● **Oswego tea**

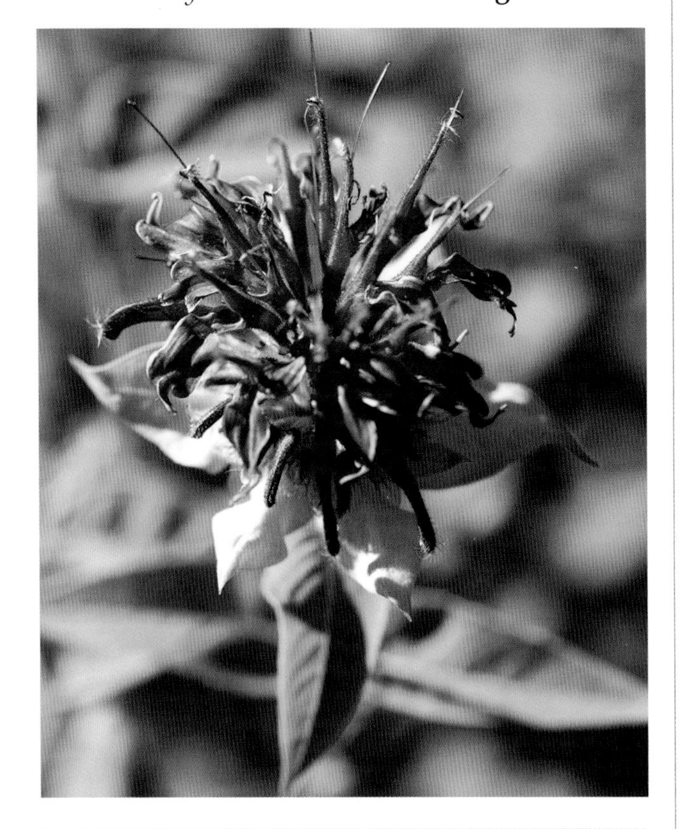

Bergamot originated in North America, where the great swathes of red bergamot flowers in the grasslands around the Oswego River near Lake Ontario earned it its name of 'Oswego tea'. The Cherokee Indians as well as the Chippewa, Fox and Ojibwa Indians were the first to use it to ease digestive and respiratory symptoms. Its superb health benefits became more widely known after the famous Boston Tea Party in 1773, when the citizens of Boston rebelled against taxes imposed on tea and the monopoly given to the East India Company. Disguised as Indians, they raided three British ships in Boston Harbour, tossing a shipload of English tea overboard. Bergamot or Oswego tea became the fashionable tea to drink.

CULTIVATION

Bergamot is easy and rewarding to grow and is so loved by bees and butterflies that no garden should be without it. It needs full sun and well-composted soil, and in midsummer it is spectacular with its bright flowering spikes ranging from 80 cm to 1 m in height. Once spent, these need to be cut off and the plant tends to look a bit lost, so it is best planted in a mixed border. It forms a cushion-like perennial clump that needs to be divided every three or four years. Do this in winter by thrusting two forks back to back into the centre and splitting it in that way. Plant out into well-composted soil and by midsummer you will have tall spikes of bright, fragrant flowers again. There are many bergamot varieties, with flowers ranging in colour from mauve to deep magenta, and from bright pink to purple. All have the same uses.

MEDICINAL USES

Bergamot is a most comforting tea for the elderly, taken last thing at night. Bergamot health tea helps settle the digestion, eases muscular aches and joint pains, and acts as a sedative that disperses fears and helps to regulate the sleep pattern. Taken with chamomile tea (add one flowering head or one leaf to chamomile tea), bergamot also helps to calm and unwind, digest rich food and ease the day's tensions. For digestive problems, colic, nausea, bloated distended stomach, vomiting, flatulence and belching, make the standard brew tea (¼ cup bergamot flowers and leaves steeped in a cup of boiling water), and add four cloves per cup. Sip slowly and chew one of the cloves gently every now and then. A teaspoonful of this brew can be given to a fretting baby and to children who have eaten too many sweet things.

Bergamot health tea

SERVES 1

If you enjoy the taste of Earl Grey tea, you can make your own by adding one or two bergamot leaves and a bergamot flower to a pot of ordinary Ceylon tea. This will infuse, giving it that typical Earl Grey taste. (Note that commercial Earl Grey tea is not made with bergamot, but with the dried rind or essential oil of the bergamot orange, Citrus bergamia*.)*

1 bergamot flower, calyx discarded
1 bergamot leaf
1 teabag of your favourite tea
1 cup boiling water
Honey and lemon to taste

Pull the petals out of the calyx and infuse with the leaf and your favourite tea for a few minutes in boiling water. Strain, sweeten with honey and add a slice of lemon. Serve either hot or cold and sip slowly. If served cold, make ice cubes with the top petals of the bergamot flower, and add a little lemon juice. This tea will relax you and clear a stuffy head.

Bergamot massage cream

Use this cream to ease aches, muscular strains and stiff sore muscles and to soften dry wind- or sun-burned skin.

1 cup good aqueous cream
1 cup fresh bergamot flowers and leaves
10 cloves, lightly crushed
6 drops clove oil
2 teaspoons vitamin E oil

Simmer the aqueous cream, bergamot and cloves, stirring frequently for 20 minutes. Cool for 10 minutes and strain. Discard the leaves, flowers and cloves. Add the clove oil and vitamin E oil, stir well, and spoon into a screw-top glass jar. Warm the cream before applying by standing the jar in a bowl of hot water. Apply the cream frequently, and in the case of sprains and sore muscles, keep the area warm with a hot-water bottle wrapped in a soft towel.

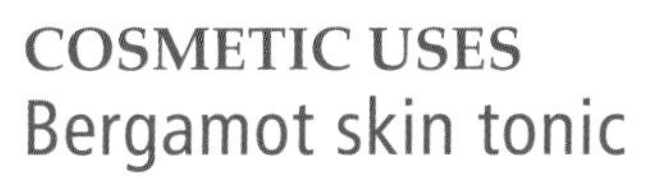

COSMETIC USES
Bergamot skin tonic

Use this tonic for itchy, dry skin and sunburn.

1 cup bergamot leaves and flowers
1½ litres water

Boil the bergamot in the water for 10 minutes. Cool and strain. Use as a splash or spritz, or add to the bath.

CULINARY USES
Bergamot and peach jelly

SERVES 4–6

This was one of my children's favourite puddings, which I made often during summer using a basket of ripening peaches that needed to be eaten, and a whole row of bright bergamot in flower.

10 peaches
3 tablespoons gelatine
1 cup warm water
1 litre unsweetened peach and orange juice or peach and mango juice
Honey if desired
1 cup bergamot flowers, stripped off their calyxes

Peel and slice the peaches. Mix the gelatine with warm water until dissolved. Stir the gelatine into the fruit juice, adding a little honey if it is not sweet enough. Add the peaches, and finally toss the bergamot flowers stripped off their calyxes into the mixture. Pour into a glass bowl and set in the fridge. Once set, serve with whipped bergamot cream or custard decorated with bergamot flowers.

Roasted okra with bergamot flowers

SERVES 4

The secret of this extraordinary lunch dish is to use very young and tender okra pods. Serve the dish with roast chicken and roast potatoes.

20 very young okra pods
Olive oil
Sea salt and black pepper
½ cup chopped bergamot petals
Juice of 1 lemon
Parmesan cheese
Tabasco sauce

Trim the stalks off the okra pods. Dip pods individually into olive oil and lay them on a baking sheet. Sprinkle with salt, black pepper, chopped bergamot petals and lemon juice. Roast for 20 minutes or until they start to crisp. Sprinkle with parmesan cheese and a few drops of Tabasco sauce. Serve hot.

Bergamot cream

250 ml thick cream
1–2 tablespoons icing sugar
½ cup bergamot petals

Whip the cream with the icing sugar. Fold the bergamot petals in lightly. Spoon into a pretty glass bowl and decorate with bergamot flowers.

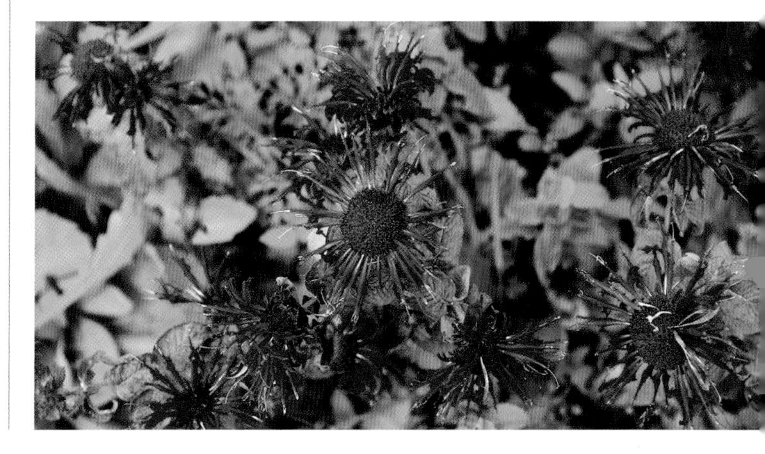

Borage

Borago officinalis

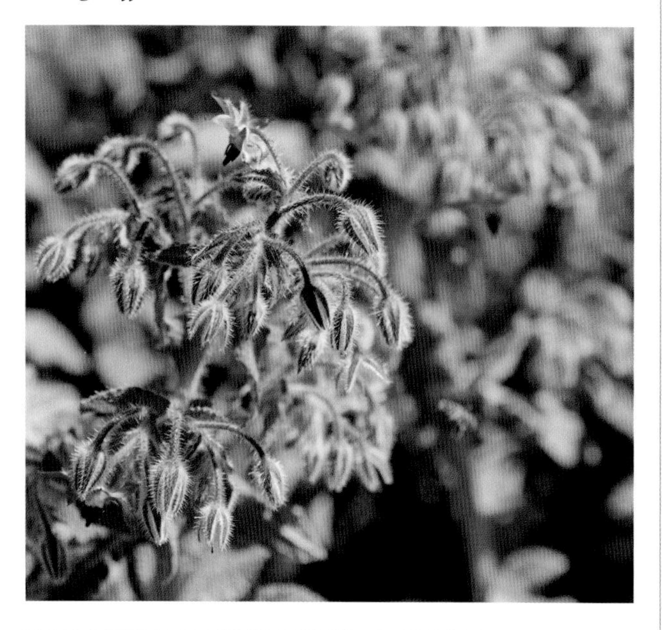

A hairy weed native to the Mediterranean regions, borage is a robust and prolific annual that grows with ease all over the world. It is an ancient, much-revered herb, and has an important place in both food and medicine. Through the centuries its calming and stress-relieving qualities have been well recognised, and the crusaders took it on their pilgrimages to give them courage and induce calmness of mind. In Elizabethan times, borage flowers were added to drinks like claret cup to prevent drunkenness while adding to the merriment. Traditionally the flowers were made into syrups and wines, taken for coughs and colds and also for anxiety and fear, which is why borage has been important through the ages for treating grief and depression.

CULTIVATION

The exquisite blue, star-shaped flowers make a wonderful show in summer and attract bees and butterflies to the garden. They have a fresh, cucumber-like flavour and can be added to cordials, Pimm's cup, salads and desserts. The plants are prolific, and both leaves and flowers benefit from picking. Borage readily seeds itself and needs space in the garden as it can grow up to 80 cm in height and about 60 cm in width. It needs richly composted, well-dug soil in full sun and thrives with a good twice-weekly watering. Even in the dry area where I live it seems to survive against all odds, sending up its blaze of beautiful blue and reseeding itself everywhere, even in winter. The tiny seedlings are easily transplanted.

MEDICINAL USES

A tea made from borage leaves and flowers will reduce high temperatures by inducing sweating and will act on flu and colds quickly and reliably. Rich in potassium and calcium, the tea is both a tonic and a blood purifier. To make borage tea add ¼ cup fresh flowering tops and leaves to a cup of boiling water. Allow the tea to stand for five minutes, then strain and sip slowly. With its high mucilage content it soothes respiratory ailments, chronic coughs, bronchitis, pleurisy, tight chests and whooping cough, easing and breaking down mucous. Make no more than one cup of borage tea a day; divide it up and take a little throughout the day.

Borage also has a comforting emollient action due to its soothing saponins and tannins, which is helpful for sore, inflamed skin.

> CAUTION: Like comfrey, borage contains pyrrolizidine alkaloids, so it should not be taken internally too often. The flowers and seeds, from which borage oil is made, are the safest parts of the plant.

Borage lotion

Use this lotion for eczema, psoriasis, sunburn, rashes and itches.

1 cup borage leaves and flowers
3 cups water

Boil the borage leaves and flowers in the water for 10 minutes. Leave the lotion to cool, then strain and pour into a spritz bottle and spray frequently over the area or dab on often. It will soothe a wide range of skin conditions.

CULINARY USES

Borage sangria

SERVES 6–8

I was once lucky enough to find an ancient recipe made by monks in England, who called borage 'the Good Herb'. My modern version of this ancient drink has drawn many a favourable comment, especially when served warm on a cold winter's night.

3 thumb-length sprigs fresh rosemary
2 cups borage leaves, stems and flowers, roughly chopped
4 tablespoons honey
4 cups good red wine
2 cups pure apple juice
2 lemons, thinly sliced
1 naartjie, thinly sliced
Borage flowers

Crush the rosemary and borage leaves, stems and flowers and pour the honey and wine over them. Stir well and leave to stand for about an hour. Add the apple juice and the fruit and stir well. Cover and refrigerate for a day and a night. Strain the following day. Keep chilled. Serve either hot or cold before dinner and float several borage flowers on it before serving.

Hearty borage winter health soup

SERVES 6–8

Borage survives the coldest winds, so you will always be able to find something fresh and green during the winter frosts. This is my winter standby and I make a big pot every few days as it keeps well in the fridge. Soak the pulses overnight beforehand.

1 cup butter beans, soaked overnight
1 cup pearl barley, soaked overnight
1 cup lentils, soaked overnight
1 cup split peas, soaked overnight
3 large onions, finely chopped
Sunflower oil
2 sweet potatoes, grated
6 celery stalks and leaves
6 carrots, finely grated
2 cups borage leaves, finely chopped
4 tomatoes, skinned and chopped
Sea salt and cayenne pepper to taste
2 tablespoons soy sauce
2 teaspoons Marmite
Juice of 1 lemon
2 litres water or stock

Drain and rinse the soaked beans, barley, lentils and peas. Brown the onions in the oil. Add the sweet potato and celery and stir-fry. Once they start to brown, add all the other ingredients. Mix well and simmer gently, adding more water if necessary. Keep covered and on low heat, and adjust the flavouring as preferred. Cook for about one hour or until the beans are tender. Serve with fresh brown bread and butter.

COOK'S NOTE

This soup is rich in vitamins and is filling and satisfying. Ring the changes by using green peppers, mushrooms, finely shredded cabbage or kale, spring onions, grated pumpkin or butternut, or squash.

Borage fritters

SERVES 4–6

These fritters make a delicious snack served as an appetiser or as a side dish to stews or roasts.

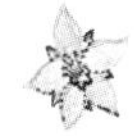

12 borage leaves
Sunflower oil

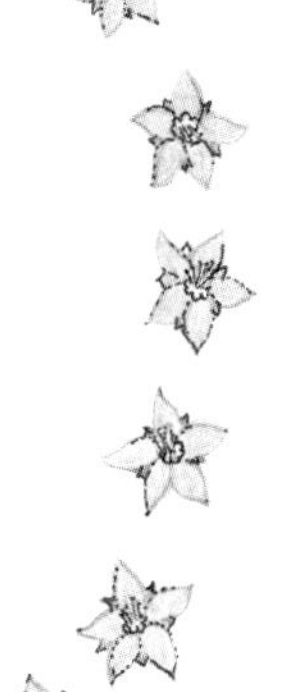

Batter
1 cup flour
1 cup milk
1 egg, beaten
½ cup water
1 teaspoon grated nutmeg
1 teaspoon crushed coriander
Sea salt and black pepper to taste

Mix all the batter ingredients together until a runny consistency is achieved. Heat the oil in a frying pan. Dip each leaf into the batter and lay it carefully in the hot oil, turning when necessary. When they are golden brown, remove the leaves from the oil with tongs and drain on crumpled paper towel. Serve hot.

COOK'S NOTE

Set borage flowers in an ice tray, one flower per ice cube. In a cooldrink the ice will melt, leaving the flower to be enjoyed, as it tastes fresh and delicious when chilled.

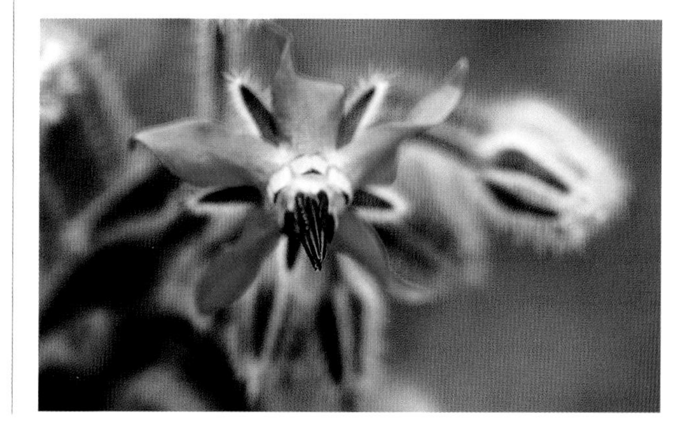

Broccoli

Brassica oleracea

Broccoli is the flowering head of an easy-to-grow winter annual. It is a member of the huge and vital cruciferous family of cabbages, kales and cauliflowers that developed from the ancient wild cabbages in Europe and the Mediterranean area.

It is incredible to think that for well over 2 000 years broccoli has been planted as a food crop. We have the Romans to thank for their dedication in selecting the best plants and saving the seed year by year that put broccoli in a class of its own.

By the 16th century broccoli had become so much a part of the Mediterranean diet that broccoli trade began, and in this way it gradually spread throughout the world. Monks in medieval England created the first medicinal gardens and grew food crops among the medicinal herbs. They treated the sick with these plants, and broccoli, onions, celery and other green herbs such as thyme, shallots and some of the spinaches, were cooked into nourishing 'gruels' and broths that became well known for relieving coughs, colds, flu, bronchitis and 'wasting illnesses'.

Broccoli is listed in ancient herbals and pharmacopoeias as a medicine and food. It was also recorded as being a good food for the spirit, lifting despair, depression and anxiety. Broccoli featured strongly in these medications and broths, and its role in the diet was recognised in restoring physical and emotional wellbeing.

It was only in 1923 that the D'Arrigo brothers, originally from Italy, began the first plantings of broccoli in California. In 1929 the brothers began advertising this extraordinary health food, and the broccoli industry took off and has never looked back!

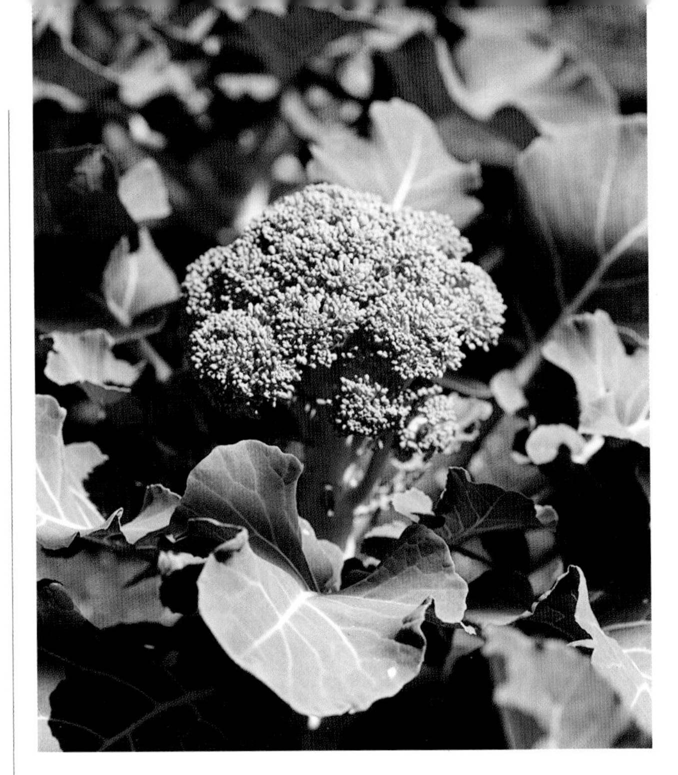

CULTIVATION

Best grown as a winter annual, broccoli thrives in a deeply dug richly composted bed in full sun. Start the seeds off in seed trays (they germinate easily) and when big enough to handle, about 10 cm in height, prick the tiny plants out and plant into moist rows, spaced 50 cm apart. Do not let them dry out. Keep them shaded with dry leaves for the first few days.

The florets form quickly and can be reaped at a fairly young stage. Water the plants well twice-weekly. Allow some to set seed as in the heat of the summer aphids and black fly are a problem, and in order to save the crop broccoli needs to be heavily sprayed with chemicals. This is why winter-grown broccoli is so important. Chemically sprayed broccoli will not build up health, it will break it down, and heavy spraying is the only way that commercial farmers can produce crops. So rather grow broccoli sprouts in the summer months and grow your own broccoli through the cooler months. Sow the first seeds in March and continue through to early August. After that grow your own organic seed sprouts throughout the summer. Broccoli seed, especially organically grown seed, has become worth its weight in gold! Save all you can from your own plantings.

MEDICINAL USES

Broccoli is an excellent source of vitamins C, A, K, B_6 and E, as well as folic acid, magnesium, calcium, potassium and phosphorus. With this amazing array of health boosters, broccoli has been considered a superfood for centuries.

Make 'monks' broccoli broth' as a winter health builder and have it daily. I make this soup every week and keep any excess in the fridge. Warm up a cupful when on the run and squeeze in extra lemon juice if feeling tired or if a cold is threatening. In cases of breast cancer, lung cancer, colon cancer, cancer of the throat, oesophagus, pharynx, larynx, stomach and prostate, this soup should be part of the daily diet.

Broccoli is essential for smokers. It is low in calories, high in lutein, and is essential for obesity, toxaemia, high blood pressure, kidney ailments and constipation.

And given our exposure to cell phone, computer and chemical radiation, broccoli is a lifesaver. Start growing it today!

Broccoli sprouts are extremely valuable for children. Teach them to grow their own and to eat them on sandwiches and in salads daily. Chop the organically grown broccoli leaves into stir-fries – it boosts the immune system!

Monks' broccoli broth for colds, flu and cancer protection

SERVES 6

I have perused many ancient herbals and have found this to be closest to the gruel or broth served by the monks as a health booster.

½ cup olive oil
2 cups chopped onion
2 cups thinly sliced leek
2 cups chopped celery
2 large broccoli heads
1 cup pearl barley
2 cups buckwheat greens, flowers included
2 cups mustard greens, flowers included
2 cups spinach
2 cups radish, finely chopped, leaves included, or 2 cups grated turnip, leaves included
Juice of 2 lemons and a little lemon zest
Sea salt to taste
Red pepper or paprika to taste
2 litres rich stock

Pour the olive oil into a large heavy stainless steel pot. Brown the onions and leeks. Add the remaining ingredients, stirring all the time. Simmer until everything is tender. Add more lemon juice and salt, if needed. Remember that this is a health soup for coughs, colds, flu, bronchitis, cancer protection and for age-related ailments such as macular degeneration of the eyes, digestive problems and circulatory ailments. So do not add other flavourings or sauces.

Broccoli contains vitamin C – 73 mg to 100 g of broccoli. It is also rich in vitamins A and B_2 predominantly with calcium, iron and potassium, and is used to clear toxaemia, ease hypertension, clear a toxic liver and to get the digestive system up and running. Steam 2 cups daily and eat with lemon juice.

CAUTION: Do not eat broccoli if you have an underactive thyroid; it will exacerbate the problem.

CULINARY USES

Steamed broccoli florets and leaves

SERVES 4–6

This is a real comfort food and one that is good for the entire family. Use a bamboo steamer if possible as it gives the broccoli a fresh taste.

1 head broccoli

Cheese sauce

3 cups milk (full-cream or low-fat)
2 tablespoons cornflour
½ teaspoon salt
½ teaspoon paprika
1 egg, beaten
1½ cups grated cheddar cheese

Steam a whole head of broccoli, broken into florets, as well as the lightly chopped surrounding leaves. It steams in about 15 minutes to tender perfection.

While the broccoli is steaming, make a rich white sauce. Simmer 2½ cups of the milk in a heavy-bottomed pot. As it begins to boil, stir in the cornflour that has been dissolved in the remaining half cup of milk. Add the salt, paprika and beaten egg. Stir in, whisking all the time, on very low heat (do not stop or take your eyes off it for a minute). As it thickens, stir in one cup of the cheddar cheese, mixing it in quickly. Spoon the hot broccoli into an ovenproof glass dish. Pour the cheese sauce over it, sprinkle with the remaining half cup of grated cheese and a grinding of black pepper and keep it warm in a low oven until ready to serve. This will melt the cheese and keep it piping hot. Serve with Sunday roast chicken, roast potatoes and garden-picked winter peas.

COOK'S NOTE

Fresh broccoli florets in a winter salad of butter lettuce, celery stalks and leaves, rocket, mustard greens and baby spinach, with a good squeeze of lemon juice, will keep winter colds and flu away. For variety, add sprinklings of sprouts and lots of chopped parsley. It will give you energy you didn't know you had!

Buckwheat

Fagopyrum esculentum

Although buckwheat is not truly a grain, it is classified as such in most cook books. Sometimes called 'Saracen corn', it originated in Asia and was brought to Europe by the crusaders. Today it is still widely grown, primarily for its remarkable mineral and vitamin content and its exceptionally high rutin content. Rutin is of utmost importance in strengthening the walls of blood vessels, in the treatment of high cholesterol, and for varicose veins, thread veins and the capillaries in the retina of the eye. The creamy white flowers are equally rich in rutin, and are tender and appetising served on all sorts of savoury and sweet dishes.

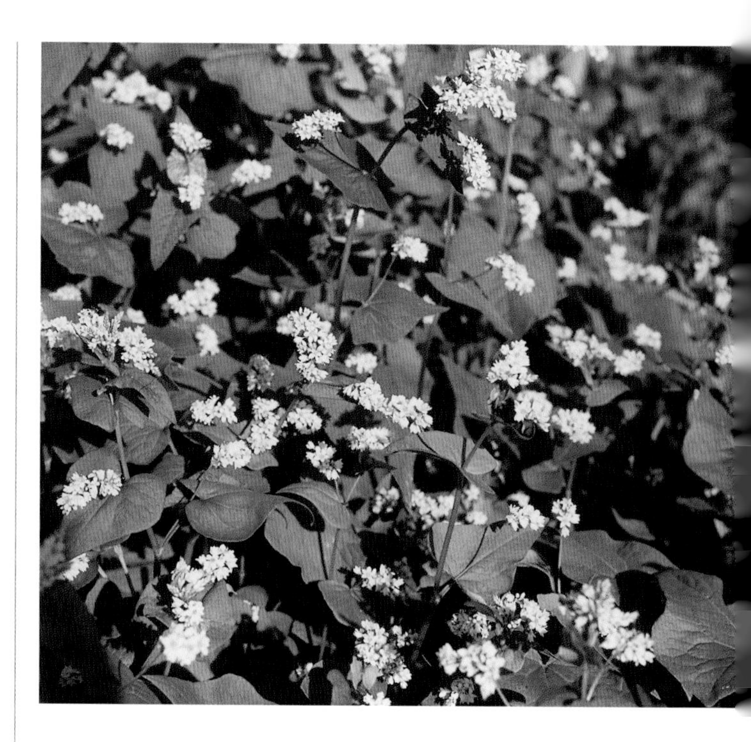

CULTIVATION

Modern research has found this humble plant to be one of the most important medicinal plants known to humankind, and as it is so easy to grow and delicious to eat, no garden or cook should be without it. It needs well-dug, well-composted soil in full sun. Seeds can be sown directly into the soil, which needs to be kept moist for the first few weeks. Tender whole seedlings can be pulled up and eaten even in the earliest stages. Sow the rows 30 cm apart and sprinkle the heart-shaped seed thinly in shallow drills. It will grow quickly to about 60 cm in height. You can grow 2–4 crops a season, starting in early August, as it is such a fast-growing annual.

MEDICINAL USES

Buckwheat is exceptionally rich in bioflavonoids, which is why it is essential in treating circulatory problems, cold hands and feet, chilblains and haemorrhoids. It also strengthens the inner wall of the tiniest capillaries and disperses small bruises that appear for no apparent reason. Buckwheat contains all eight essential amino acids, which helps to tone the whole body. It is rich in vitamin C, calcium, magnesium, beta-carotene, phosphorus, zinc, manganese, folic acid and potassium, making it an excellent all-round tonic for the whole body, and for circulation and the heart in particular.

Buckwheat restores health and vitality to those in deep depression due to its remarkably high vitamin and mineral content. Post-flu depression and postnatal depression respond immediately to buckwheat tea. Arthritis and gout in the crippling inflammatory stages respond equally well to buckwheat tea and buckwheat flour and groats in the diet. To make buckwheat tea, pour a cup of boiling water over ¼ cup fresh flowers, leaves and stems. Allow the tea to stand for five minutes before straining. Take one cup daily for two weeks, then take a break for four or five days before starting again.

CAUTION: Medical science suggests that people with allergies or those who have cancer should not eat buckwheat as it is high in vegetable protein and can cause a reaction.

Hulled buckwheat salad

For inflammation associated with arthritic pain (gout and muscular pain included), hulled buckwheat is now accepted as being an effective anti-inflammatory.

1 cup hulled buckwheat
3 cups water
1 teaspoon celery seeds
1 teaspoon fennel seeds
½ cup fennel flowers
1 cup buckwheat leaves and flowers
Fresh lemon juice

Prepare hulled buckwheat the same way you would cook rice, but without salt. Cook all the ingredients in a heavy-bottomed pot, simmering until tender. Drain, add fresh lemon juice and enjoy it as a salad, either hot or cold.

CULINARY USES

Buckwheat cake

SERVES 6

This cake keeps well and is the ideal lunchbox treat.

1 cup sunflower oil
4 eggs
1 cup liquid honey
1½ cups buckwheat flour
½ cup buckwheat flowers, broken into small pieces
2 teaspoons ground cinnamon
2 teaspoons ground allspice
4 teaspoons baking powder

Preheat the oven to 180°C. Line a cake tin with oiled greaseproof paper. Whisk the oil, eggs and honey together until creamy. In another bowl, mix the buckwheat flour with the flowers, cinnamon, allspice and baking powder. Add the oil, egg and honey mixture and beat lightly until well blended. Pour into the prepared cake tin and bake on the middle shelf for 30–35 minutes or until lightly browned. Serve with tea or coffee or as a dessert with apple purée or sliced peaches and cream.

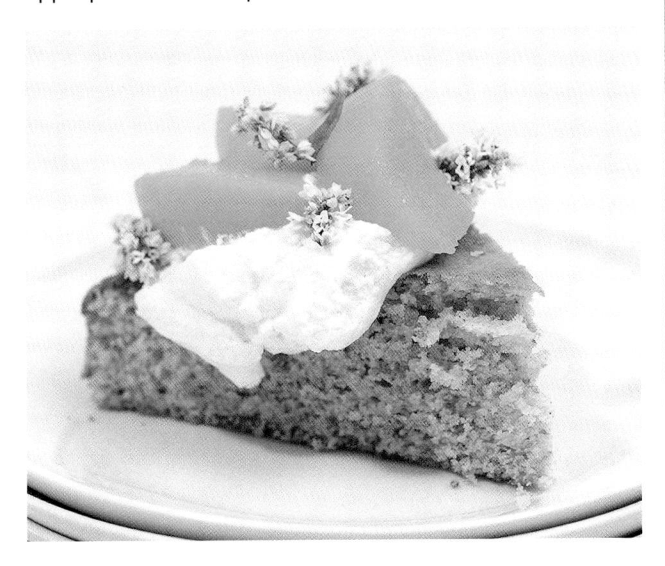

Buckwheat flower salad

SERVES 6

This attractive salt-free salad is so loaded with nutrients that it should be served daily! Onion or garlic can also be added.

2 cups buckwheat flowers
2 cups buckwheat leaves
2 cups thinly sliced cucumber
1 butter lettuce
2 cups chopped celery
1 cup thinly sliced radishes
2 cups carrot parings (pare with a potato peeler)
2 cups diced avocado
1 cup chopped green and red sweet peppers
½ cup chopped parsley
1 cup chopped fresh pineapple

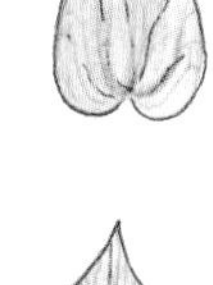

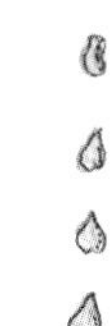

Dressing
Juice of 1 lemon
½ cup sesame seeds
½ cup olive oil
½ cup honey
½ cup grated ginger root

Mix the dressing ingredients together in a screw-top jar and shake well. Mix the salad ingredients together in a glass bowl and add the dressing while mixing. Serve immediately, decorated lavishly with buckwheat flowers.

Buckwheat flower stir-fry

SERVES 2–4

I love stir-fries and make them often, especially after a hard day when there is little energy left to make a big meal. Use whatever ingredients you have for variety. Serve with buckwheat groats (cook them as you would cook rice) or brown rice, or even just brown bread and butter. It makes a nourishing, healthy meal.

1 medium-sized aubergine
1 large onion, finely chopped
2–4 tablespoons olive oil
2 cups chopped buckwheat flowers
2 cups peeled and grated potato
2 cups thinly sliced mushrooms
2 cups grated or thinly sliced courgettes
1 tablespoon fresh thyme
1 tablespoon chopped mint
Sea salt and black pepper to taste
Juice of 1 lemon

Peel and slice the aubergine finely and soak in cold, salted water while you prepare the rest of the ingredients. Fry the onion in the olive oil until it starts to brown. Add the buckwheat flowers and stir-fry, then add the potato. Add a little more oil if necessary and once the potato starts to brown, add the aubergine slices (pat the aubergines dry before adding). Stir-fry well. Add all the other ingredients, shaking the pan and stirring continuously. Serve hot on rice with a green salad and squeeze more lemon juice over the stir-fry.

Bulrush

Typha latifolia ● **Cattail**

The bulrush is a cosmopolitan aquatic genus that has become a loved and valued plant in all its varieties worldwide. It is different from the bulrush mentioned in the story of Moses in the Bible, *Cyperus papyrus*, which is a member of the sedge family.

Several kinds of bulrush have been used through the centuries in many countries as both food and medicine, and in China a much-respected medicine is made, known as pu huang, from the long brown flowering spikes of the following: *Typha angustifolia*, *T. davidiana*, *T. orientalis* and *T. bungeana*. All are used interchangeably with *T. latifolia* as hormonal compounds known as phytoecdysteriods.

Around the world bulrushes have been used in folk medicine since the earliest centuries and almost every river has its succulent edging of this valuable plant. Each year I am amazed that in a deep furrow along the sandy road to my small farm, a stand of bulrushes blooms in abundance through the scorching hot months, before fading into virtual obscurity through the dry winters. Just a trickle of runoff rainwater starts the first new blades again, and before long in even the driest summer, there are sufficient flowering stems for the medicine-seeking sangomas.

The young flowering spikes are gathered for flower arrangements before they mature, but the majority are left so that pollen can be gathered. Many tribes harvest the unripe flowering spikes while still tender and cook them as a vegetable, especially during times of scarcity in North Africa, North America, parts of Europe and Asia (native lands of the bulrush). Traditional recipes utilise the inner stems, roots, rhizomes and young shoots in often strange but fascinating ways.

CULTIVATION

The garden staff at the Herbal Centre sometimes grow bulrush rhizomes in a big pot filled with compost, and lower it into a pond. Eventually the pot is turned out, washed well, and the base of the stalks and the thick rhizomes are peeled, washed and simmered in boiling salted water. Pieces of rhizome and tufts of new growth are replanted into fresh compost in the large pots and again sunk into the pond.

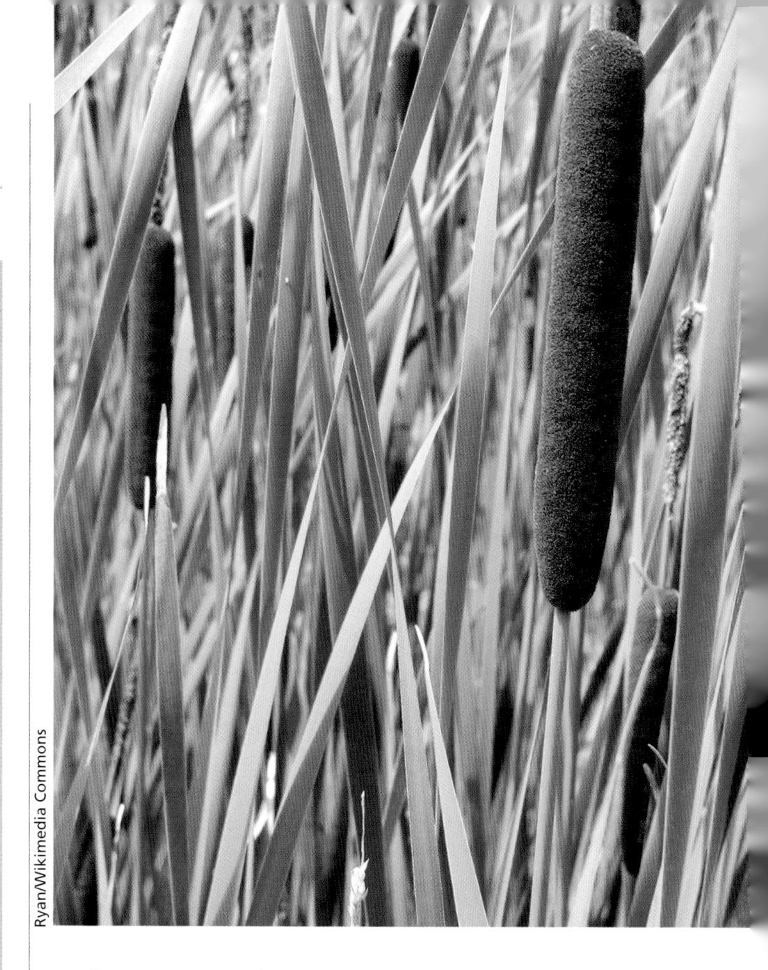

Ryan/Wikimedia Commons

In rivers, new plants can be dug out of the muddy submerged clumps, and scattered seed will take hold in every moist and hospitable place. Many farmers destroy bulrush beds as the water courses, dams and streams can become strangled by this tenacious plant.

In South Africa, *T. capensis* is the name given to the common bulrush, or *T. latifolia capensis*, or *T. capensis* syn *T. latifolia* subsp. *capensis*. Today around 15 species are found worldwide; all retain the name *Typha* and are basically similar and used for the same things.

MEDICINAL USES

All parts of the bulrush are used, the pollen being the most valuable medicinally. However, the young shoots, boiled or eaten fresh, are an excellent diuretic and also control excessive menstrual bleeding, improve circulation and promote healing of bruises, wounds, scrapes and cuts.

Dried pollen on the flowering spike is used as a treatment over wounds and bleeding cuts, and can be used on cattle too, which I learned from the staff on my husband's cattle farm! Dried flowering spikes can be packed over wounds to assist quick healing, and replaced daily.

In Europe, the bulrush is a valuable medication, listed in the pharmacopoeias of many countries, and made into medicines for tapeworms, diarrhoea, angina pains, postpartum pains, cancer of the lymphatic system, painful or copious menstruation, abnormal uterine bleeding, and for haemorrhaging wounds. Bulrush tea is taken internally and used externally in a poultice or dressing. To make bulrush tea, pour a cup of boiling water over ¼ cup chopped and well-washed leafy stem bases. Stir frequently, pressing down the pieces of succulent leaf base, for five minutes, then let the tea stand and cool for a minute or two, strain, and sip slowly. Take the tea two or three times a day. However, always ask your doctor before starting a home treatment, especially where there is angina and internal bleeding.

I learned from women on the farm how they used bulrush flowers in various ways. During their monthly menstrual cycle the women packed handfuls of stored, dried bulrush 'pollen' into small cotton or calico pouches they had sewn, making soft 'sanitary towels'. In the case of abscesses, boils and sprains, a poultice of warm honey mixed with the bulrush 'fluff' made a valuable dressing bound in place with bulrush leaves. This is still used today by farm workers in some rural areas, and the rhizomes are still used for reproductive problems in men and women, taken as a tea and eaten as a vegetable.

Today a registered medication for hormonal treatment is made by metabolising the flavonoids, volatile oils and hormonal compounds in the ripe 'flowers' of the bulrush into either oestrogenic or androgenic substances that are medically registered.

A bulrush decoction can be taken to ease menopausal symptoms. To make the decoction, cut young flowering stems into thumb-length pieces, place the pieces in a saucepan with enough water to cover, and simmer for one hour. Strain the liquid and refrigerate it. One cup is taken per day.

COSMETIC USES

Bulrush cream

Use this cream to treat dry skin and lips, and brittle nails during menopause.

2 cups good aqueous cream
2 cups young bulrush flowering tips
1 cup tender bulrush leaf bases
2 teaspoons vitamin E oil

Place the aqueous cream, flowering tips and leaf bases in a double boiler and simmer for 40 minutes. Remove from the heat, allow to cool and then strain. (The discarded shoots and flowers can be tied in cloth and used for washing.) Add the vitamin E oil to the cream and mix thoroughly. Spoon into a sterilised glass jar and massage frequently into the skin and nails. The rural farm workers used sunflower oil simmered with the bulrush flowering tips a decade ago. Now aqueous cream is more readily available and is far more easily applied and absorbed!

> WARNING: Bulrush stimulates the uterus and should therefore not be used in any form during pregnancy.

CULINARY USES

As a young bride on a remote farm, I was shown how to cook bulrush shoots, the tender bases of the young leaves and the unripe flower spike. The pollen of the ripe flower was added to flour to enrich it substantially and a delicious 'scone' was cooked in a pan on the open fire.

Bulrush stew

SERVES 6–8

I recall sitting by the fire as a young woman, tentatively tasting this unusual stew, and being so surprised by the rich flavour and succulent wholesomeness of it all that I make it to this day.

4 large onions, chopped
½ cup sunflower oil
4 cups bulrush shoots, chopped tender stems and young flowers
4 cups dried beans (haricot, sugar or kidney), soaked overnight and cooked
4 cups spinach leaves or pumpkin vine tips
2 teaspoons salt
Vinegar to taste

Brown the onions in a little sunflower oil. Add the chopped bulrush shoots and stems and stir-fry for a minute. Add the cooked beans and the spinach leaves or pumpkin vine tips. Add enough water to cover, then simmer until everything is tender. Add salt and a dash of vinegar just as you serve it.

Burdock

Arctium lappa

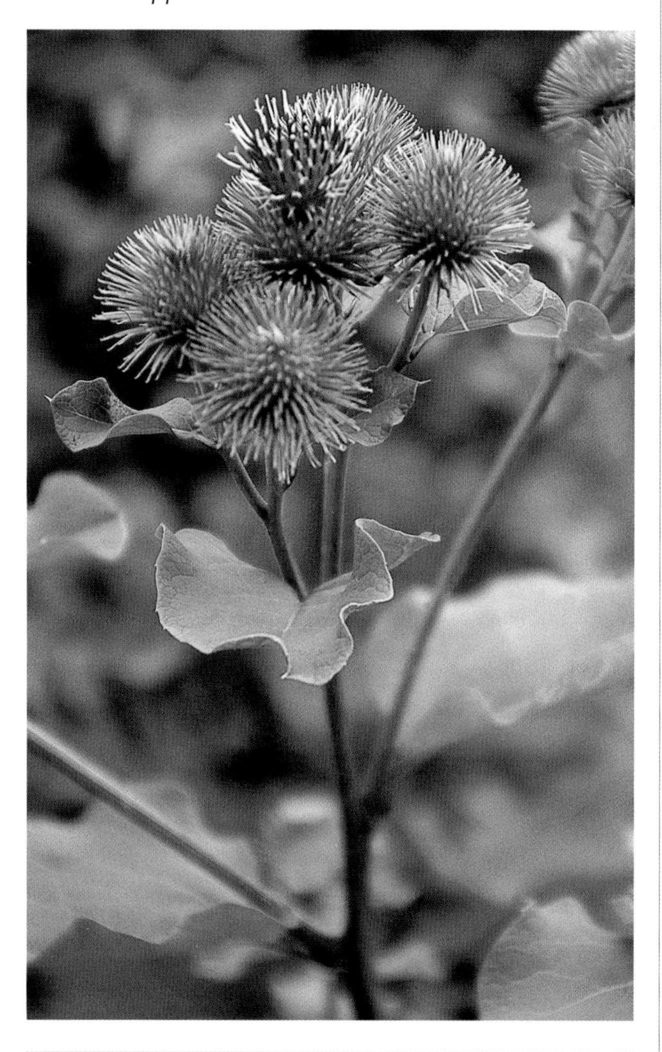

This rather unusual herb originated in Europe and parts of Asia, where it is much respected as both a food and a medicine. It grows in temperate regions throughout the world and is being commercially propagated in China for its medicinal seeds. Both Western and Chinese medicine have researched and documented the medicinal uses of burdock, and its ancient uses are being scientifically proven. It is a superb skin treatment for recurring ailments such as weeping eczema, psoriasis and allergic rashes. It has a cleansing effect on the whole body, from the liver to blood circulation, the kidneys and respiratory organs, and it has antibiotic, antiseptic and diuretic properties.

CULTIVATION

I have established burdock as an easy-to-grow biennial, and it flourishes, surprisingly, in the heat of the African sun just the way it does in the bitter winter winds and frost of Europe. It needs a deeply dug, rich, well-composted loamy soil in full sun, and I find that it takes afternoon shade quite happily. It needs a deep watering twice or even three times a week and thrives if the leaves are sprayed. In its second year it will send up a flowering head of many small, rounded capsules with a small crown of purple stamens and masses of burs, hence its name. These hook into everything and so get transported easily for germination.

MEDICINAL USES

Once widely used in cleansing, detoxifying remedies, burdock has been used through the centuries to lower blood sugar levels, break up kidney stones and as a treatment for acne, boils and abscesses. Crushed flowers and buds pounded to a pulp and warmed were applied to the area, even over the kidneys, and held in place with a large, warmed burdock leaf, bound with bandages. Burdock tea is excellent for easing the itch and heat in measles and for soothing and relaxing muscle spasms. It also appears to have antitumour action and will reduce the swelling and discomfort in mumps. To make a standard brew, pour a cup of boiling water over ¼ cup fresh buds and flowers and a small piece of leaf and stem. Allow the tea to stand for five minutes, then strain and sip slowly.

Burdock contains a rare and precious ingredient, arctiin, which is a smooth-muscle relaxant, and it makes a wonderful healing cream.

Cleansing burdock tea

SERVES 1

This is excellent as a cleansing, rejuvenating tea, also good for acne and boils. The Chinese add a few burdock seeds.

1 cup boiling water
1 burdock flower
1 piece burdock leaf, about 3 cm square
Cinnamon stick
Honey
Powdered ginger

Pour the boiling water over the flower and piece of leaf. Stir with a cinnamon stick and let the tea draw for five minutes. Strain, sweeten with a touch of honey and a pinch of powdered ginger, and sip slowly. Add one dandelion flower if you are taking the tea for acne or boils. They combine exceptionally well.

Burdock healing cream

This cream can be used to soothe sprains, arthritic joints, rashes, eczema and psoriasis.

1 cup burdock (flowers, buds, pieces of leaf and stem)
1 cup good aqueous cream
1 teaspoon vitamin E oil

Mix the chopped herbs well with the aqueous cream. Simmer for 15 minutes in a double boiler with the lid on. Cool and strain. Discard the burdock and mix in the vitamin E oil. Pour into a sterilised screw-top glass jar and store in a cool place. Apply frequently to stiff muscles, strains and rashes.

Burdock vinegar for acne

1 bottle apple cider vinegar
2 cups burdock flowers, chopped

Warm (but do not boil) the vinegar. Place the chopped flowers and their attached stems in a large glass jar and pour the warmed vinegar over it. Every part of the flowers needs to be submerged. Leave it to draw for 10 days, giving it a daily stir, then strain. Discard the flowers, then bottle and label the vinegar. Use a dash in the rinsing water after washing the face and dab on spots and pimples frequently.

CULINARY USES

Burdock bud syrup

MAKES 2 LITRES

This makes a most refreshing drink, served hot or cold.

20 very young burdock buds
2 cups burdock stems, peeled and cut into 3 cm lengths
4 litres cold water
4 cups dark brown treacle sugar
2 teaspoons ground cinnamon
½ teaspoon ground cloves
1 cup thinly sliced ginger root

Trim the buds and stems with a sharp knife to remove all the rough bits. Place the buds and stems in two litres of the water, bring to the boil and simmer for 10 minutes. Discard the water and boil up again with the remaining water, again simmering for 10 minutes. Add the sugar, cinnamon, ground cloves and thinly sliced ginger root. Keep the lid on and simmer gently for a further 10 minutes. Remove from the heat, cool and strain. Bottle the syrup and keep in the fridge. Dilute ¼ glass syrup and top up with iced water and crushed ice and a thin slice of ginger. Sip slowly.

COOK'S NOTE

In ancient cultures, young tender burdock flower buds were combined with dandelion or chamomile flowers to make a warming and cheering wine, which can also be made from burdock flowers alone. The root can be cooked as a vegetable, and the peeled and fried stems make a tasty snack.

Burdock flower cleansing soup

SERVES 4–6

This is a most unusual soup, very fresh and very green. It is so rich in vitamins and minerals that I try to make it every few weeks, especially if I have been eating out a lot. It is a superb detoxifier, of particular importance after an anaesthetic or after a lot of X-rays, or if you have been plagued by boils or bad skin conditions and feel overloaded nd burnt out. It will get rid of all sorts of toxins and acidity.

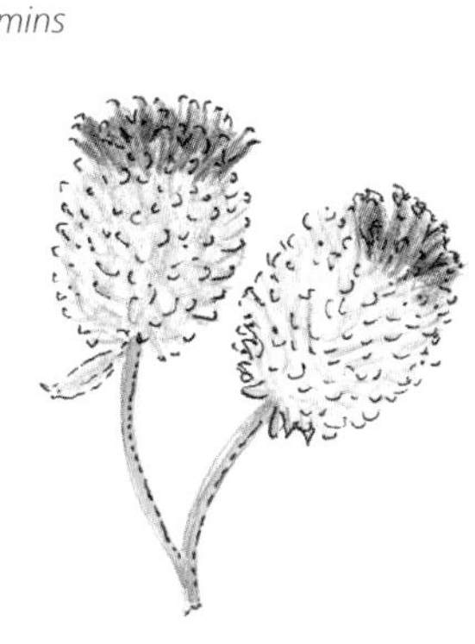

1 butter lettuce, roughly chopped
3 cups chopped celery stems and leaves
1 cup chopped fresh parsley
1 cup torn-up burdock leaves and stems
1 cup trimmed young burdock buds
2 thinly sliced onions, green tops included
2 cups fresh lucerne leaves, stripped off their stems
1 cup pearl barley, soaked overnight
3 grated carrots
2 litres water
Juice of 1 lemon
Sea salt to taste

Bring all the ingredients to the boil in a heavy-bottomed pot. Turn down the heat and simmer gently with the lid on until the barley is soft, usually about 40 minutes. Top up with water if necessary. Liquidise to make a smooth soup, and serve piping hot.

Calamint & emperor's mint

Calamintha ascendens • *C. officinalis* • *Micromeria* species

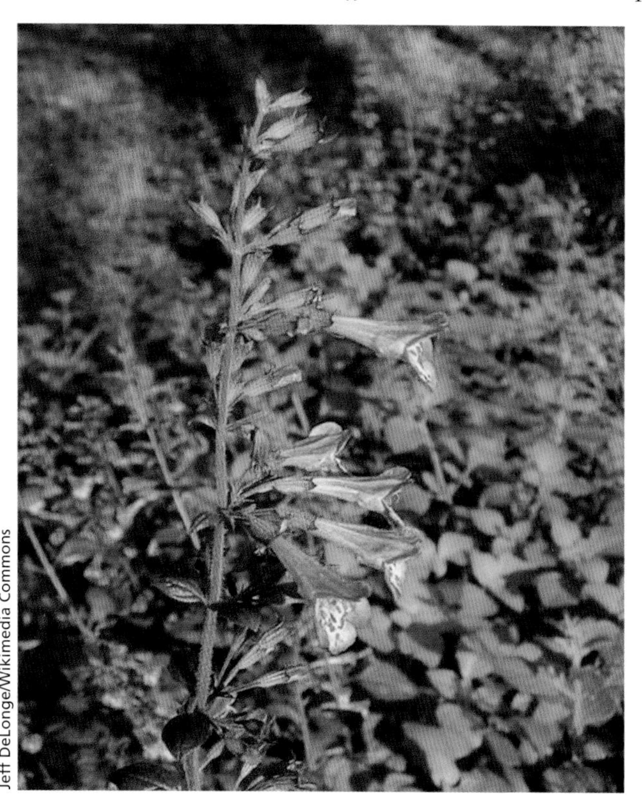
Jeff DeLonge/Wikimedia Commons

Calamint

Calamint originated in Europe and Asia, extending from the British Isles eastwards towards Iran. It flourishes in poor soil and is a familiar sight along roadsides. It was greatly esteemed in ancient times for its medicinal properties and the Greeks used it to clear coughs and ease digestive disorders, while leaf poultices were used to treat bruises and sprains. Calamint tea induces sweating and in medieval times it was revered as a detoxifier and cleanser, and was used as a treatment against the plague. Modern scientific research has verified the presence of a powerful oil rich in pulegone in the plant, and research is still being conducted into its use as an expectorant in respiratory ailments. Simply taking a deep breath and inhaling the pungent peppermint-like aroma is enough to open sinuses and clear a blocked nose. In days gone by calamint was believed to have magical protective properties and bunches of fresh calamint were hung in the doorways of homes to protect the occupants, giving rise to the name 'protection plant'.

CULTIVATION

Calamint and emperor's mint are confusingly similar in appearance and fragrance, and are used medicinally to treat the same ailments, yet they are not related at all. Both are delightfully fragrant and pretty creeping perennials, with slightly hairy, oval, thumbnail-sized leaves and tiny white or mauve flowers. The difference lies in the propagation – calamint has a creeping rootstock that can be divided at any time of the year once the soft flowering spikes have been cut back, while emperor's mint sows itself freely all around the mother plant. Both take sun and light shade. Calamint has only been cultivated since the 17th century and once you have it in your garden it will always reseed itself.

MEDICINAL USES

The sprays of tiny white flowers last well in water and if crushed and tucked under the pillow they will ensure a good night's sleep as the strong peppermint aroma opens the nose and clears the sinuses.

A tea made from calamint is still favoured in Europe today to help relieve colic, wind and indigestion. To make the tea, pour a cup of boiling water over ¼ cup fresh flowering sprigs. Allow the tea to stand for five minutes, then strain, and sip it slowly. This tea is particularly soothing when you have overeaten, or when you feel nauseous or chilled. Use the same tea for a fretting child or a colicky baby, giving a teaspoonful of the warm tea at a time. For a cough, tight chest, flu or a bad cold, use the same brew but add the juice of one lemon and three teaspoons of honey. It will encourage sweating and in this way bring down a fever; it will also act as an expectorant and clear the nose and lungs.

CAUTION: Avoid both calamint and emperor's mint if you are pregnant, as they are very strong herbs.

Calamint steam treatment for blocked nose and sinuses

3 litres boiling water
2 large cups fresh flowering calamint sprigs

Pour the boiling water over the calamint sprigs in a large bowl; make a towel tent over your head, and bend over the steaming bowl. Keep your eyes shut and inhale the steam deeply. It is an excellent treatment to open the nose, loosen phlegm and act as an expectorant.

Mango and calamint smoothie

SERVES 2

To aid digestion and ease heat build-up after sports exertion.

1 large ripe mango, peeled
½ small pineapple
3 teaspoons calamint flowers and leafy sprigs
½ spanspek melon
1 cup crushed ice

Peel and cut the fruit into pieces. Liquidise fruit, flowers, sprigs and ice in a blender. Pour into a glass and sip slowly. Do not eat anything within 30 minutes of drinking the smoothie.

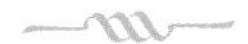

CULINARY USES

Calamint after-dinner tea, and refreshing iced tea

Serve this tea in place of after-dinner coffee, in small cups, or add fresh sprigs to filter coffee. The same tea cooled and mixed with equal quantities of fresh unsweetened fruit juice, particularly litchi juice, served with crushed ice and a sprinkling of calamint flowers, will refresh and revive you after a long day. With a little dash of white wine it makes a party-time treat and a tonic as well!

1 cup boiling water
¼ cup fresh calamint sprigs, leaves and flowers

Pour the boiling water over the calamint sprigs, leaves and flowers and allow the tea to stand for five minutes before straining. Serve hot and sip slowly.

Calamint or emperor's mint conserve

Use this delicious sugar to flavour puddings, herb teas and after-dinner coffee.

10 flowering sprigs of calamint or emperor's mint
Dark brown caramel sugar

Pick the flowering sprigs and crush them lightly with a rolling pin. Sprinkle layers of dark brown caramel sugar under and over the sprigs and seal in a wide-mouthed jar. After a week remove the sprigs and seal the jar again. Use this sugar to flavour puddings, herb teas and after-dinner coffee. Alternatively, place 10 flowering sprigs in one bottle of runny honey, such as orange blossom honey. Leave it for one week, standing in the sun. Strain and taste. If it is not strong enough, repeat. Serve with calamint tea.

Peach and calamint dessert

SERVES 4–6

This light, fragrant dessert is perfect after a heavy meal.

12 large yellow peaches, peeled and sliced
2 apples, peeled and roughly chopped
2 tablespoons thinly sliced fresh ginger root
1 cup sultanas
Sugar to taste
½–¾ cup tiny calamint flowers, pulled out of their calyxes
2 cups apple juice
A little water
2 sprigs fresh calamint leaves

Simmer all the ingredients together until the peaches and apples are tender. Discard the calamint sprigs. Serve hot or cold with whipped cream sprinkled with more of the tiny mauve or white calamint flowers.

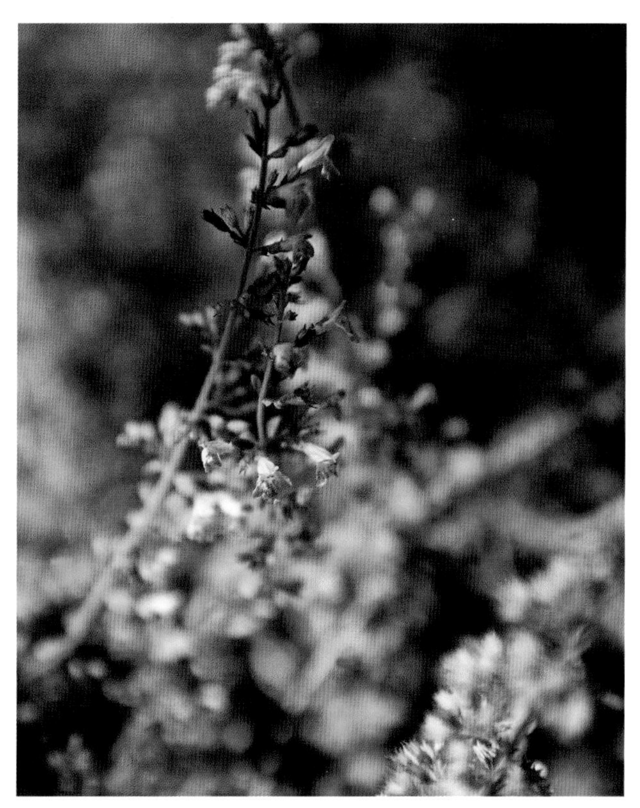

Emperor's mint

Calendula

Calendula officinalis

Calendula is often confusingly referred to as 'marigold' in overseas herbal books. However, South Africans know marigold (*Tagetes* sp.) as that strong-smelling, pungent, insect-repelling mainstay in our summer gardens, often planted among vegetables to keep them insect-free. Do not use any *Tagetes* species for medicinal or culinary purposes in any way – they do not have the same properties as calendula.

Calendula officinalis has no insect-repelling properties, but this old-fashioned winter-flowering herb is an amazing medicinal plant, its therapeutic properties having been well documented since the earliest times. An old 12th century Herbal suggested that merely looking into the brilliant bright orange calendula flowers would clear up eye ailments, improve the eyesight and clear the head!

CULTIVATION

Growing calendulas is remarkably easy. Sow the seeds in late summer and plant out the little seedlings in well-dug, richly composted soil in full sun about 25–30 cm apart. Keep them moist until they have settled, after which they will need to be watered two or three times a week. You will be rewarded with masses of flowers all through the winter and well into spring and early summer. Calendula is a winter annual, so grow a row to save for the summer ahead. Dry the petals on brown paper in the shade. Turn daily, and when fully dry store in a glass jar with a tight lid. You'll find many uses for the petals.

MEDICINAL USES

Calendula has anti-inflammatory properties, relieves muscle spasm, prevents haemorrhages, is astringent and antiseptic, helps to heal wounds, regulates menstruation, helps to relieve gastric disturbances, colitis, fevers and infections, and is detoxifying and mildly oestrogenic. Quick relief from the above ailments can be obtained by drinking a cup of calendula tea. To make the tea, pour a cup of boiling water over ¼ cup fresh calendula petals and leave to stand for five minutes before straining. When cooled, the tea can be used as a lotion for skin problems such as acne, eczema, oily skin, psoriasis, rashes, grazes, stings, bites and even sunburn. Calendula petals can be used to make an exceptional healing massage oil, and calendula cream is a classic remedy for cuts, grazes, wounds and skin irritations.

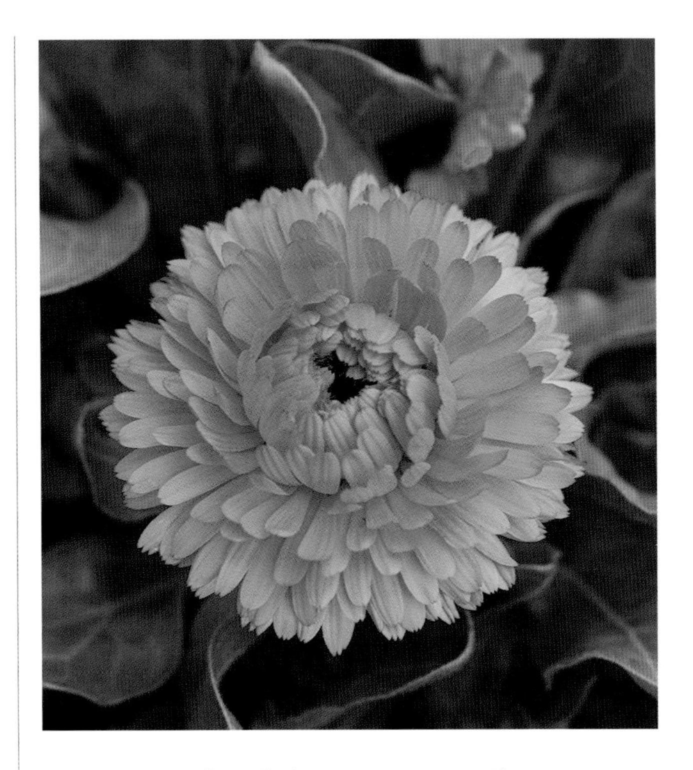

Healing calendula massage oil

This is one of the most comforting oils for chilblains, haemorrhoids and broken capillaries.

Calendula petals
Almond oil

Warm equal quantities of calendula petals and almond oil for 15 minutes, stirring continuously. Strain and bottle in a sterilised glass jar. Massage into the affected area frequently during the day. A teaspoonful or two added to the bath will also soften and moisturise dry skin, and it is soothing and calming for nervous tension and menstrual pain.

Calendula antiseptic cream

Calendula cream is antiseptic, antifungal, anti-inflammatory and astringent. It is easy to make and no home should be without it.

1 cup calendula petals
I cup good aqueous cream
2 teaspoons vitamin E oil

Heat the petals and aqueous cream in a double boiler for 20 minutes, stirring frequently. Strain and discard the petals, and mix in the vitamin E oil. Pour the cream into a sterilised glass jar, seal and keep in a cool place.

CULINARY USES

Calendula omelette

SERVES 1

This is a quick and easy supper dish and full of goodness. Make individual omelettes and serve immediately.

½–¾ cup grated cheddar cheese
¼ cup parsley
½ cup fresh calendula petals
2 eggs
2 tablespoons water
A pinch of salt
Black pepper

Mix the grated cheese, parsley and calendula petals and set aside. Whisk the eggs well with the water and seasoning. Heat a little olive oil in a frying pan and pour in the egg mixture. Allow to set for about three minutes, tipping the pan to ensure that the omelette cooks evenly. Spread the cheese mixture over one half of the omelette and allow it to settle for a minute or two. As soon as the omelette is cooked, flip one side over to cover the cheese mixture, and slide it onto a hot plate. Decorate with triangles of buttered toast and sprinkle with more calendula petals. Serve immediately.

COOK'S NOTE

Calendula is used as a natural yellow food colouring in the food industry. The bright orange petals can be added to many foods, from drinks and jams to curries, desserts, rice dishes and pancakes. I sprinkle the fresh petals on dishes all through the winter (never use the green parts – it is only the petals that have medicinal properties).

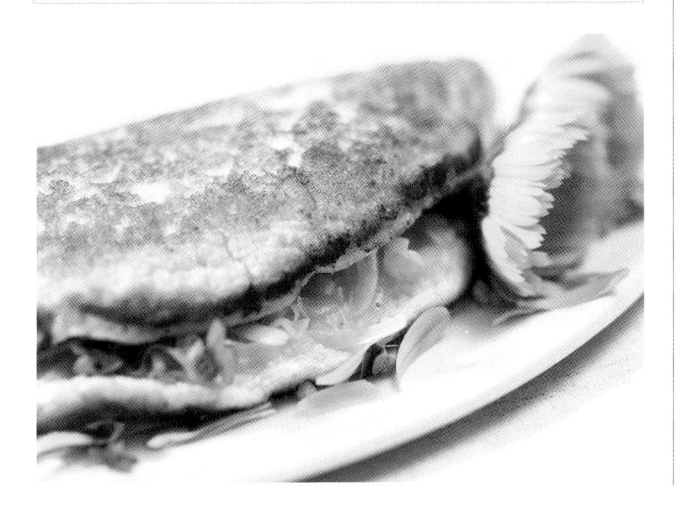

Calendula curry

SERVES 6–8

This nourishing, hearty standby dish freezes successfully and keeps well in the fridge. If you are vegetarian, substitute mushrooms for the meat.

500 g diced lean beef (topside or rump)
2 cups chopped onions
½ cup sunflower oil
2 cups diced carrots
2 cups chopped celery
3 cups chopped tomatoes
2 cups chopped green peppers
3 cups peeled, diced potatoes
1–2 cups calendula petals
½ cup honey
½–¾ cup fruit chutney
2 tablespoons curry powder mixed with a little milk
1 litre water
Salt and cayenne pepper to taste

Brown the meat and onions in the oil in a heavy-bottomed pot. Add all the other ingredients. Simmer gently, stirring every now and then. Adjust the flavour if necessary and add more water if it boils away. Simmer until the meat is tender. Sprinkle with more calendula petals and serve piping hot, with brown rice and peas.

Calendula custard

SERVES 4

This was my children's favourite dessert served either hot or cold, on its own or with apple tart, stewed rhubarb or peaches.

1 cup calendula petals
1 litre hot milk
Piece of vanilla pod or 1 teaspoon vanilla essence
3 eggs
1 cup sugar
1 tablespoon cornflour
1 teaspoon cinnamon
1 teaspoon allspice

Bruise the petals well to release the bright yellow colouring. Heat the milk in a double boiler and add the petals, keeping the mixture just under boiling point. Add the vanilla. Beat the eggs with the sugar, cornflour, cinnamon and allspice, and whisking carefully and continuously, add this mixture to the simmering milk. Remove the vanilla pod. Whisk gently until the custard thickens. Serve with whipped cream and sprinkle with calendula petals.

Californian poppy

Eschscholzia californica

The fact that this glorious orange flower is edible comes as a great surprise to many people. I learned about its remarkable healing properties from an American Indian visitor to my herb gardens, who inspired me to know and grow more of this old-fashioned plant that has been so taken for granted. Centuries ago, American Indians used the flowers, and to some extent the leaves, as a painkiller, particularly for toothache. A leaf and a couple of petals would be well chewed and the tooth packed with the softened leaf. It has tremendous analgesic, antispasmodic, calming and sedative properties, and is valuable in treating both physical and psychological problems in children as it is gentle and safe.

CULTIVATION

Usually treated as an annual, the Californian poppy is a gorgeous sight in spring with its brilliantly coloured flowers and finely cut grey-green leaves. It thrives in any soil as long as it is well-drained, and has adapted to withstand all sorts of climates around the world, far from its native habitat in western North America. It needs full sun and thrives on a twice-weekly watering (slightly more in hot weather), and thereafter can literally be forgotten about! It benefits from picking as the more you pick the more flowers it produces. Sow seed in boxes in autumn and keep them warm, protected and moist throughout winter. Transplant seedlings in late winter to a well-dug, well-composted bed in full sun, spaced 40 cm apart. The mature height of the plant is about 30 cm.

MEDICINAL USES

Although similar in effect to the opium poppy (*Papaver somniferum*), the Californian poppy has a very different effect in that it is not narcotic and it does not disorientate like the opium poppy.

Researchers are looking at the promising effect it has on bedwetting in highly strung children, as well as in cases where there is difficulty establishing a good sleep pattern, and in those with anxiety, nightmares, sleep-walking and panic attacks.

The easiest way to take Californian poppy as a medicine (other than in food) is as a comforting tea. Combined with chamomile to enhance relaxation and encourage sleep, it is an easily assimilated and very gentle medicinal nightcap that is completely safe for children. To make Californian poppy tea, pour a cup of boiling water over three petals and a small leaf of the Californian poppy, and add a tablespoon of fresh chamomile flowers. Allow the tea to stand for five minutes, then strain and sweeten with a touch of honey. For a child aged under three years, give half a cup; for children aged over three years and for adults, sip a full cup slowly just before going to bed.

NOTE: Chamomile and the Californian poppy flower at the same time of the year.

Californian poppy muscle-relaxing cream

This cream is calming, relaxing and relieves pain and spasm, making it particularly useful for strains, sprains, aching shoulders and stiff necks.

1 cup good aqueous cream
1 cup fresh Californian poppy petals and buds
4 or 5 Californian poppy leaves
2 teaspoons vitamin E oil
10 drops rose-scented pelargonium or lavender essential oil

Simmer petals, buds, leaves and aqueous cream in a double boiler. Stir frequently, pressing the petals down into the cream. After 30 minutes, cool and strain. (The petals can be tied in a facecloth and used in the bath with soap to massage aching legs and back.) Mix the vitamin E oil into the aqueous cream and add the rose-scented pelargonium essential oil or lavender essential oil, as these oils ease muscle tension and spasm. Spoon into a sterilised glass jar with a well-fitting lid and label. Use liberally for aches and muscle spasm, and on children with bruises and restless legs.

Californian poppy poultice

This poultice makes a very comforting treatment for sprains, bruises, aches and painful muscles in winter, when this plant flowers in abundance. We dry petals for use during the rest of the year.

Fresh Californian poppy flowering sprays, stems and leaves
Hot water
½–¾ cup Californian poppy muscle relaxing cream (see above)
Pure cotton cloth and towel

Soften and warm the flowering sprays, stems and leaves in hot water. Then mix in the Californian poppy muscle relaxing cream. Apply this mixture to the affected area, as warm as is comfortable. Cover with a cotton cloth, then a towel and place a hot-water bottle over the area (or use a heat lamp). Keep the area warm while relaxing for 15–20 minutes. Remove the poultice and massage in the soothing cream. The resultant relaxation and pain release can be enhanced by drinking a cup of Californian poppy tea. To make this tea, pour a cup of boiling water over ¼ cup of fresh petals and one leaf, leave it to stand for five minutes, strain, sweeten if desired with a touch of honey and sip slowly.

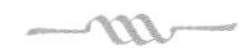

CULINARY USES

Californian poppy spring fruit salad

SERVES 4–6

This fruit salad is a delight as the warmer days tumble together! It is wonderful made with early peaches, but can be made with any fruit in season.

Brown sugar to taste
2 cups well ripened mulberries, stalks removed
2 cups thinly sliced strawberries
4 pears, peeled and chopped
2 apples, peeled and grated
4–6 early peaches, peeled and sliced
2 papinos or small pawpaws
Juice of 1 orange
1 cup Californian poppy petals

Sprinkle the sugar over the mulberries and strawberries and let them stand at room temperature for at least two hours. Thereafter mix the remaining ingredients together, saving some of the Californian poppy petals for decoration. Serve in a pretty glass bowl with whipped cream.

New potato salad with Californian poppies

SERVES 4

Dressing
1 tablespoon balsamic vinegar
2 tablespoons olive oil
2 tablespoons good mayonnaise
2 tablespoons plain Bulgarian or Greek yoghurt
Sea salt and black pepper to taste
1 cup lightly packed Californian poppy petals

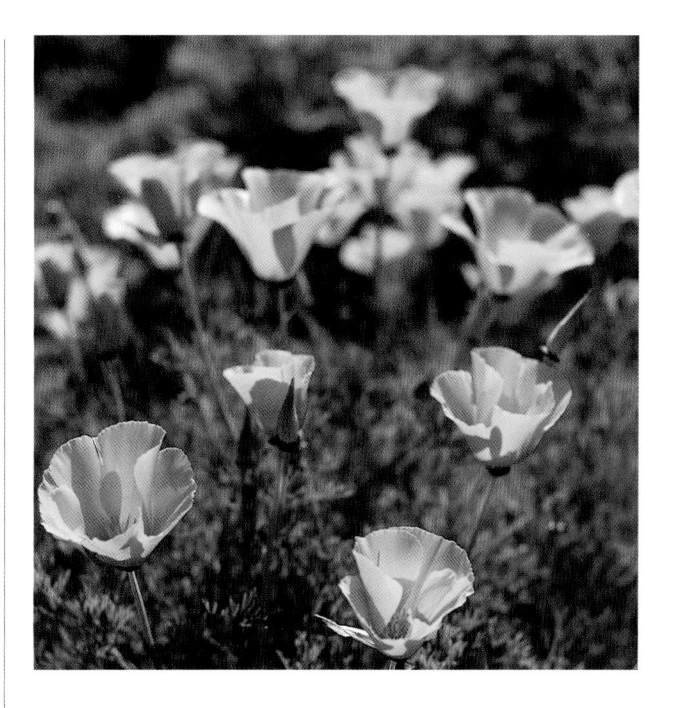

Boil the unpeeled new potatoes in salted water until tender. Leave them to cool with their skins on. Meanwhile mix the dressing ingredients together, keeping a few petals aside for garnishing. Toss the potatoes in the dressing in a glass bowl and sprinkle a little chopped parsley over the salad. Keep in the fridge until ready to serve and decorate with the Californian poppy petals.

Californian poppy and aubergine stir-fry

SERVES 4

This tasty salsa-like dish is delicious served with hot crusty bread as a starter, or with a salad as a lunch dish.

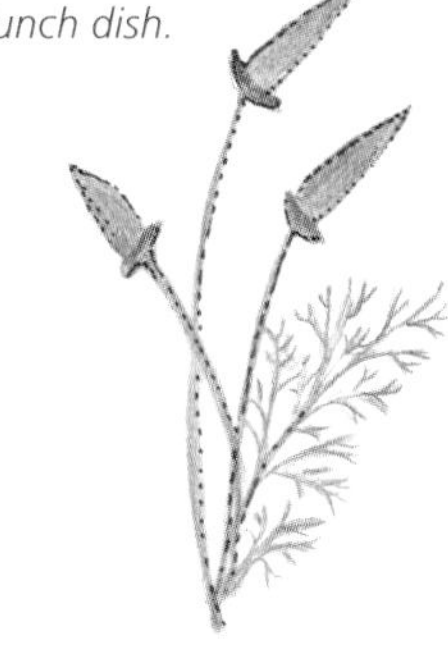

3 medium-sized aubergines
Olive oil
½ cup chopped pecan nuts
½ cup sesame seeds
½ cup Californian poppy petals
Sea salt and black pepper to taste
Juice of 1 lemon
¾ cup parmesan cheese

Peel and slice the aubergines and soak in salted water for 10 minutes before draining. Sauté them in a little olive oil until tender. Add all the other ingredients except the parmesan cheese. Mash and mix well, stir-frying continuously. Spoon the stir-fry into a serving dish and sprinkle with the cheese. Decorate with chopped parsley and a few of the Californian poppy petals.

Cape sorrel

Oxalis pes-caprae ● **Suring**

Sorrel is the common name confusingly attributed to several species of plants with acidulous (sour) sap. *Oxalis pes-caprae* has beautiful, brilliant yellow flowers in late winter and is not to be confused with the *Rumex* species of sorrel. Indigenous to the Cape of Good Hope and used in traditional Cape cooking, Cape sorrel is an easy-to-grow plant that has become a prized hothouse plant overseas, where it obligingly blooms at a completely different time of year to its native cousins. Several local tribes use fresh Cape sorrel as a salt substitute for bland foods, and when eaten with fresh grilled fish on the beach, Cape sorrel makes a succulent, never-to-be-forgotten addition to a glorious meal.

CULTIVATION

Cape sorrel grows prolifically on waste ground, tolerating icy winds and salt spray as readily as it tolerates desolate, hot sandy areas. It requires no care or attention at all, except perhaps a weekly watering during its winter flowering period. It thrives on the Cape's winter rainfall and stoically withstands the cold, wet conditions, offering a blaze of uplifting colour before the other spring flowers appear. However, its flowering period is often brief as by late spring the heat shrivels the flowers and eventually it all but disappears underground, leaving only a few dried leaves to mark the spot where it grew. With regular watering in the garden it can go on well into summer, but its dormant period is late summer to midwinter. With well-dug, well-composted soil in full sun it will flourish in the garden, but always be sure to mark the spot where it grows or in its dormant period you may be apt to forget that it is there and plant something else on top of it. Cape sorrel is a herb well worth growing.

MEDICINAL USES

Sailors in the 16th and 17th centuries calling at the Cape collected the tender, juicy, swollen roots of the Cape sorrel as a treatment for scurvy, and ate the leaves and flowers as well. The swollen root was dried and taken on long voyages as it could be rehydrated in water, and used medicinally.

The leaves can be crushed and applied to burns, scratches and grazes, and they are still used as a first-aid treatment in rural areas of the Cape today.

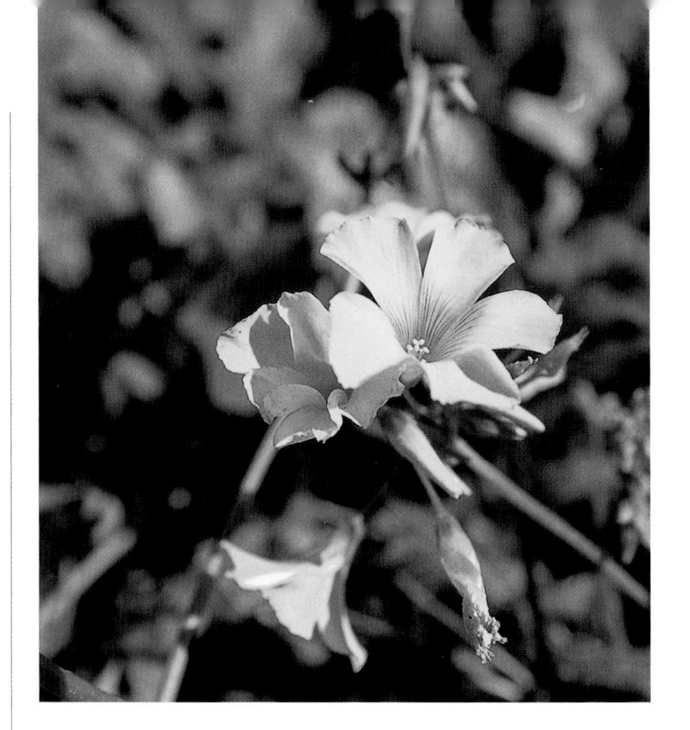

Cape sorrel poultice

This poultice is used for boils and suppurating sores.

Cape sorrel leaves
Hot water
Crêpe bandage

Warm the leaves in hot water, and bind over a boil or suppurating sore to bring it to a head, using a crêpe bandage to keep the poultice in place. Replace the poultice frequently with fresh warmed leaves.

COSMETIC USES

Sorrel flowers pounded with water and made into a paste can be spread on acne spots and pimples; this will quickly clear spots of redness and help them to dry up. Teenagers should eat a few flowers every day during the plant's spring flowering to clear their skins of oiliness and pimples, and the juice of the flowering stems can be dabbed onto spots to hasten healing.

Cape sorrel vinegar for problem oily skin

This old Cape remedy is valuable for problem oily skin. Make two or three bottles while the flowers are in bloom.

Fresh Cape sorrel flowers and a few leaves
1 bottle apple cider vinegar

Steep the flowers and leaves in the bottle of vinegar. Place in the sun for four days and shake it daily. Repeat this for four more days, then strain. Apply frequently to the problem area. Wet a pad of cotton wool with warm water and wring out. Then dip the pad into the vinegar solution and apply to skin three times a day after washing the face.

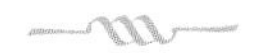

CULINARY USES

Yellow sorrel salad

SERVES 4–6

This is the first salad I make every spring, using fresh springtime ingredients; its piquant taste makes it a favourite with everyone. Serve with sorrel mayonnaise.

1 butter lettuce
2 papinos or 1 medium pawpaw, peeled and diced
2 oranges, peeled and sliced
2 cups sliced celery
2 cups watercress
2 cups finely grated carrots
2 avocados, peeled and diced
1 cup peeled grated butternut
4 hard-boiled eggs, shelled and sliced
Black pepper
1 cup Cape sorrel flowers

Line a dish with butter lettuce leaves. Lightly mix all the ingredients (except the eggs, black pepper and sorrel flowers) and spoon onto the bed of lettuce leaves. Arrange the sliced eggs on top. Grind some black pepper over the salad and sprinkle with sorrel flowers.

Sorrel salad dressing

MAKES 1 SMALL BOTTLE

This 'quick mayonnaise' is very easy to make and is far healthier than the stabilised and preserved commercial mayonnaises.

½ cup thick cream
½ cup plain yoghurt
½ cup runny honey
½ cup apple juice
2 teaspoons mustard powder
1 tablespoon finely chopped parsley
1 tablespoon finely chopped chives
Sea salt and black pepper to taste
½ cup fresh Cape sorrel flowers

Whisk the cream lightly until it holds its shape. Add the yoghurt and whisk gently. Mix the honey, apple juice and mustard powder together and add to the cream and yoghurt mixture. Add the parsley, chives, sea salt and black pepper to taste, and finally stir in the Cape sorrel flowers. Pour into a small jug, and serve with the yellow sorrel salad or with fish or chicken dishes.

Cape sorrel and pickled fish

SERVES 8–10

This is a traditional Cape dish enjoyed not only by South Africans but also by visitors from overseas who often ask for the recipe. Serve it cold with salads.

2.5 kg firm white fish – Cape salmon, kingklip or kabeljou are best
4 onions, neatly sliced
4 teaspoons salt
2 teaspoons cayenne pepper
¾ cup sugar – brown treacle sugar is best
1 tablespoon turmeric
750 ml brown grape vinegar
125 ml water
½ cup thinly sliced fresh ginger
20 coriander seeds
¾ cup sultanas
4 fresh lemon leaves
1 cup fresh sorrel flowers

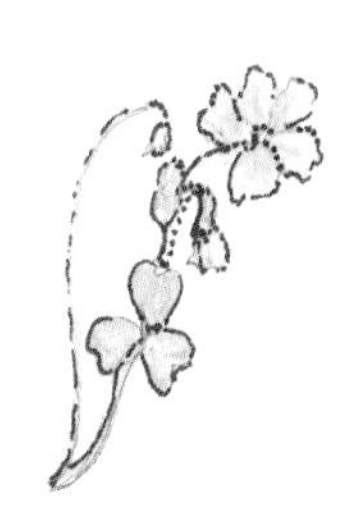

Cut the fish into small neat portions and set aside. Mix all the ingredients, except the sorrel flowers, and simmer in a heavy-bottomed pot for 15–20 minutes. Stir well, then add the fish pieces carefully so as not to break them. Simmer for another 20 minutes with the lid on. Carefully lift the fish out of the sauce and place in a glass or stainless steel dish. Pour the sauce over the fish, remove the lemon leaves, and let the dish cool. Just before serving, sprinkle with the fresh sorrel flowers. This dish keeps well in the fridge.

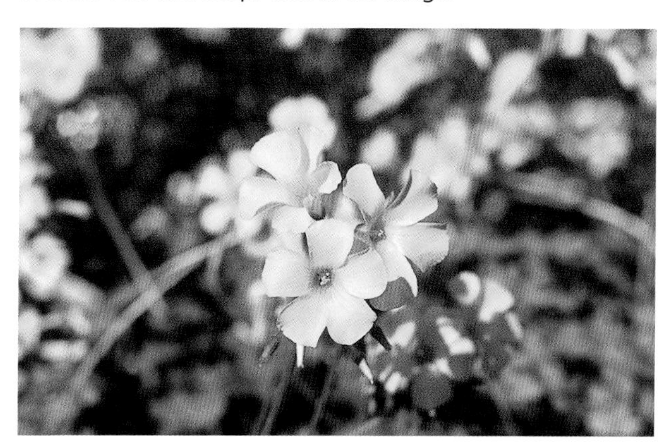

Caraway

Carum carvi

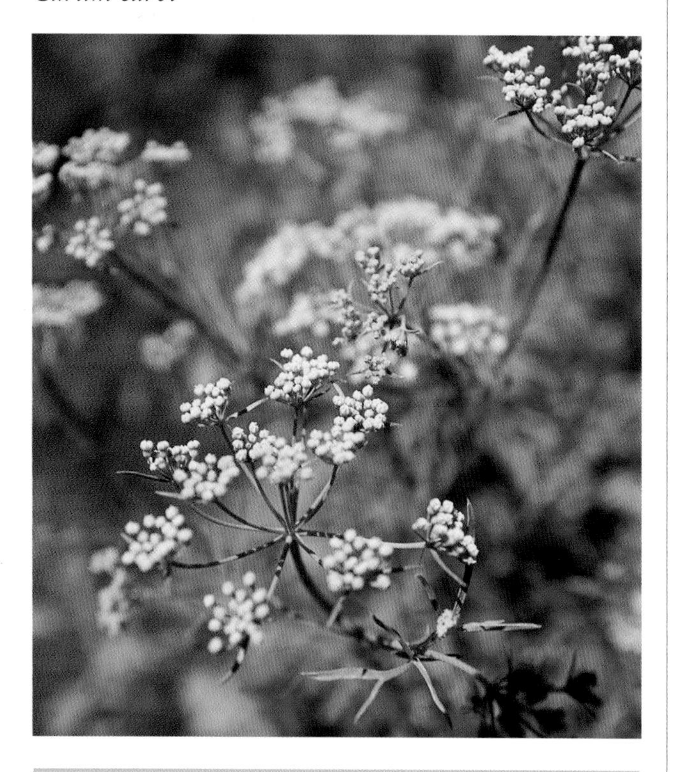

The word 'caraway' has its origins in the ancient Arabic word for seed, *karawya*. The ancient Egyptians used it in medicine and as a flavouring, and Isaiah speaks of the cultivation of caraway in the Bible. Archaeologists have found seed in small clay containers in diggings on Mesolithic sites, dating from thousands of years BC. The herb originated in Central Europe, Asia and North Africa, where it is found on waste ground and grasslands. Its tendency to self-seed prolifically meant that it became widespread and naturalised further afield. Caraway is one of the most ancient herbs and is still cultivated extensively as a food and medicine. It is now cultivated worldwide on a large scale.

CULTIVATION

Cultivated primarily for its seeds, but also for its flavour-filled leaves, roots and flowers, caraway makes a charming garden plant, and has the lace flowers typical of its Umbelliferae family origins. The flowers have the same effects as the seeds, although they are not as potent, and they can be used in fruit salads, salads and stir-fries with delicious results. Caraway needs a sunny position and loose, light soil and grows as a quick annual two or three times a season during the warm months, scattering seed everywhere. I sow the seed straight into the ground three times during spring and summer and give it a good dressing of compost three times a year.

MEDICINAL USES

Caraway is a much-respected antispasmodic; the seeds soothe and work directly on the digestive tract, easing spasms, colic, bloating, flatulence and heartburn. Some Middle East eating-houses serve a tiny bowl of caraway seeds on each table to chew on between courses or between mouthfuls. Interestingly, caraway's antispasmodic, diuretic and expectorant qualities have been confirmed by medical research, and to add to its benefits, the seeds and leaves sweeten the breath, improve appetite, counter heart irregularity and ease menstrual cramps. The standard brew for all these ailments is ¼ cup caraway flowers and two teaspoons of seeds in a cup of boiling water. Allow the tea to stand for five minutes, then strain and sip slowly. If used as a mouthwash and gargle, it will clear bad breath, gum ailments and even tighten the teeth, it is believed! A teaspoonful or two of this tea will calm and quieten a restless baby, ease indigestion and restore a feeling of wellbeing in the elderly.

Caraway is a remarkable herb; it can even be added to your dog's food and will help to counter wind and bad breath. Caraway is now being medically tested as a heart and pulse regulator and as a treatment for severe menstrual pain. The flowers and seeds are an expectorant and tonic, and are added to some patent medicines, particularly for the treatment of chronic coughs.

Caraway muscle-soothing cream

Caraway with mint is an old-fashioned muscle relaxant and I have made this cream for many years, particularly for pain and discomfort associated with menstruation. Warm the cream by standing it in a jar of hot water, then massage it in gently, and rest with the knees up and a hot-water bottle and blanket over the affected area.

1 cup fresh caraway flowers with a few leaves and stems
1 tablespoon crushed caraway seeds
½ cup fresh mint
1½ cups good aqueous cream
3 teaspoons vitamin E oil

In a double boiler, simmer the flowers, leaves, stems, seeds, mint and aqueous cream together for 30 minutes. Cool it, strain, and add the vitamin E oil. Mix well and spoon into sterilised glass jars.

A soothing tip is to stuff fresh flowering caraway sprigs into the cover of a hot-water bottle, between the bottle and the cover. The heat of the boiling water will release the fragrance and the gentle oils and help to relax painful spasms.

Make several pots of caraway flower cream in the summer. It will become a valuable pain reliever throughout the year. Keep it refrigerated in hot weather.

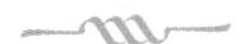

CULINARY USES

Caraway egg and potato salad

SERVES 4–6

This popular salad can be served with cold meats or cheese, or simply with crusty bread.

8 medium-sized potatoes
1 butter lettuce
A few fresh spinach leaves
6 hard-boiled eggs
1 thinly sliced green pepper
1 cup caraway flowers, broken up and stalks removed
Juice of 1 lemon
Sea salt and black pepper to taste

Dressing
2 teaspoons crushed caraway seeds
4 tablespoons olive oil
2 teaspoons dry mustard powder
2 tablespoons balsamic vinegar

Boil the potatoes, peel off the skins and dice. Tear up the lettuce and spinach leaves, and quarter the eggs. Mix everything together carefully. Place the dressing ingredients in a screw-top jar, seal and shake well. Pour the dressing over the salad and serve immediately.

Caraway flower and peach pashka

SERVES 4

This is a lighter version of the traditional Russian dessert. Use strawberries and peaches, apricots and mangoes, or any combination of your choice.

2 tablespoons clear thin honey
1 cup plain Bulgarian yoghurt
250 g smooth cottage cheese
4 cups mashed fruit, such as strawberries and peaches
2 cups caraway flowers, stripped off their stems

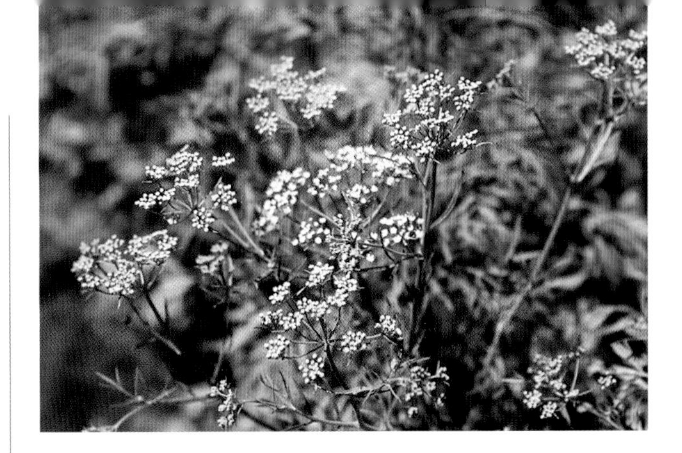

Stir the honey into the yoghurt, then mix in the cottage cheese. Add the mashed fruit and the caraway flowers. Spoon the mixture into a cheesecloth-lined clean, wet flower pot. Chill, and leave it to drain over a bowl. Take the pashka out of the mould after two hours and serve it on a glass plate decorated with fruit slices and umbels of pretty caraway flowers. Serve with caraway tea or after-dinner coffee.

Caraway fish curry

SERVES 4

Nourishing, delicious and easy, this dish is good as it is, or it can be enhanced with the addition of aubergines, mushrooms, mango or pawpaw slices.

4–6 deboned hake fillets
Sunflower oil
Juice of 1 lemon
Sea salt and cayenne pepper to taste
1 tablespoon finely grated ginger
2 teaspoons crushed caraway seeds
4 large tomatoes, peeled and chopped
4 medium onions, finely chopped
A few fresh green curry tree leaves
2 tablespoons honey
1 teaspoon ground coriander seed
1–2 teaspoons turmeric
1–2 teaspoons good curry powder
1 cup caraway flowers

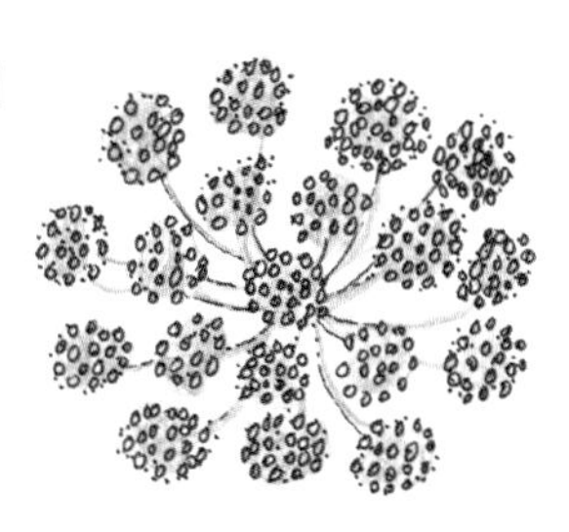

Gently fry the fish in a little sunflower oil with the lemon juice, sea salt, cayenne pepper, ginger and caraway seeds. Meanwhile soak the tomatoes in boiling water to facilitate peeling, then peel and chop. Add to the fish and simmer gently. In another pan, fry the chopped onion in a little oil until it browns. Add the curry leaves (if you have them), honey, spices and caraway flowers and cook for a few minutes, then mix into the fish and tomato mixture. Add a little water if necessary and simmer for four minutes. Serve with rice and decorate with caraway flowers.

Carnation

Dianthus caryophyllus ● **Clove pink**

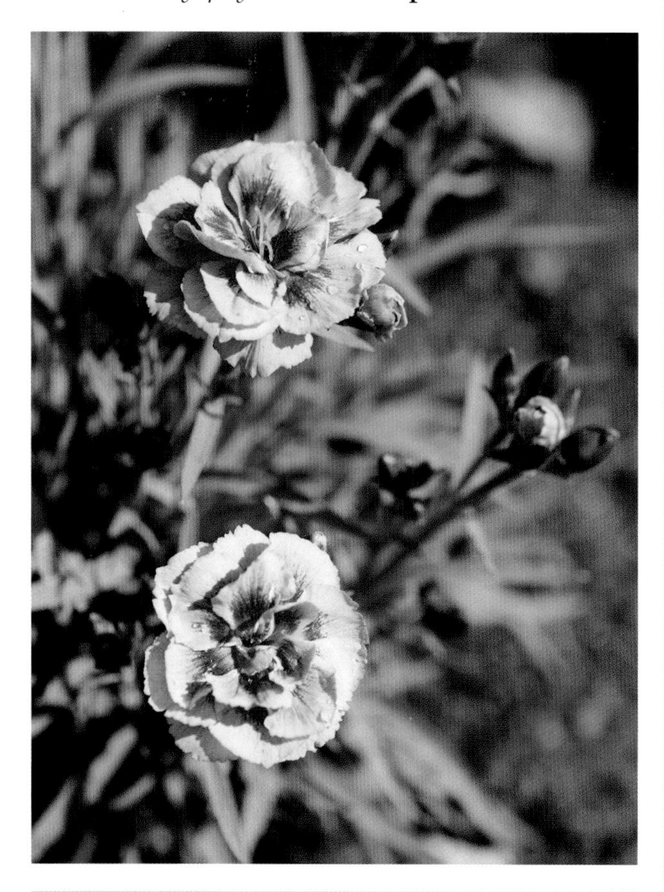

The carnation is an ancient herb, revered through the centuries for its beautiful clove-like scent and remarkable medicinal value. Native to southern Europe and India, it was a common feature in European monastery and cottage gardens, and in Elizabethan texts it was referred to as the 'gillyflower'.

The original species, *Dianthus caryophyllus*, has sadly become almost extinct through the centuries, giving way to the hybridised forms of carnation with little scent and even less medicinal value. Today carnations are available in a vast array of colours, from red, pink, salmon and magenta through to white and yellow, and even striped and flecked, but it is the old-fashioned clove-scented variety, usually pink, that is used herbally. The species *D. carthusianorum*, *D. plumarius* 'Doris', *D. deltoides* (Maiden pink) and the *D.* × *allwoodii* pinks, which are a cross between *D. caryophyllus* and *D. plumarius*, can also be used herbally.

CULTIVATION

Carnation is a short-lived perennial that needs well-drained soil. Propagation is easy, either by sowing seed or taking stem cuttings in spring. Merely strip off the little leafy tufts that form along the flowering stem, and leaving the small 'heel' still attached, strip off the lower leaves and press the cutting into wet sand. Keep it shaded and moist and it will quickly send out tiny roots.

MEDICINAL USES

For about 2 000 years the bright petals of *Dianthus* have been used medicinally to soothe and calm nervousness and anxiety, and to treat kidney and bladder ailments, skin ailments such as eczema, and constipation.

Our grandmothers made a beautifully scented simple carnation cleansing cream, which they used daily to cleanse off grime and oiliness and to moisturise dry skin areas and cracks around the lips. Carnation lotion, in turn, is a great favourite to refresh and soothe on a hot day.

Carnation tonic wine

MAKES 1 LITRE

3 teaspoons crushed coriander seeds
2 teaspoons powdered ginger
2 teaspoons powdered nutmeg
½ cup honey
4 cups good white wine
½ cup carnation petals, white heels removed
½ cup lemon balm leaves (*Melissa officinalis*)

Mix the spices into the honey. In a double boiler, warm the wine with the carnation petals and lemon balm leaves for 5–10 minutes. Add the honey and spice mixture and warm for a further five minutes. Strain, pour into a wine bottle and cork well. Keep refrigerated. Take half a cup at a time and sip it slowly. For sensitive stomachs, dilute with a little water. It can be served warm on a winter's night, or cool in summer.

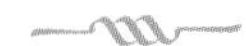

COSMETIC USES

Carnation cleansing cream

1 cup good aqueous cream
1 cup of fresh carnation petals, stripped off their calyxes
2 tablespoons glycerine
1 tablespoon almond oil
2 teaspoons vitamin E oil

Place the aqueous cream and carnation petals in a double boiler and mix in the glycerine and almond oil. Simmer for 15 minutes with the lid on, stirring every now and then. Pour through a sieve and quickly stir in the vitamin E oil. Pour into a sterilised jar with a screw-top lid.

Carnation lotion

1 cup carnation petals, stripped off their calyxes
10 cloves
1 stick cinnamon
1 litre boiling water

Add the carnation petals, cloves and cinnamon stick to the boiling water. Simmer for 10 minutes with the lid on. Cool, strain and pour into a spritz bottle. Add a few drops of carnation essential oil if desired. Shake well and spray frequently over the face, neck and arms.

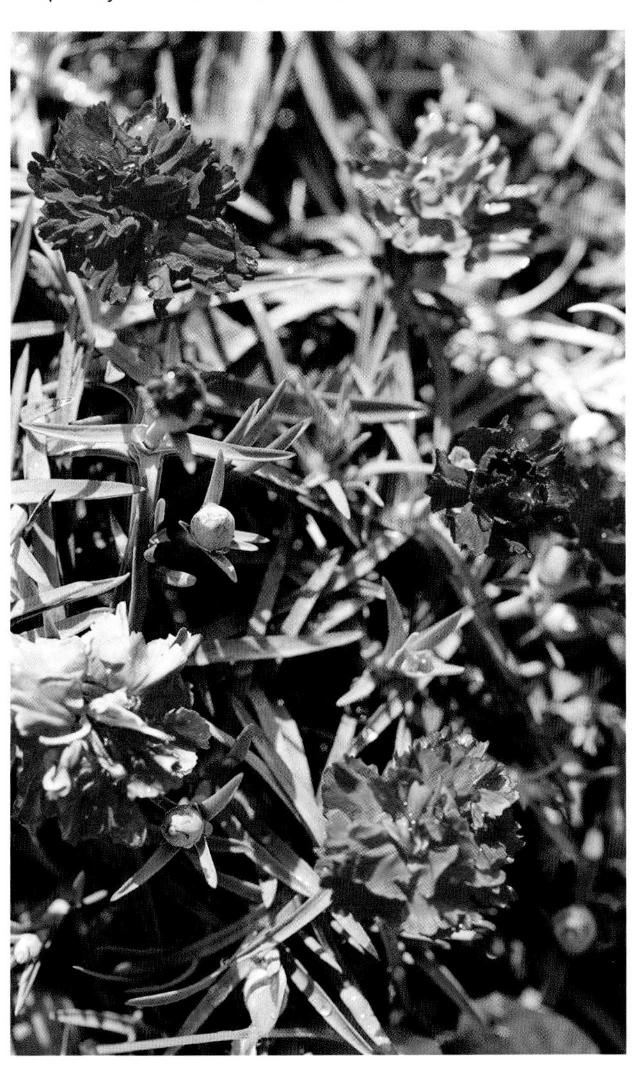

COOK'S NOTE

When cooking with carnations, remove the bitter white heel at the base of the petal (heels tend to be more bitter in some varieties than others). Use the petals lavishly in salads, cakes, desserts and drinks.

CULINARY USES

Mango nectar with carnation petals

SERVES 1

This drink is a magical midsummer experience. I serve it every year as a party drink and no one can get enough!

1 mango, peeled and sliced
1 cup unsweetened mango juice
3 mint leaves
Carnation petals, heels removed

Blend the mango flesh, juice and mint together in a liquidiser, adding a little water if it is too thick. Serve chilled in a tall glass, with carnation petals and mint leaves sprinkled on top.

Carnation pickle

This enchanting recipe dates back to 1629, from a book titled The Garden of Pleasant Flowers. *It ends with the charming line: 'This pickle now draws the highest esteem with Gentlemen and Ladies of the greatest note.' I make it as a sweet-and-sour pickle to serve with cheese.*

6 cups carnation flowers
Brown sugar
A few cloves
2 teaspoons coriander seeds
2 cups brown grape vinegar
2 bay leaves
1 stick cinnamon

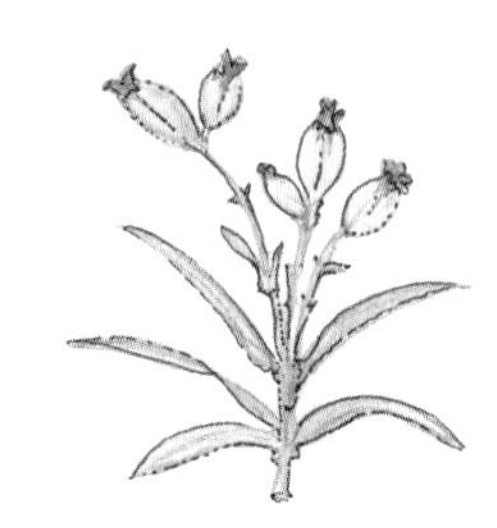

Strip the flowers out of their calyxes and remove the bitter white heels from the petals with a sharp knife. Lay a thin layer of petals in a wide-mouthed jar and sprinkle with brown sugar. Add another layer and sprinkle with sugar and a few cloves and the coriander seeds. Add more layers and more sugar. Warm the vinegar with the bay leaves and cinnamon for 10 minutes. Pour the hot vinegar over the carnation petals. Seal and allow the pickles to stand for two weeks before eating. A peeled, sliced cucumber, pickling onions, or green peppers and even sweet corn cut off the cob, can be added to the recipe, in alternating layers with the carnation petals.

Carpet geranium

Geranium incanum • **Wild geranium** • **Bergtee** • **Vrouetee** • **Creeping geranium**

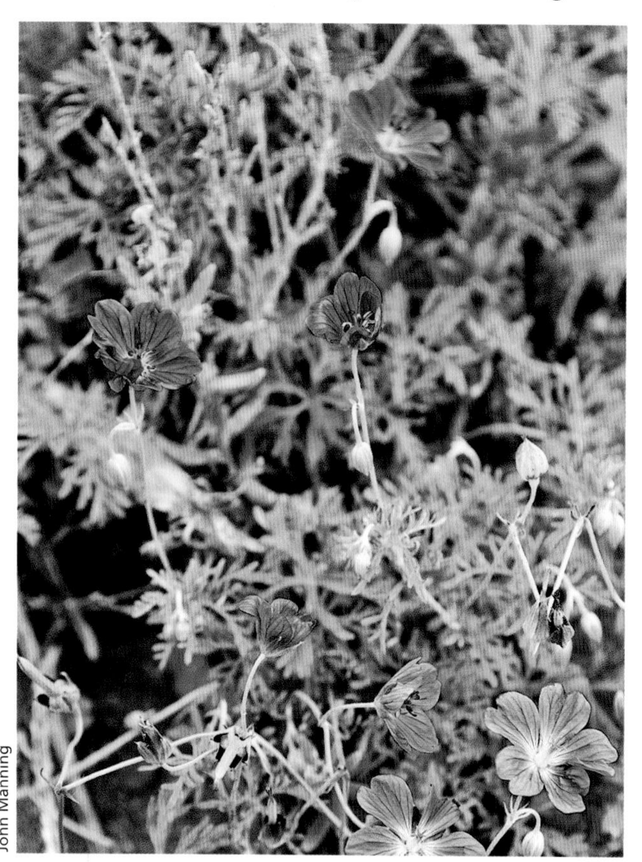

John Manning

While all the plants previously known as geraniums are now correctly known as pelargoniums, only one small, rather unobtrusive plant is still called geranium, and that is South Africa's pretty, feathery-leafed groundcover, the carpet geranium. Used for centuries by most South Africans, this much-loved indigenous plant is now sold in nurseries around the world as far afield as Australia. In Europe and Britain it is known as creeping geranium and it is grown in hanging baskets and window boxes, with its feathery silvery leaves and small bright magenta flowers cascading attractively.

I look on the carpet geranium as a childhood friend. My grandmother grew great swathes of it in her terraced seaside garden in Gordon's Bay in the Cape when I was a child, and we used it in many ways: we drank a pleasant-tasting tea made from it on most mornings, and dipped the flowers, wet with rain or dew, into icing sugar and served them as sweets to our friends.

CULTIVATION

The carpet geranium is not fussy as to soil type and requires little more than a place in the sun, the odd spade or two of compost every now and then, and never much more than a weekly watering. Pull off rooted tufts to propagate, and keep them shaded and moist until they are established. This pretty groundcover is undemanding and deserves far more space in our gardens.

MEDICINAL USES

Traditionally, a tea made from the leaves and flowers was taken to ease bloating, diarrhoea, excessive and irregular menstruation, colic, indigestion and flatulence. It is called *vrouetee* because this is the best tea for expelling the afterbirth, starting milk flow for the newborn, and easing cystitis and other bladder infections in women. To make the tea, steep ¼ cup flowers in a cup boiling water for four or five minutes. Strain and sip slowly.

We underestimate the value of carpet geranium, and as it forms part of our history, it should be planted more widely. In my hot mountainside gardens I have struggled to keep it going, particularly on the very dry, baking days when everything wilts. Some gardeners may need to consider partial or light shade.

In the early days of the Cape, plant sellers traded *vrouetee* for other plants and seeds. Over a cup of *vrouetee* women shared stories and supported one another. Sitting on a couple of bricks around a fire and sipping this pleasant brew brought great comfort in many ways.

As a young mother, I sat with a group of women in the Cape and shared in their cups of comfort on the busy Grand Parade. From them I learned to treat cystitis with several cups of *vrouetee* and how the flowers of the carpet geranium could be melted into oil or aqueous cream and used to soothe rash or itchiness under the breasts or around the panty line. The flowers need to be finely chopped and pressed down well in either almond oil or olive oil (more recently I mixed grape seed oil with aqueous cream, ½ cup of each). Simmer for 30 minutes, then strain. Bottle in a glass jar with a well-fitting lid. I was also told by those amazing women never to wear synthetic underclothes and only to wear cotton close to the skin, and I have done so ever since.

COSMETIC USES

Carpet geranium can be used to make an age-old lotion for itchy skin and oily hair, and when mixed with oats, it makes a superb scalp treatment for dandruff, flaky scalp and psoriasis of the scalp, soothing and softening the irritated area.

Carpet geranium lotion for itchy skin and oily hair

2 cups *Geranium incanum* leaves, sprigs and flowers
1 cup rose-scented pelargonium flowers and leaves
2 tablespoons aniseeds
2 litres water

Boil the carpet geranium with the other ingredients in the water for 10–15 minutes. Strain, and use as a lotion on dry itchy skin, as a rinse on hair that becomes oily very quickly and as a spritzer spray on sunburnt skin and heat rashes.

Carpet geranium and oats scalp treatment

1 cup oats (the large-flaked non-instant kind)
1 litre carpet geranium lotion (see recipe above)

Simmer the oats in the geranium lotion for five minutes until the oats start to soften. Remove from the heat and cool until pleasantly warm. After shampooing and rinsing the hair, carefully spread handfuls of the warm oats and geranium-lotion mixture onto the scalp, massaging it in well. Wrap your hair in a towel and relax for 10 minutes, then rinse thoroughly with warm water to which a little apple cider vinegar has been added.

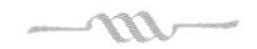

CULINARY USES

Crystallised carpet geranium flowers

My grandmother taught me the wonderful art of crystallising violets when I was a child, and I have since experimented with many other flowers. Carpet geranium is one of the best! The flowers should have a bit of stalk still attached.

1 cup carpet geranium flowers
2 egg whites, softly beaten but still fairly runny
Castor sugar

Dip each flower into the egg white and paint inside and out with a paint brush, holding it by its little stalk 'handle'. Have a baking tray ready, lined with greaseproof paper and sprinkled with a little castor sugar. Dip each flower into the castor sugar and sprinkle some sugar over it, so that all surfaces are coated. Arrange the flowers on the baking tray, place in a preheated warming drawer, and turn off the heat. Leave the flowers there until they are dry. During winter or damp weather, switch the warming drawer on for about 10 minutes every now and then, and then switch off again. Store the flowers in a sealed container and use to decorate cakes and desserts.

Fragrant carpet geranium tea

SERVES 1

This pleasant tea is a real comfort on days when one is feeling rushed and harassed. In hot weather it can be made into a refreshing iced tea by cooling the same infusion and adding about ¾ cup fresh fruit juice (grape or litchi is wonderful) and an ice cube.

1 cup boiling water
1 thumb-length sprig peppermint
¼ cup carpet geranium leaves and flowers
1 cinnamon stick
2 teaspoons honey

Pour the boiling water over all the ingredients. Allow the tea to stand for five minutes, then strain and sip slowly. Alternatively, allow the tea to cool and make into iced tea as described.

Pear and carpet geranium stir-fry

SERVES 4

This delicious, quick-and-easy dessert proves to be popular with everyone.

6 large ripe pears, peeled, cored and cut into pieces
2–3 tablespoons butter
3 tablespoons brown sugar
½–¾ cup chopped pecan nuts
½ cup carpet geranium flowers

In a wok or frying pan, stir-fry the pears in the butter and add the sugar and pecan nuts, stirring for about five minutes. Just before serving, add the carpet geranium flowers. Spoon the dessert into individual glass bowls. Serve warm with whipped cream, decorated with more fresh carpet geranium flowers.

Catmint

Nepeta mussinii ● *N. cataria* ● **Catnip**

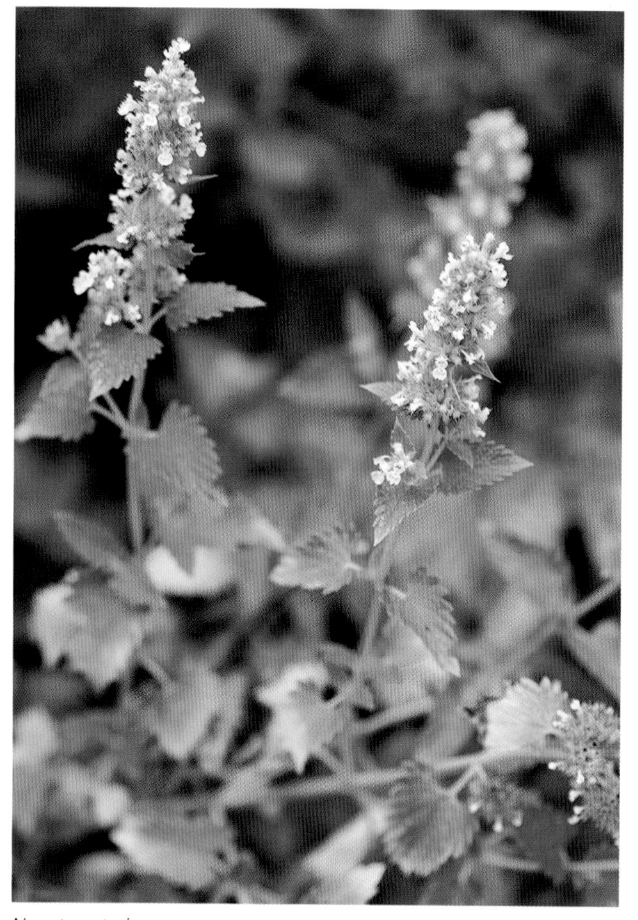

Nepeta cataria

A pretty perennial border plant dating back to antiquity, catmint has been around for centuries as an insect repellent, a medicine, a charm, and a salad for cats! It is native to Europe and Asia and has subsequently been naturalised all over the world. The tiny mauve flowers and the flowering spikes are recorded in ancient pharmacopoeias as a gentle yet profound medication, especially for children but also for adults as a calming, quietening drink at the end of a hectic day. In the Middle Ages, catmint syrup or catmint honey was sold in the market places as a medication for coughs, colds, sore throats, intestinal cramps and sleeplessness. Interestingly, while catmint is a calming herb for humans, it sends cats into a frenzy of delight, acrobatics and joy!

CULTIVATION

Catmint requires full sun and deeply dug well-composted soil for its flowering spikes to create a show. It reaches 15 cm in height, and from its basic clump-forming habit it can spread 50 cm in width, forming a neat attractive cushion. It thrives with a deep twice-weekly watering and needs to be cut back twice-yearly right down to the base of the stems and given a good dressing of compost lightly dug in around it.

Catnip helps to keep aphids, whitefly, red spider and even fungal attacks away from special plants, and it remains a favourite old-fashioned flower in the most modern of gardens. It makes a pretty companion plant to roses, fruit trees, beans, broccoli and cauliflowers and can be planted between spinach and lettuce rows.

MEDICINAL USES

Catmint tea is a respected drink for stress, anxiety, coughs, colds, flu and indigestion. It is also a calming and safe medication for children who sleep fitfully and bed-wet. To make the standard brew tea, pour a cup of boiling water over ¼ cup fresh flowering sprigs. Let the tea stand for five minutes, stir frequently, strain, sweeten with a touch of honey, and sip slowly. The tea has been found to ease insomnia and ensure sleep without nightmares. It also reduces anxiety, tension and heart palpitations, eases indigestion, flatulence, colic and diarrhoea, relieves headaches, and releases muscular cramps and pains. It has been unquestionably found to have a sedative effect in all age groups. Because of its pleasantly calming effects, catmint tea is listed today in medical texts and modern pharmacopoeias as a relaxant herb, equally safe for toddlers and the aged.

Through the years I have created what I call 'peace pillows' or 'sleep pillows', which are small pillows filled with the relevant dried herbs and soft foam, with a washable pillowslip. The pillow is small enough to tuck into the neck or the small of the back while sitting or it can be placed under a bigger soft pillow to give support where it is needed.

Catmint pillow for insomnia and anxiety

Plain white cotton fabric (for the inner slip)
Pure cotton fabric in a design (for the pillowcase)

Select pure, soft cotton fabric. Do not be tempted by synthetic non-crease fabrics as these do not 'breathe' and will become hot and uncomfortable. The priority is to find pure cotton and to wash off the starchy 'covering' of the material before commencing.

Cut the plain white cotton folded double 35 x 24 cm. Sew a double seam all around it, about 1 cm from the edge, leaving an opening of 12 cm at one end in order to stuff in the herbs and foam. Make a pillowcase from the pretty cotton (slightly bigger than the inner slip) and leave a longer flap at one end to fold over like an ordinary pillowcase.

Filling

- 1 cup dried lavender sprigs (Margaret Roberts lavender retains its scent well)
- 1 cup dried catmint flowering sprigs
- 1 cup dried rose-scented pelargonium leaves
- ½ cup cloves
- ½ cup chopped dried lemon peel
- ½ cup dried lemon zest
- 1–2 teaspoons lavender oil

Mix the lavender sprigs, catmint and pelargonium together. Then make the scented fixative mixture with the cloves, dried lemon peel and zest, and spoon it into a big glass jar. (To make the zest, peel the lemon with a potato peeler and dry it in the sun.) Add the lavender oil to the clove and lemon peel mixture, shake well and leave overnight.

The next morning add more lavender oil if needed and let it blend well overnight. Mix the now headily fragrant fixative into the lavender, rose-scented pelargonium leaves and catmint. Keep in a sealed container overnight, then mix it with foam chips to make a soft and comfortable filling. Stuff the pillow and sew up the side. Keep it in a large plastic bag to keep in the fragrance.

To refresh the pillow, make a small cotton bag filled with the fixative, sew it up securely, open the end of the inner pillow slip and push the new fragrant fixative into the centre of the pillow.

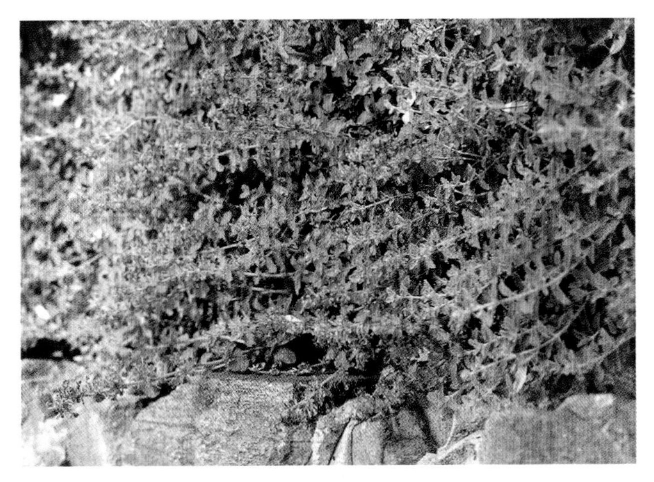

Nepeta mussinii

CULINARY USES

Catmint honey

- 6 catmint flowering sprigs
- 6 crushed cardamom pods, husks removed
- 1 jar runny honey

Push the catmint and cardamom into the jar of honey – wild flower or orange blossom honey is perfect for this recipe. It is a slow process, but you need to push the sprigs to the bottom. They will slowly rise in the honey, so open the jar every now and then and press the catmint down again. The catmint imparts a delicious flavour with the cardamom seeds. This delicious honey can be used as a sweetener for hot teas. The soothing and calming qualities of the catmint will be released into the tea.

Catmint spicy rub

This delicious rub is perfect for spicing up chicken breasts, big brown mushrooms, roast potatoes, sweet potatoes and pumpkin.

- ¼–½ cup dried catmint flowers, stripped off their stems
- ½ cup crushed coriander seeds
- ¼ cup caraway seeds, crushed
- 1 teaspoon chopped chilli (mild or hot, depending on how you like it)
- ¼ cup dried thyme leaves and flowers
- 1–2 teaspoons crushed Himalayan salt or crushed coarse sea salt
- 2 teaspoons paprika

Mix the ingredients together thoroughly and store in a screw-top jar. Rub about one tablespoon of the mixture onto chicken or vegetables before grilling or roasting. You will find many uses for this exceptional flavouring – try adding about two teaspoons to a savoury pancake batter for a different taste!

COOK'S NOTE

Tiny catmint flowers pulled out of their calyxes were an ancient and edible decoration used on desserts, cakes, fruit salads, soups and stews, while catmint tea was a favourite drink in Europe long before coffee and Ceylon tea were introduced.

Cauliflower

Brassica oleracea var. *botrytis*

The cauliflower has to be among the most spectacular and delicious of all the flowers to find a place in this book! Originating in the Mediterranean area and Asia Minor, records show that it has been a valuable food and surprisingly an equally valuable medicine since the sixth century BC. It was grown as a food crop in Turkey and Egypt in about 400 BC and from there it spread to Greece, Italy and France as a favoured delicacy, cooked in milk. As the spice trade progressed, finely grated nutmeg was considered to be the perfect match with cauliflower, and is still popular with it today!

The medieval monks grew cauliflower in their cloister gardens to make a delicious soup with onions, leeks and celery to treat coughs, colds and pneumonia, and by the 14th century it was listed in the first medical texts and pharmacopoeias as a medicinal plant. During the winter months the monks pickled cauliflowers in vinegar flavoured with strong-tasting seeds like dill, fennel, fenugreek and mustard seeds, for use during the winter months. Cauliflower was introduced to England around 1586 as 'colewort' and was made into a gruel to treat lung infections and severe coughs.

I was entranced by beautiful botanical drawings displayed in the ancient monastery collections at some of the abbeys in Britain and Europe. Cauliflower stood out in its pale magnificence, painted as a winter medicine with mustard seeds alongside it!

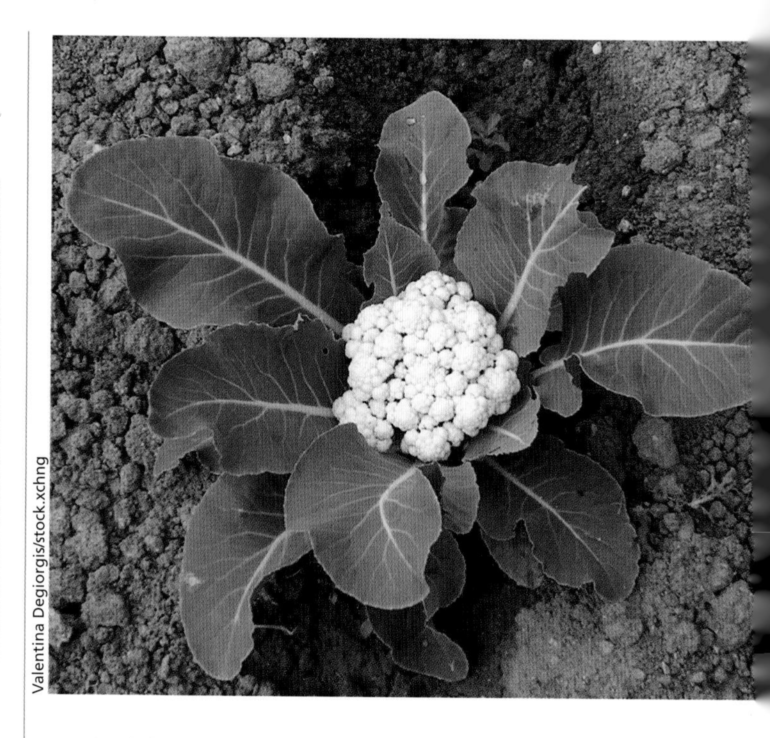
Valentina Degiorgis/stock.xchng

CULTIVATION

I plant cauliflower as a winter annual as the summers are generally too hot in South Africa and aphids love all the brassicas in the summer months! (I am a dedicated organic gardener and do not spray any kind of poisonous insect repellent, so I grow the brassicas only in the cold months.)

At the end of summer sow seed in seed trays and keep them moist. Transplant into compost-filled bags once they are big enough to handle. Keep moist and protected, and move the bags of young cauliflowers out into the sun for increasing periods each day until they are about 12 cm in height. Plant out in full sun, spaced 50 cm apart, in rows that have been deeply dug and richly composted. Flood with water two or even three times a week if the winter days are warm.

Cauliflowers look spectacular in the flower garden too. Last winter, Flanders poppies and chamomile (self-seeded) came up in my cauliflower rows, which looked breathtaking. I left them growing happily together, and interestingly, had masses of butterflies in the early, still cold, spring days!

MEDICINAL USES

Cauliflower is rich in vitamins B_3, B_5 and C, as well as folic acid, potassium, iron and fibre. The entire cabbage family is rich in immune-boosting and cancer-fighting components and is vital in the diet, especially in soups and broths for treating coughs, colds, bronchitis, pneumonia. A potent and remarkable juice can be made from cauliflower together with other important immune-boosting plants. It is of particular value during winter to ward off flu and bronchitis. I was given the recipe or 'formula' below by a homeopathic doctor:

Immune booster juice

SERVES 1–2

2 cups fresh lucerne sprigs and flowers
2 cups buckwheat leaves and flowering tops
2 cups red clover flowers and leaves
2 cups fennel bulbs and leaves, sliced
2 cups violet leaves and flowers (garden violet, p. 200, not African violet)

2 cups cauliflower florets and leaves
2 cups broccoli florets and leaves
3–4 fresh organically grown carrots
2–3 peeled apples
2 beetroots, peeled and quartered
3 cups fresh young barley grass or wheatgrass

Push all the ingredients through a juice extractor. The apples, carrots and beetroot supply the juice, so alternate them with the other ingredients when juicing. They also add sweetness. Half a glass a day is ideal, made fresh every day. Remember that fruit and vegetable juices always need to be taken fresh as after two hours they lose their optimal potential. I use a spiral juicer to extract every precious drop from the wheat and barley grass and the leafy plants. This juice is also excellent as an anticancer drink. I am privileged to have been given this remarkable recipe and to be able to pass it on.

Chicken and cauliflower 'hot pot'

Quick and easy to make, this wonderful soupy 'stew' fights colds, flu and bronchitis.

1 organic chicken
2 large onions, finely chopped
Olive oil for browning the chicken
4 carrots, sliced

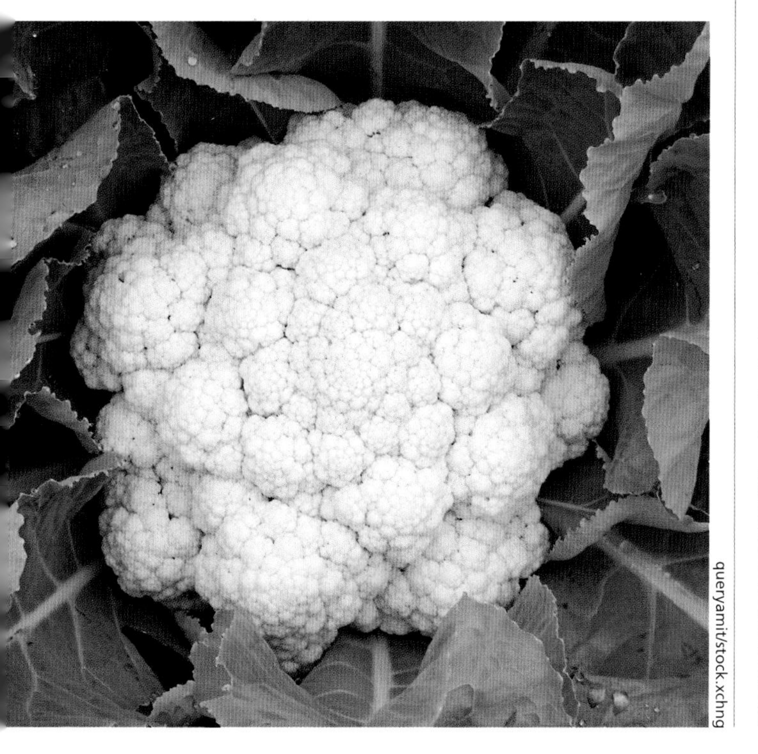
queryamit/stock.xchng

1 medium-sized cauliflower and leaves
3 cups chopped celery
3 cups shredded green cabbage leaves
1 cup chopped parsley
2 tablespoons fresh thyme
Water (enough to cover chicken)
Sea salt and red pepper to taste
Juice of 2 lemons

Brown the chicken and onions in the oil, turning. Add all the other ingredients and simmer until the chicken is soft and tender, usually 1–1½ hours. Add more water as needed. Finely shredded cabbage and cauliflower leaves, midribs discarded, make a very tasty, tender and delicious base to the hot pot. Keep the hot pot well chilled, take out what is needed and heat well. Serve with fresh chopped parsley and another squeeze of lemon juice.

CULINARY USES

Cauliflower pickle

MAKES 1 LARGE JAR

When there are too many cauliflowers maturing at once, they can be pickled, the way the monks did. This is a tasty way of preserving them. Serve with salads, cold meats and cheese through the summer.

1 fresh cauliflower, cut into florets
3 cups white grape vinegar
4 tablespoons honey
1 tablespoon mustard seeds
1 tablespoon coriander seeds

Cut the cauliflower into neat florets and pack them into a wide-mouthed jar. Boil the vinegar with the honey, mustard seeds and coriander seeds (dill seeds, caraway seeds, cumin seeds and aniseed are also delicious, so vary them). Simmer the vinegar for 10 minutes and pour over the cauliflower until fully covered. Seal well and store for at least one month before eating.

COOK'S NOTE

Eat raw cauliflower, straight from the garden, washed, then dipped in homemade mayonnaise with paprika. It makes a feast to remember, and it is so good for you! Raw cauliflower florets can also be dipped in batter and fried lightly in olive oil as a gourmet treat and snack food served with pre-dinner drinks.

Chamomile

Matricaria recutita • *Chamaemelum nobile*

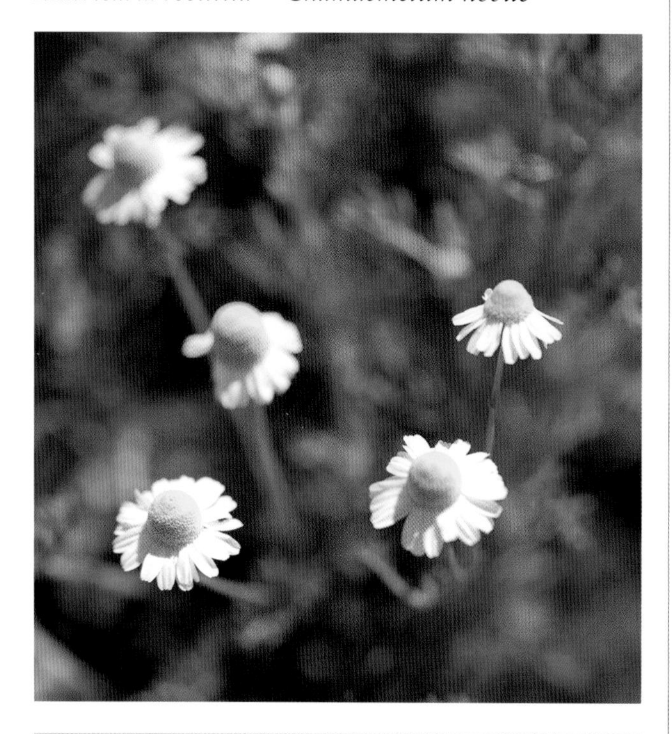

Two species of chamomile are used medicinally and they have identical properties. German chamomile, *Matricaria recutita* is a spring annual with small, daisy-like white flowers and fine feathery leaves, while *Chamaemelum nobile*, often called lawn chamomile, is a perennial that is lower-growing (about 10 cm in height) and spreading, with similar flowers and leaves. Both are indigenous to Europe and both are superb medicinal plants; their flowers, fresh or dried, have been valued for centuries for their amazing healing properties.

CULTIVATION

Growing annual chamomile is easy. Sow seed in mid-autumn where it is to grow in full sun in well-dug, well-composted soil. Keep it moist (I sprinkle a light cover of leaves over the area) and water lightly twice a day until the tiny, feathery seedlings push through. Transplant them in the very early stages when they are big enough to handle, but after that they do not like to be moved. Chamomile is essentially a cool-weather plant and will flower prolifically in spring, reaching a height of 25–30 cm. If left to go to seed it will come up year after year.

MEDICINAL USES

Chamomile is cultivated in Europe for homeopathic medicines and current research confirms its ancient uses: it is excellent for digestive problems such as acidity, gastritis, bloating, colic, hiatus hernia, peptic ulcer, Crohn's disease and irritable bowel syndrome. It helps with morning sickness in pregnant women and eases sore nipples in lactating mothers (drunk as a tea or applied as a lotion). Tense, aching muscles and menstrual cramps are quickly soothed with a cup of hot chamomile tea. It also soothes away stress, anxiety and panic attacks, and it is anti-allergenic, effective against hay fever, catarrh, asthma, eczema and skin rashes.

Chamomile flowers contain an aromatic oil that gives them their typical scent, and they have powerful antiseptic and anti-inflammatory properties. A superb gargle, douche and eyewash can be made using fresh or dried flowers. In the case of tired, red, irritated eyes, soak a clean facecloth in the warm brew, cover the eyes with it and lie down for a few minutes. Use the same brew as a gargle for a dry, strained throat, especially if you are a public speaker or a singer.

Chamomile eyewash, douche and gargle

1 cup fresh chamomile flowers
or ¾ cup dried chamomile flowers
1½ litres water

Simmer the flowers in the water for 10 minutes. Strain, add a cup of cold water, and mix well. Use as a douche or wash to clear any infections, irritations and itchiness. Store excess in the fridge and warm it a little each time you use it, but never warm it in a microwave.

Chamomile tea for insomnia

SERVES 1

This old-fashioned tea is an age-old remedy for insomnia.

1 teaspoon dried or 2 teaspoons fresh chamomile flowers
1 cup boiling water
1 clove

Place dried chamomile flowers in a little sieve and pour the water through them until almost level with the edge of the cup. (Fresh flowers can be added straight to the water.) Add a clove to the water and allow the tea to stand for five minutes. Remove the flowers and the clove, sweeten with a touch of honey and sip slowly.

Chamomile cough syrup

This is a superb cough mixture for tight chests or a soothing drink for restless children. It also makes a delicious drink, either hot or cold.

4 cups fresh chamomile flowers or 2 cups dried flowers
½–2 cups honey
1 stick cinnamon
10 cloves
Juice of 3 lemons
A few thin slivers of lemon rind
1 large sprig lemon balm mint (*Melissa officinalis*)

Simmer all the ingredients together for 20 minutes in a covered pot. Remove from the heat and allow the syrup to cool. Strain and pour into clean bottles, cork well and label. To help relieve a cough, dilute two teaspoons of the syrup in a little hot water and take frequently. As a drink, dilute ¼ cup syrup in one cup of warm or ice-cold water and sip slowly.

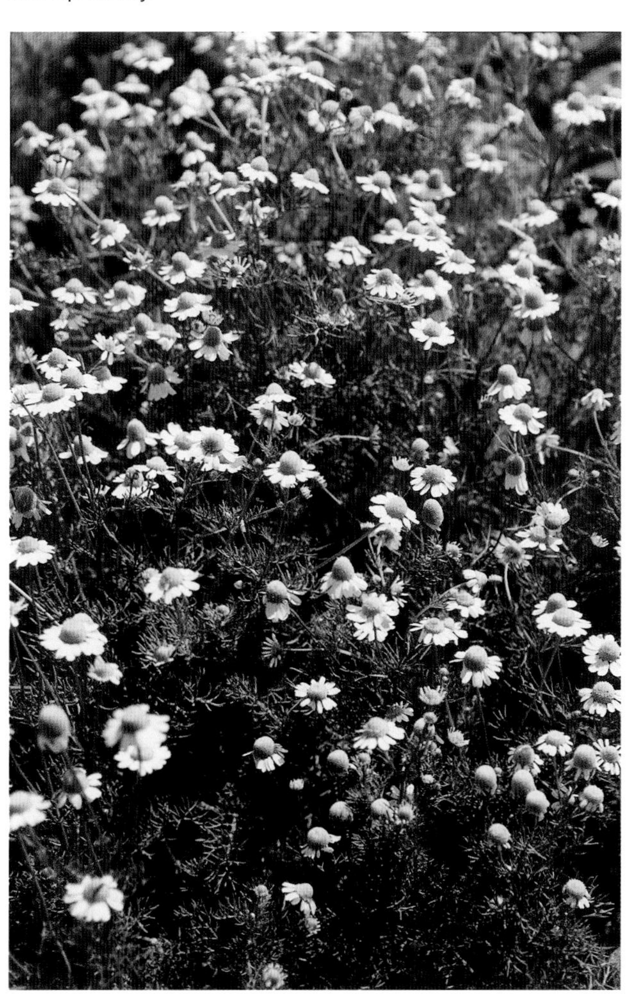

CULINARY USES

Chamomile fruit jelly

SERVES 4–6

This superb summertime dessert for the whole family is especially good at the end of a hectic day when the children are stressed. Grape, apple, mango or litchi juice may be used instead of orange juice, and pieces of fruit may be set into the jelly too.

1 litre chamomile tea
½–¾ cup runny honey
4 tablespoons gelatine
Juice of 6 oranges

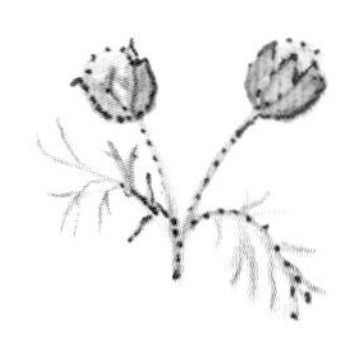

Make the chamomile tea by pouring a litre of boiling water over three tablespoons of fresh chamomile flowers or 1½ tablespoons dried flowers; leave to draw for 10 minutes, then strain. Mix the honey into the warm chamomile tea and taste, adding a little more if necessary. Dissolve the gelatine in one cup of hot water and add to the tea, then add the orange juice. Stir well, pour into a pretty glass bowl and leave to set in the fridge. Serve with custard or cream.

Honey, fruit and chamomile loaf

We dry apple slices, apricot halves and peach slices in our endlessly working driers, then chop a selection and mix with sultanas for this loaf, which is delicious and keeps well.

1¼ cups mixed dried fruit
1 cup chamomile tea
1 tablespoon honey
1 cup low-fat milk
¼ cup fresh chamomile flowers
2¼ cups wholewheat flour
2 teaspoons baking powder
¼ teaspoon salt
½ teaspoon bicarbonate of soda

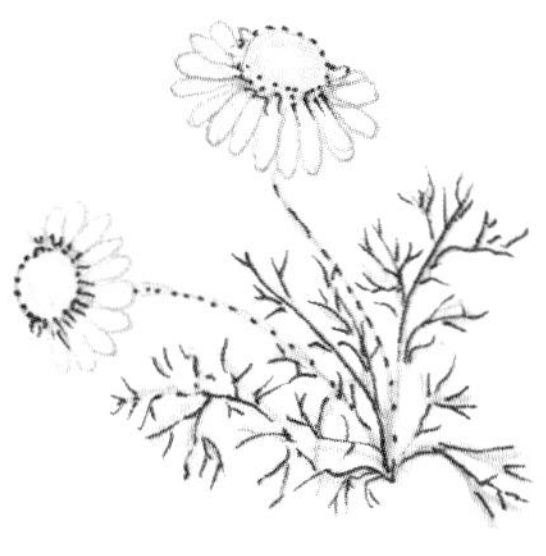

Soak the mixed dried fruit in the chamomile tea for an hour, then strain. Mix the honey into milk and heat with the flowers. Let it stand for an hour, then strain. Preheat the oven to 160°C. Grease and line a loaf tin with baking paper. Sift the flour, baking powder, salt and bicarbonate of soda together into a mixing bowl. Add the softened fruit with the strained warm milk, little by little, alternating and mixing it well. Spoon into the lined loaf tin and bake for 45 minutes or until a skewer inserted into the middle of the loaf comes out clean. Cool for a few minutes, then turn the loaf out carefully onto a wire cake rack. Once cooled, slice carefully and spread with a little butter. It tastes best served with a cup of chamomile tea.

Chicory

Cichorium intybus

A deep-rooted, hardy perennial that sends up a beautiful blue flowering branch in summer, chicory was once a common sight in Europe and Western Asia along roadsides and in marshy places. It has become naturalised all over the world. Records of herbal uses of chicory date back to the first century. In about AD 60, Pliny the Elder made a mixture of chicory juice, rose oil and vinegar to treat headaches, and modern research into chicory's detoxifying properties indicates that he was on the right track. Since the earliest times chicory root has been dry-roasted and ground to make a coffee substitute, or peeled, scrubbed and either boiled as a vegetable or roasted with onions and potatoes.

CULTIVATION

The chicory root stump or crown may be dug up and trimmed before flower production, then stored in a warm, dark place to develop young buds called chicons. These are eaten in salads, or as a vegetable. Witloof is traditionally the favourite variety to plant, but seedlings of other varieties are now also on sale at nurseries. These should be planted in rows spaced 30 cm apart. If planting from seed, sow them in rich, well-composted soil, in full sun in rows spaced 30 cm apart. Alternatively, sow them initially in seed trays until they are big enough to handle, then plant out in rows.

MEDICINAL USES

Chicory has a mildly bitter taste and the root is similar medicinally to the root of the dandelion, *Taraxacum officinale*, exerting a cleansing action on the liver, stomach, kidneys and urinary tract. As a treatment for gout, rheumatic conditions and general aches and pains of the joints, chicory was once considered to be particularly appropriate for the elderly, and was also used as a gentle laxative for children. Today doctors find that chicory tea aids digestion, clears toxins, reduces inflammation, has a tonic effect on the liver and gall bladder, and flushes the kidneys. If the same tea is used as a wash or added to the bath during an attack of cystitis, it gently soothes any external discomfort and itch. To make the tea, pour a cup of boiling water over ¼ cup mixed leaves and flowers and leave to stand for five minutes; it can be sweetened with a touch of honey if desired. Usually one cup a day will do the trick. The tea is slightly laxative and safe for children made as a standard brew; give children under 10 years of age half a cup at a time.

Mothers in medieval France and England grew chicory in their cottage gardens and used the herb for purging and for flushing out the bladder. Today's research verifies these uses: chicory cleanses the bladder and colon, clears infections, acts as a strong tonic and increases the flow of bile.

CAUTION: Excessive and continued use of chicory may impair the function of the retina in the eyes due to its exceptionally powerful action.

Chicory flower bath

This ancient remedy has been used for centuries to ease varicose veins and haemorrhoids and to reduce anal inflammation and itching.

3 cups chicory flowers and stems
10 chicory leaves
3 litres water

Simmer the flowers, stems and leaves in water for 20 minutes. Strain and add to the bath. Alternatively, soak small towels in the warm brew and apply to the area, carefully wrapping it in place, to bring comfort and relief. Soak the towels in the hot liquid now and then and reapply.

This marvellous brew has also been used for gout pains and rheumatic, hot and swollen joints. It can be cooled and reheated as needed. Cooled chicory flower water has astringent properties and has been applied to thread veins on the face with cotton wool.

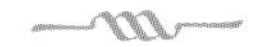

CULINARY USES

Chicory and tuna salad

SERVES 4

Use mustard greens, spinach, rocket, butter lettuce or any other green leaves of your choice in this salad.

1 tin tuna in brine
2 cups green beans
2 cups green leaves
1 sweet pepper, thinly sliced
Sea salt and black pepper to taste
Juice of 1 lemon
1 cup good mayonnaise
1 teaspoon mustard powder
½ cup finely chopped spring onions
1 cup chicory flowers

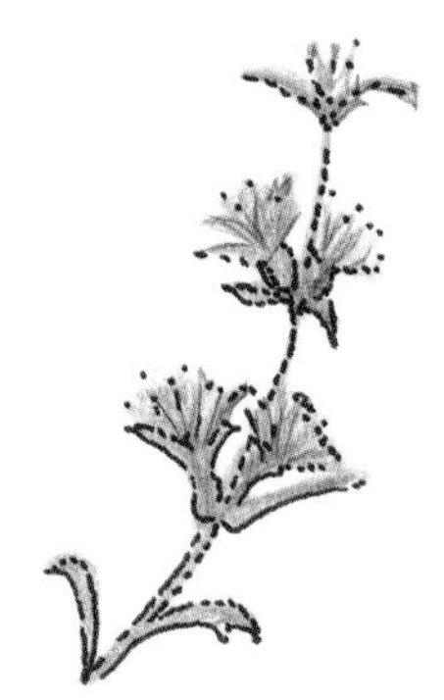

Break up the tuna. Steam the beans lightly and refresh in cold water, then cut them up. Shred the green leaves into small pieces. Mix all the ingredients together and decorate with blue chicory flowers. Serve with crusty bread as a lunch dish.

Chicory stir-fry

SERVES 4

Apple is an excellent complement to chicory in this thoroughly tasty and nutritious stir-fry. It must be served immediately.

2 medium-sized onions, chopped
2 cups thinly sliced leeks
Olive oil
2 cups thinly sliced brown mushrooms
2 apples, peeled and coarsely grated
½ cup parsley
2 sticks celery, chopped (leaves included)
1 cup chicory flowers
1 cup peeled and coarsely grated sweet potato
Sea salt and cayenne pepper to taste
Juice of 1 lemon
½ cup sesame seeds
1 dessertspoon Worcestershire sauce

Brown the onions and leeks in the olive oil, then add the mushrooms and stir-fry briskly. Add the apples, parsley, celery, chicory flowers and sweet potato and season with salt and cayenne pepper. Finally, add the lemon juice and sesame seeds, followed by the Worcestershire sauce. Stir-fry until tender, and serve piping hot with brown rice.

COOK'S NOTE
Remember that chicory is a bitter herb and that the apple takes away some of the bitterness. However, like dandelion, chicory is so good for you that it is worth using often.

Pickled chicory flowers

MAKES 2 JARS

This is an old-fashioned recipe made with hot spicy vinegar and onions. Keep a jar close at hand for a quick and tasty addition to soups, stews and stir-fries. (Pickled flowers may be used in the stir-fry recipe above in place of fresh chicory flowers.)

4 cups chicory flowers
4 cups onion rings
2 cups good grape vinegar

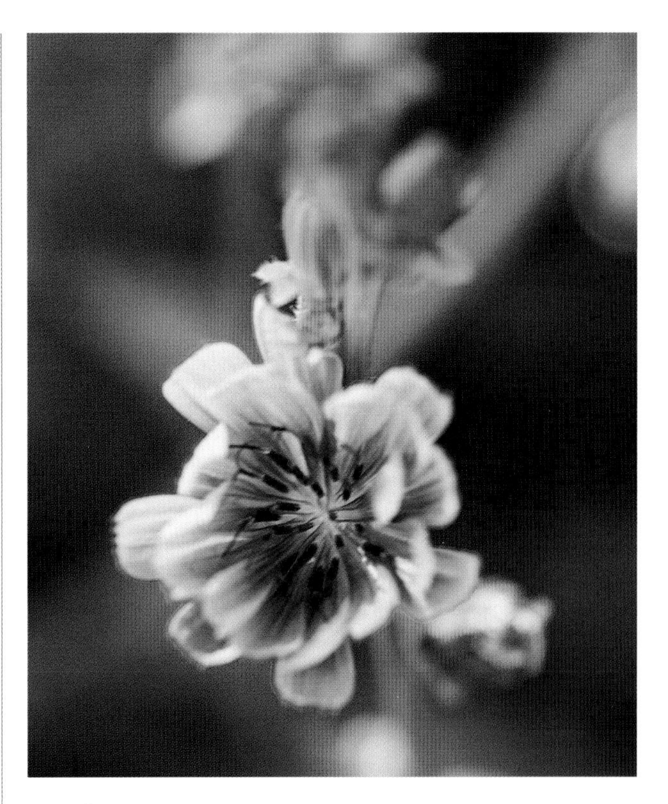

1 cup honey
2 tablespoons coriander seeds
1 bay leaf

Fill two wide-mouthed glass jars with chicory flowers and onion rings. Boil up the vinegar with the honey, coriander seeds and bay leaf. Pour this over the chicory flowers, seal and leave for 10 days.

Chicory and pear dessert

SERVES 4

The end of summer is the time to make this delicious dessert, when chicory is in full bloom and pears are ripening. You can serve it with custard or ice-cream in place of the whipped cream.

6–8 pears
1½ cups water
¾ cup soft brown sugar
3 crushed cardamom pods
1 cup chicory flowers

Peel and core the pears and cut into small pieces. Bring the water to a brisk boil, add the pears, sugar, cardamom pods and chicory flowers and simmer gently for five minutes. Remove from the stove and cool. Serve in individual glass bowls with whipped cream and decorate with fresh blue chicory flowers.

Chives

Allium schoenoprasum

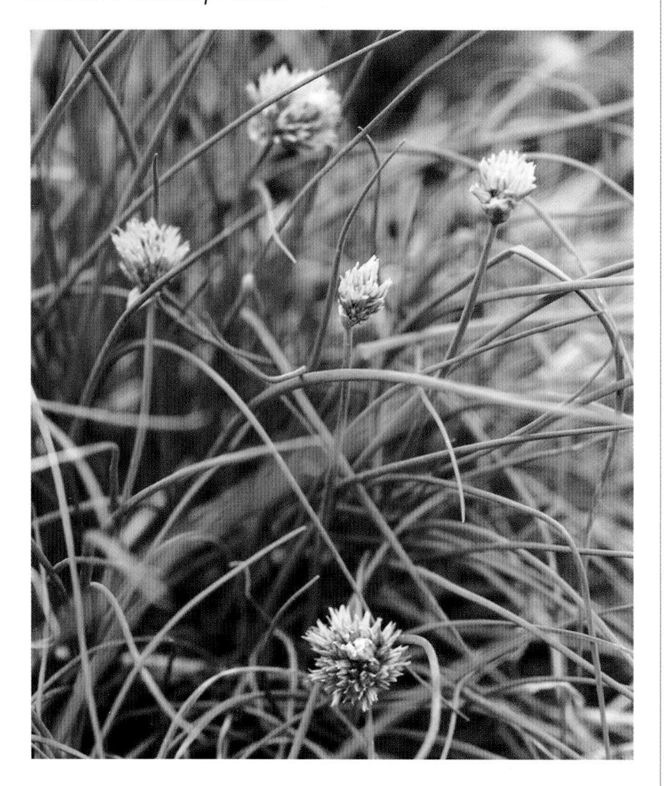

There is much speculation today about where this remarkable plant originated, but it is likely that Marco Polo found it on his travels to China, where it had probably been in use for a few thousand years. He brought it back to the West, and today it is widespread and one of the most popular culinary plants. A member of the onion family along with garlic, leeks and spring onions, chives contain sulphur, which accounts for their pungent smell and flavour.

CULTIVATION

Chives, garlic chives and wild garlic all need well-dug, richly composted soil in full sun and a deep twice-weekly watering. Chives die down in winter, at which time they can be divided into small clumps and replanted. Wild garlic and garlic chives can be divided at any time of the year. Plant chives 20 cm apart as a path edging as they only grow to about 20 cm in height. Wild garlic and garlic chives need 40–50 cm between them, and their pretty flowering heads will reach about 50 cm in height.

MEDICINAL USES

Chives have marvellous medicinal properties and from the earliest times were used in the treatment of chest ailments, bladder and kidney infections and to cleanse the blood. Modern research verifies their age-old uses: chives lower blood pressure and cholesterol, build up resistance to infection, treat respiratory disorders and assist the digestive tract and urinary system. All *Allium* species contain mild natural antibiotics, and although chives are not as potent in this regard as garlic, for example, their benefits are still quite astonishing.

Fresh chives also ease and promote digestion, and chopped and sprinkled onto food they stimulate the appetite. Chopped chive flowers with grated carrots, celery and parsley make a health-booster salad, and together with dandelion flowers and leaves, they fight flu and colds exceptionally well. A large daily helping of all these superb health-boosting, immune-building herbs will go a long way towards helping us cope with the pressures of modern living.

One of Europe's favourite cough remedies remains a mixture of fresh grated ginger root with equal quantities of chopped chive flowers and a little bit of honey. This remedy goes back to the time when ginger was traded as a magical spice.

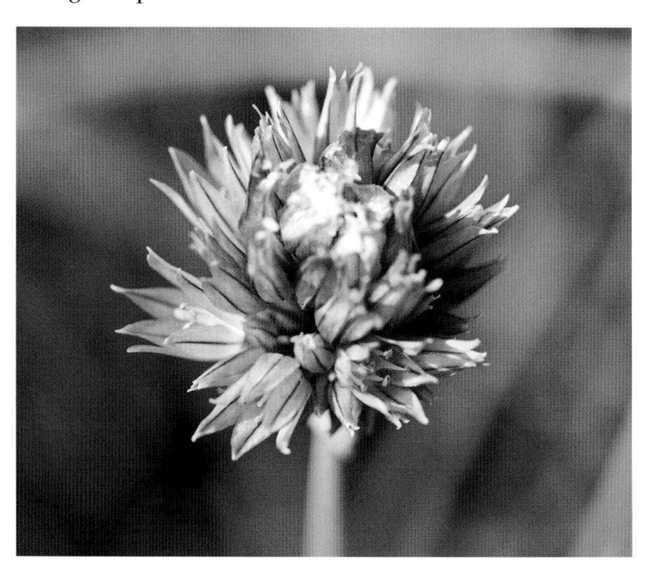

Old chive remedy for colds

Our great-grandmothers used this pungent remedy to boost resistance and fight coughs, colds and flu.

1 onion
A few chive leaves and flowers
Brown sugar

Slice the onion and chive leaves and flowers, cover them with brown sugar, and leave them to stand for 4–6 hours, well covered. Strain off the juice and take a teaspoonful at a time. To soothe a sore throat, add a little lemon juice to the mixture. Chives can also be chopped with onions and mixed with a little grated fresh ginger root, lemon juice and chopped parsley; in the old days this mixture was spread onto fingers of bread and given to children suffering from a cough or cold.

CULINARY USES

Chive blossom vinegar

This pretty pink vinegar is delicious as a salad dressing, and a dash added to stir-fries, grills, braais or stews enhances all the flavours. Make it in spring when the blossoms are abundant. You can also add peeled garlic cloves, chopped onions, coriander seeds and a bay leaf, or even a fresh cayenne pepper.

1 bottle white grape vinegar
Chive flowers, including garlic chive flowers

Fill the bottle of vinegar with chive flowers and place it in the sun for five days, shaking it daily. Strain the vinegar and discard the flowers. Pour into an attractive bottle and add fresh chive flowers for identification. (The pungent taste of the chives means that you only need to keep the vinegar in the sun for one five-day period, whereas with other herb vinegars the process is repeated for optimum flavour.)

COOK'S NOTE

Chive, garlic chive or wild garlic flowers can be used interchangeably in the recipe above. Chives have a tonic effect and improve the appetite, so use lavishly.

Creamed spinach and chive flower supper dish

SERVES 4

This is a nourishing and delicious vegetarian dish that everyone enjoys, and it helps to keep colds and flu at bay.

Large bunch chopped spinach (to make 4 cups when cooked)
2 cups chopped onion
1 cup chive flowers
2 tablespoons butter
3–4 tablespoons cornflour
500 ml milk
1 cup plain Bulgarian yoghurt
Sea salt and black pepper to taste
2 teaspoons mustard powder
1 cup grated cheddar cheese

Cook the spinach, onion and chive flowers in a little salted water for about six minutes. Strain well. In another pan, melt the butter, mix in the cornflour and add the milk and yoghurt slowly, whisking continuously. As it thickens, add the seasoning, mustard powder and cheese. Mix the white sauce into the spinach and onions, spoon into a baking dish, top with more grated cheese and brown under the grill for a few minutes. Serve hot, decorated with chive flowers, together with crusty brown bread.

Chive and garlic chive health salad

SERVES 4–6

This tasty salad will boost the immune system and is satisfying enough to have as a lunch dish served simply with brown bread and butter.

3 cups thinly sliced English cucumber
1 whole head celery, thinly chopped
2 ripe avocados, cut into squares
½ cup chopped parsley
½ cup stoned olives
2 cups watercress or land cress, lightly chopped
2 cups finely grated carrots
1 cup chive flowers
1½ cups chopped onion mixed with chopped garlic chives
1 cup mozzarella cheese, cut into small squares or coarsely grated

Dressing
½ cup lemon juice
½ cup olive oil
2 teaspoons mustard powder
½ cup honey
Cayenne pepper
Small pinch sea salt

Mix the salad ingredients together lightly in a bowl. Place all the dressing ingredients in a screw-top jar and shake well. Pour the dressing over the salad and decorate with garlic chive flowers.

COOK'S NOTE

Chive leaves can be chopped and scattered over a variety of dishes ranging from salads to soups, and the flowers can be used in salads, pasta dishes and stir-fries, adding immune-boosting benefits.

Clover

Trifolium pratense

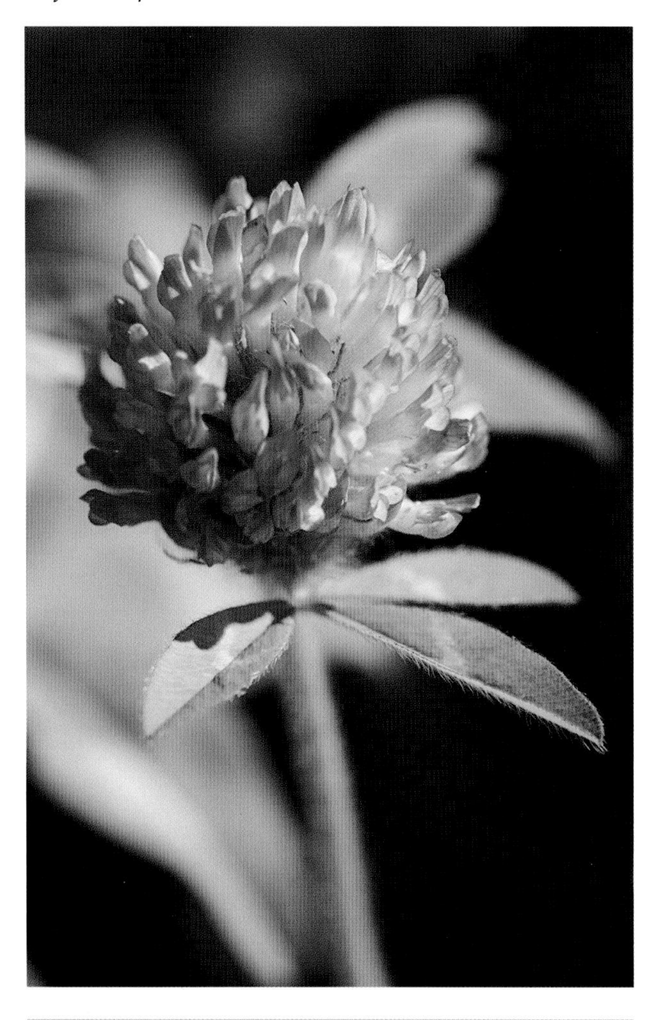

It may come as a surprise that both red and white and clover (*Trifolium pratense* and *T. repens*) are herbs with astonishing medicinal value that have been esteemed for centuries. Medieval Christians associated clover's three-lobed leaves with the Holy Trinity, and monks in Europe grew it in their physic gardens to cure all manner of ailments, from kidney stones to conjunctivitis, arthritic pains and dry coughs.

Clover is native to Europe and Asia and is used all over the world in animal fodder. It is an excellent companion plant for pasturing crops as it replenishes the soil with both nitrogen and boron (a mineral often lacking in over-cultivated soil), as well as other trace elements.

CULTIVATION

Clover is a short-lived perennial and is very easy to grow. Little tufts can be pulled off the mother plant and planted out in moist soil. All it requires is richly composted soil in full sun and a deep twice-weekly watering, and it offers an abundance of honey-scented flowers in return.

MEDICINAL USES

Around 1930, red clover flowers were used as an anticancer treatment, and some doctors are still prescribing it today for breast, ovarian and lymphatic cancers. It was once widely used in the treatment of bronchitis, whooping cough, arthritis and gout, and to soothe psoriasis and eczema, taken both internally and applied externally as a healing cream. Country children have rubbed crushed clover flowers onto bee stings and insect bites to soothe the affected area. Crushed red clover flowers and leaves can be used as a compress over inflamed joints, and together with a cup of clover tea, even severe aches will be soothed. To make the tea, pour a cup of boiling water over ¼ cup red clover flowers and leaves. Allow the tea to stand for five minutes, then strain and sip slowly. The cooled tea also makes a superb eyewash for conjunctivitis and irritated red eyes. In the case of a cough, bronchitis and whooping cough, mix a good squeeze of lemon juice, two teaspoons of honey and a pinch of ginger powder into the tea.

Clover cream

Use this cream for bites, itches, rashes, eczema and psoriasis.

1 cup clover flowers
1 cup good-quality aqueous cream

Simmer the clover flowers in the aqueous cream in a double boiler for 20 minutes, giving it an occasional stir. Strain the cream, pour it into a sterilised jar and seal. Keep it refrigerated and apply as a soothing treatment.

Clover compress for arthritic joints and gout-inflamed areas

This compress is soothing for arthritic joints and gout-inflamed areas.

Clover flowers and leaves
Hot water
Crêpe bandage

Crush the clover flowers and soak them in hot water. Drain them and bind in place over the affected joint with a crêpe bandage. Leave the compress on overnight.

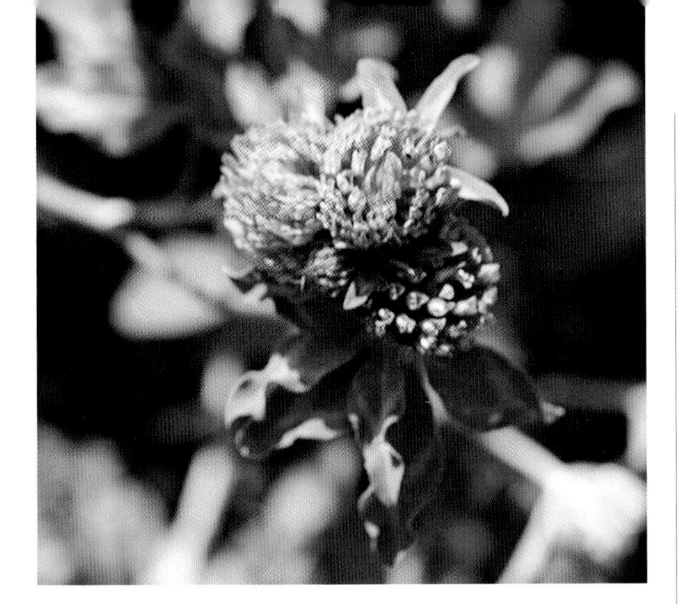

Clover douche to soothe vaginal itching

2 cups clover flowers and leaves
2 litres water
½ cup apple cider vinegar

Boil the clover flowers and leaves in the water for 15 minutes, with the lid on. Set the liquid aside to cool, then strain and add the apple cider vinegar. Use it lukewarm as a douche or use it as a wash lotion externally. Its emollient qualities will quickly soothe the irritated area.

CULINARY USES

Red clover stir-fry

SERVES 4

Olive oil
2 medium-sized onions, chopped
1 cup green pepper, chopped
2 cups sweet potato, coarsely grated
1 cup celery stems and leaves, chopped
1 cup red clover flowers
Salt and black pepper
Soy sauce
Juice of 1 lemon

Heat the oil in a large pan and fry the onions until golden. Add the green pepper and stir-fry, then the sweet potato and fry some more. Add the celery stems and leaves and the red clover flowers. Season to taste with a touch of salt, black pepper, soy sauce and lemon juice. Serve piping hot with roasted chicken and rice.

Lentil and clover risotto

SERVES 4

This vegetarian dish is quick and easy to make, and full of healthy goodness.

1 large onion, finely chopped
2 tablespoons olive oil
1 cup finely chopped green pepper
2 cups cooked lentils
1 cup cooked brown rice
1 cup mung bean sprouts
1 cup clover flowers
1 tablespoon finely chopped parsley
Juice of 1 lemon
Sea salt and black pepper to taste

Fry the onions in the oil until golden brown. Add the green pepper and stir well, then add the remaining ingredients and stir-fry. Add a little water and cook through quickly with the lid on for six minutes. Serve piping hot, decorated with clover flowers, together with a salad.

Cauliflower and clover cheese

SERVES 4

This is a nourishing supper dish, with the clover lending its delicious honey-like taste to the cheese sauce.

1 large or 2 small cauliflowers
500 ml milk
1 cup clover flowers
2 eggs, well beaten
2 tablespoons flour
Sea salt and cayenne pepper to taste
½ cup cold milk
1 cup strong cheddar cheese, grated

Break the cauliflowers into florets and boil in salted water for 20 minutes. Heat the milk with the clover flowers to boiling point, and then turn down the heat. Whisk the eggs with the flour, salt and cayenne pepper and add the half cup of cold milk. Gradually add this mixture to the hot milk and clover, and stir briskly while it thickens, being careful not to let it burn. Finally, add the cheese, keeping some aside for the top.

Drain the cauliflower well and place it in an ovenproof dish. Pour the cheese sauce over it and sprinkle the top with additional cheese. Place the dish under the grill to melt the cheese, and serve it piping hot, decorated with clover flowers.

Coriander

Coriandrum sativum

Coriander has been used as a medicinal and culinary herb for over 2 000 years. Native to Europe and the Middle East, it is mentioned in the Ebers papyrus dating back to about 1500 BC, in Sanskrit texts, and in the Bible, where it is one of the bitter Passover herbs. The Chinese recorded its use during the Han Dynasty, between 202 BC and AD 9.

All parts of the plant have a pungent aroma and may be used in cooking. The broader lower young leaves, called *dhania*, are much loved in Indian cuisine. In parts of Europe the root is eaten as a tasty vegetable, and the seed can be used in curries, chutneys, soups, sauces, vinegars and vegetable dishes. The pretty lacy mauvish-white flowers, typical of the Umbelliferae family, can be added to salads, stir-fries, fruit salads and stewed fruit. The Romans combined coriander seeds with cumin and vinegar and used it as a preservative for meat, very similar to the blend of spices we use for making biltong!

CULTIVATION

Growing coriander is simple and rewarding, since three or four crops can be achieved before the first frosts of winter. It needs full sun and a light, well-drained soil with a good dressing of compost. It requires a good twice-weekly watering and thrives in heat and dryness. Sow the seed directly into the ground where it is to grow, about 20 cm apart, keeping the soil moist and protected with a thin layer of dry leaves until the seedlings are strong enough to withstand the full sun. They grow up to 60 cm in height.

MEDICINAL USES

This strongly aromatic annual is an exceptional remedy for colic, flatulence, digestive upsets, gripes and bloating. Apart from being a superb antispasmodic, it is a wonderful remedy for anxiety attacks and tension when taken as a tea. It also cleanses the breath after eating garlic (merely chew a flower or two or a few seeds) and helps rheumatic aches and pains, both as a tea and as a lotion. To make coriander tea, pour a cup of boiling water over either ¼ cup fresh leaves and flowers or one teaspoon of dried seeds. Leave the tea to stand for five minutes before straining, and sip slowly for all the above ailments.

Ancient Chinese coriander remedy for aching joints

1 cup fresh coriander leaves, flowers and twigs
  (or 3 tablespoons seeds)
1 litre water

Boil the fresh coriander leaves, flowers and twigs in the water for 10 minutes; if there is no fresh green plant available, use three tablespoons of seeds boiled in a litre of water for 15 minutes. Strain and pour into a sterilised bottle. Soak a cloth in the lotion and bind over inflamed areas and painful, aching joints, or use as a spritz to cool the inflamed area and to remove the itch from insect bites and rashes.

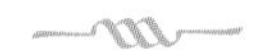

CULINARY USES

Aubergine and coriander flower lunch dish

SERVES 4

I learned this superb way of serving aubergine from an Indian chef.

4 medium-sized aubergines
2 large onions, thinly sliced
2 tablespoons olive oil
3 large tomatoes, skinned and chopped
Juice of 1 lemon
2 tablespoons freshly grated ginger root
1 tablespoon coriander flowers, without stems
1 teaspoon crushed coriander seed
1 large green pepper, thinly sliced
Sea salt and pepper to taste
2 tablespoons honey

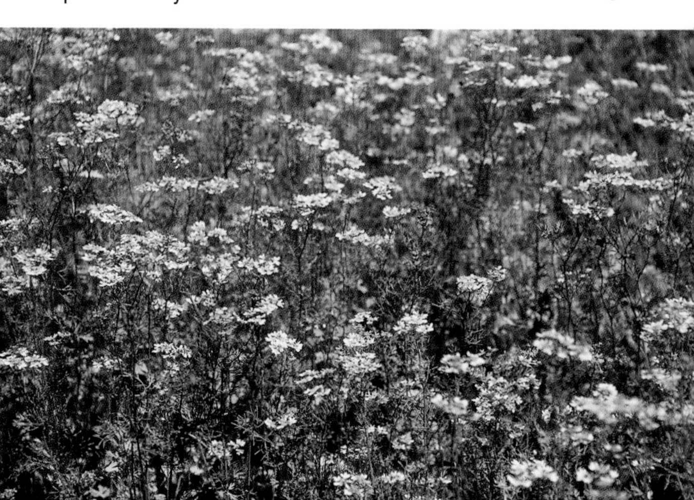

Peel and slice the aubergines, sprinkle well with salt, and cover with a heavy weight to allow them to release their bitter juices for about 20 minutes. Sauté the onions in the oil until lightly brown. Rinse the aubergines and add to the onion along with the tomatoes, stir-frying them together. Add the remaining ingredients and stir well, then cover with a well-fitting lid and turn down the heat. Simmer gently for about seven minutes. Serve with brown rice and decorate with coriander flowers.

Leek, kale and coriander flower soup

SERVES 4–6

Made at the end of autumn with the last of the coriander flowers, this warming soup is a marvellous immune system booster, keeping coughs and colds at bay.

1 large onion, finely chopped
2 tablespoons olive oil
4 thinly sliced leeks
4 cups finely chopped kale or cabbage
4 large potatoes, peeled and grated coarsely
1½ litres good chicken stock
½ cup coriander flowers, without stems
Juice of 1 lemon
Sea salt and black pepper to taste
125 ml thick cream

Lightly brown the onions in the olive oil. Add the leeks and stir-fry until they become soft and lightly browned too. Then add the kale, particularly the green outer leaves, and the potatoes. Stir-fry briefly. Add all the other ingredients and stir well. Cover and simmer for 15 minutes, stirring every now and then. Serve piping hot with a sprinkling of parsley and more coriander flowers.

Green bean and potato salad with coriander flowers

SERVES 4–6

I serve this quick-and-easy salad on summer picnics with cold chicken and everyone loves it!

4 cups young green beans
4 cups tiny new potatoes
1 medium-sized onion, finely chopped

Dressing

3 tablespoons brown grape vinegar
2 tablespoons olive oil
2 tablespoons coriander flowers, stripped off their stems

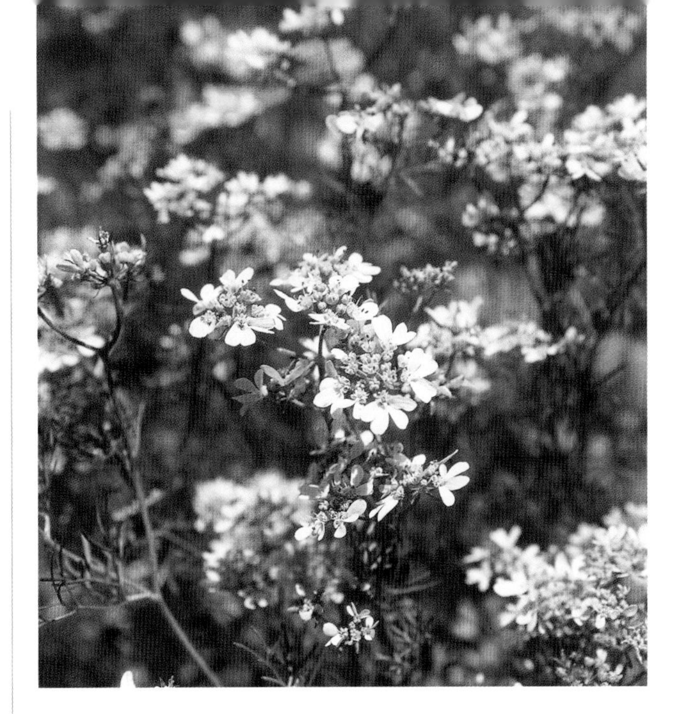

1 teaspoon crushed coriander seed
1 tablespoon chopped parsley
2 teaspoons mustard powder
½ teaspoon cayenne pepper
1 tablespoon brown sugar or honey

Cut the beans into 1 cm pieces and cook lightly. Quarter the potatoes and steam until tender. Mix both together with the finely chopped raw onion. Place all the dressing ingredients in a screw-top jar and shake until everything is well mixed and the sugar is dissolved. Add a little sea salt to taste. Pour the dressing over the vegetables and decorate with coriander flowers. Keep the salad refrigerated before serving.

OTHER USES

Fresh coriander insect repellent

The best time to make this valuable insect repellent is when the coriander is in full bloom and little green seeds are beginning to form.

Several coriander plants (including roots)
1 teaspoon tea tree oil

Wash the coriander plants well and chop into pieces. Place them in a large pot and cover with water. Simmer for 15 minutes with the lid on. Then cool and strain. Pour the potent brew into a spray bottle and add the tea tree oil. Shake well and spray to repel mosquitoes and flies, especially around the braai area.

Cornflower

Centaurea cyanus

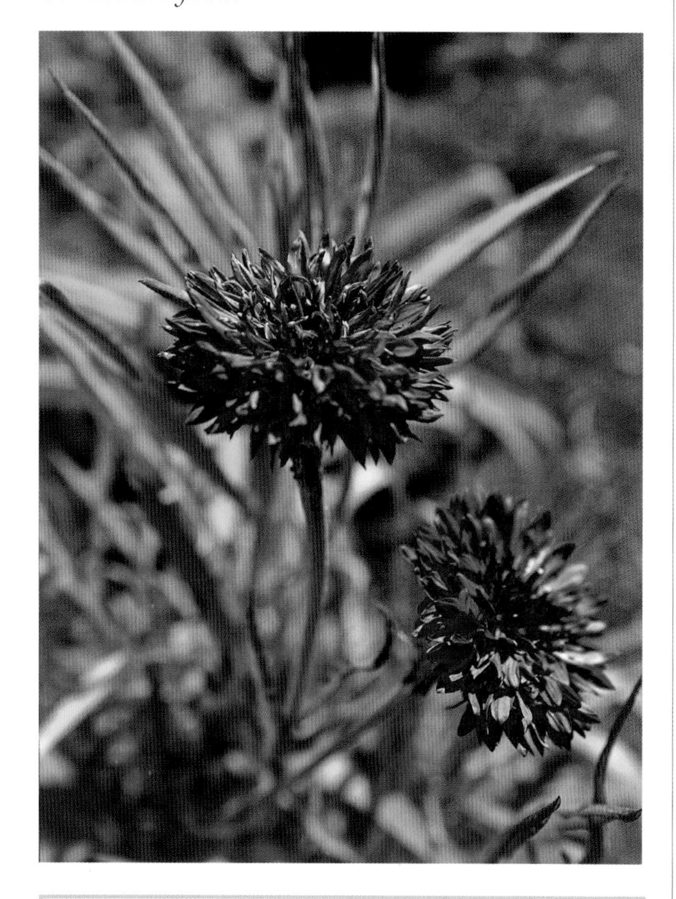

The cornflower is indigenous to Europe and now grows wild in all temperate regions, often in cornfields, which is how it got its name. The beautiful blue flowers and the leaves are both used medicinally, while use of the flowers in cooking is an ancient practice that ought to be revived. The brilliant blue petals can be added to cakes, fritters, biscuits, tarts, custards, and cheese and pasta dishes.

Monks in 12th century England, Ireland and later Wales and France made cornflower wine, which was used to treat a wide variety of ailments ranging from stomach problems, kidney and bladder ailments, tremors, vertigo and liverishness, to flu, chest ailments, coughs and excessive mucous. A cornflower infusion was used as a tonic after a severe illness, and even given to children. Modern research verifies these ancient uses as the petals and leaves have been found to contain small amounts of natural antibiotics.

CULTIVATION

I have found that cornflowers grow best as a winter annual. I sow the seed in late summer and plant the seedlings out in full sun, 50 cm apart, before winter. They grow quickly and establish themselves well in lightly composted, well-drained soil, with a good twice-weekly watering. The plants grow to about 50 cm in height. The more flowers you pick, the more are produced, right through winter and spring, until they succumb to the hot weather in midsummer.

MEDICINAL USES

In France, cornflowers are still called *casselunette*, which means 'break the spectacles', as a cornflower lotion or poultice is believed to strengthen the eyes and ease eye strain.

The flowers can also be made into a bitter tonic tea to improve resistance to infection and to ease rheumatic conditions such as aching joints and stiffness. To make the tea, pour a cup of boiling water over ¼ cup leaves and flowers; allow the tea to stand for five minutes before straining. Drink one cup a day. Cornflowers also make an excellent poultice for inflamed rheumatic joints and stiff swollen ankles.

The flowers retain their exquisite royal blue colour and are beautiful in bath preparations as they soothe and soften the skin.

Cornflower poultice for inflamed rheumatic joints

3–4 cups fresh cornflowers
5 cups hot water

Steep the cornflowers in hot water for five minutes, then spread them on a cloth and apply as hot as can be tolerated to the affected area. Repeat at least three times.

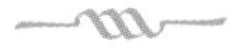

COSMETIC USES

Cornflower eye lotion

1 cup boiling water
1 tablespoon fresh blue petals

Pour the boiling water over the petals. Allow the lotion to stand for eight minutes before straining, and use as an eyebath to revive tired eyes.

CULINARY USES

Cornflower pasta salad

SERVES 4

Delicious hot or cold, this is an easy and popular lunch dish, and it brightens up any meal.

2 cups farfalle (pasta bows)
4 medium-sized ripe tomatoes, thinly sliced
2 ripe avocados, sliced
8–10 slices mozzarella cheese
½ cup cornflower petals, pulled out of their calyxes
½ cup chopped parsley
¾ cup chopped basil

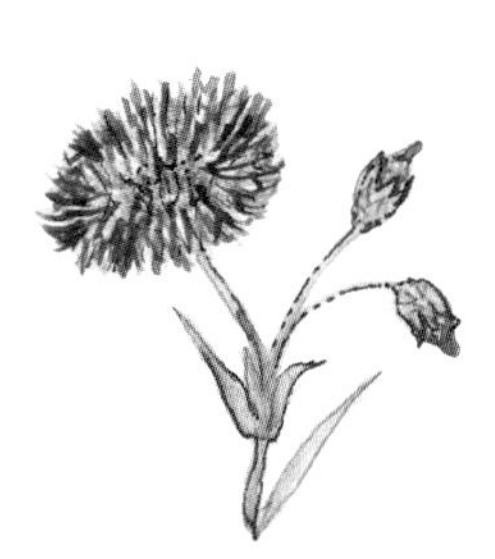

Dressing

3 tablespoons olive oil
3 tablespoons balsamic vinegar
2 teaspoons wholegrain mustard
2 tablespoons honey
½ cup sunflower seeds
½ cup sesame seeds

Cook the pasta in salted water until *al dente*, then drain, rinse and cool. Place the pasta in the centre of a flat dish and arrange the tomato, avocado and mozzarella slices all around it. Keep the cornflower petals, parsley and basil aside for the top.

To make the dressing, blend the olive oil, vinegar, mustard and honey in a blender. Add the sunflower and sesame seeds and whirl for another two minutes. Pour the dressing over the pasta, and sprinkle the dish with the cornflowers, parsley and basil. To serve the dish hot, add a little grated mozzarella cheese and pop it under the grill until it sizzles before sprinkling with the cornflowers, basil and parsley.

Butterscotch and cornflower sauce

SERVES 4–6

Served over rice puddings, plain yoghurt, ice-cream or custard, this sauce is so easy to prepare – and it turns an ordinary dessert into party fare! Try it over baked apples or bread-and-butter pudding, or as a topping on a plain vanilla cake.

250 ml cream
½ cup honey
250 ml golden syrup
4 tablespoons butter
One stick cinnamon
½ cup cornflower petals

Pour the cream into the top of a double boiler and warm. Add the honey and syrup, then the butter, cinnamon and cornflower petals pulled out of their calyxes. Simmer gently on low heat, stirring every now and then, for 45 minutes. Once the sauce starts to thicken, stir well and serve hot over any dessert.

Strawberry and banana dessert with cornflowers

SERVES 4

This has to be one of the quickest desserts I know and it is much loved by children. I make it in spring when strawberries and cornflowers are at their best.

4 cups strawberries, hulled and sliced
4 bananas, thinly sliced
Juice of 1 orange, mixed with a little honey
Whipped cream
Desiccated coconut
½ cup cornflower petals

Sprinkle the strawberries with sugar, and place layers of bananas and strawberries in individual glass dishes, ending with strawberries on the top. Pour the orange juice and honey over them. Top with a dollop of whipped cream and sprinkle with coconut. If you are lucky enough to find a fresh coconut, drain off the milk by piercing the three soft holes, saw it in half, and then grate the precious flesh and use it instead of desiccated coconut. It is superb! Finally, decorate with the beautiful blue cornflowers.

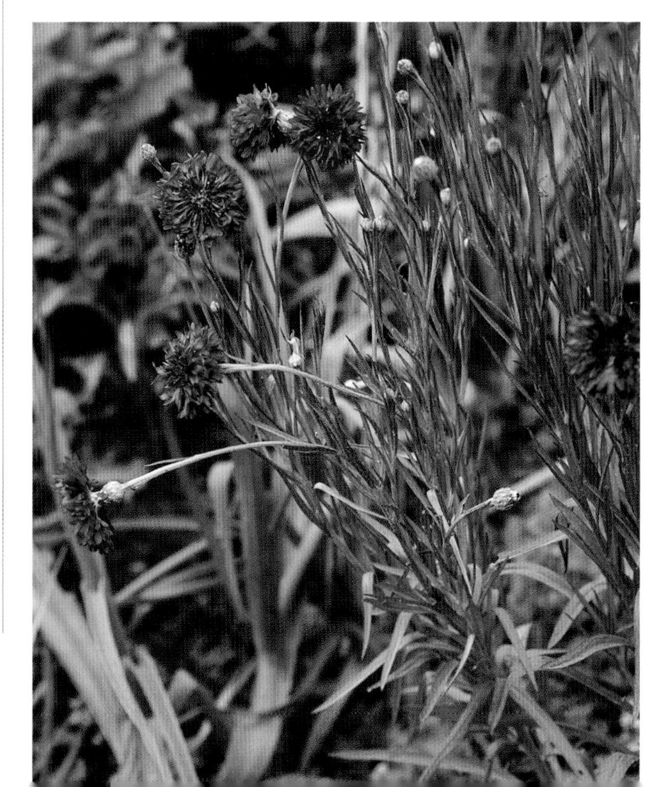

Crab apple blossom

Malus floribunda • *M. pumila*

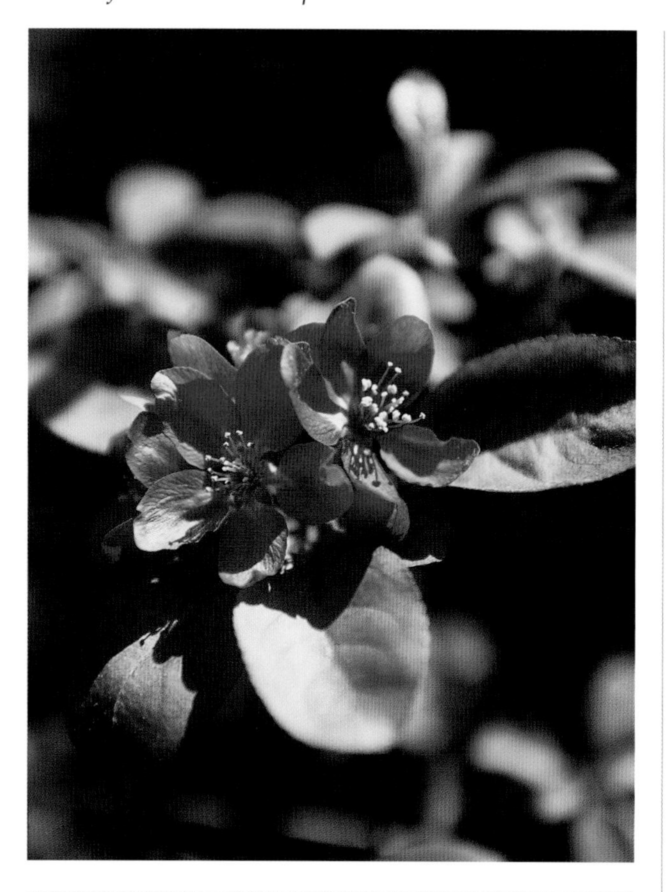

Crab apples grow wild in the hedgerows of Britain and Europe and have been used in both medicine and cooking since ancient times. Cider recipes using crab apples date back many hundreds of years, and although the sour fruit are pretty inedible, they make delicious jellies.

Some crab apple species are grown as garden ornamentals, their lovely white, pink and cerise flowers heralding spring and drawing bees and butterflies. The fruit of these ornamentals vary in colour from dark russet to crimson, orange and golden yellow. I have seen a row of large urns planted with crab apples pruned into lollipops down a suburban driveway, and marvel at their attractiveness in every season: their show of blossoms in spring, their neat greenness in summer, their flush of bright fruit and glorious coloured leaves in autumn, and their bare sculptured shapes underplanted with a blaze of violas in winter.

CULTIVATION

Planted as a hedge or as a specimen shrub or small tree, crab apples do well in richly composted soil in full sun, and can be espaliered against a wall or clipped into a charming topiary. They do exceptionally well in colder areas, but also adapt to seaside gardens and even gardens that are more tropical. Because they are so slow growing, they make perfect container subjects and it seems a pity that they are not used more in landscaping as they need so little attention. Prune in late winter.

MEDICINAL USES

In ancient herbals the crab apple was revered as a medicine for boils, abscesses, splinters and wounds, and for coughs and colds and a host of other conditions ranging from acne to kidney ailments. Many dishes made with apples and apple blossom are of medieval origin, and crab apples, roasted, drenched in honey and dried, were used by monks and physicians as a treatment for diarrhoea, dysentery and gallstones. In the spring they gathered the blossoms and preserved them in vinegar for drawing poultices and for bee stings and other insect bites.

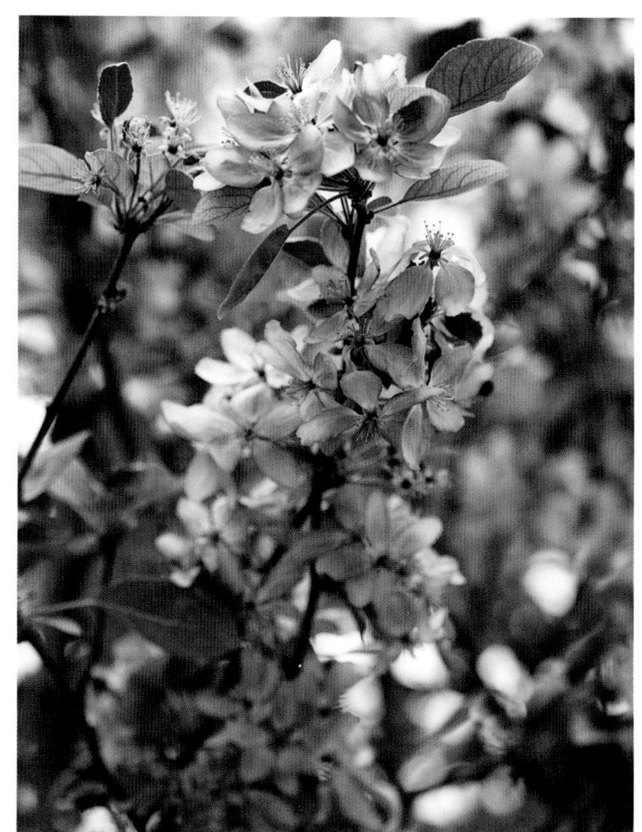

Crab apple blossom vinegar for bee stings and mosquito bites

Crab apple blossoms
1 bottle white grape vinegar

Press as many blossoms as possible into the bottle of white grape vinegar. Keep in a dark place for seven days. Strain and repeat with more fresh blossoms and buds. Strain after another seven days and keep near at hand for summer insect bites. In the case of a wasp, hornet or bee sting, soak a pad of cotton wool immediately in crab apple vinegar and hold it over the sting for 10 minutes. Keep dabbing with vinegar for another 30 minutes and you will find that it hardly swells at all. Use the same vinegar to relieve mosquito bite itches.

CULINARY USES

Crab apple verjuice

Make this in autumn and store it sealed, until spring, when crab apple blossoms are at their most glorious. That is the secret ingredient!

2 cups ripe crab apples
1 cup apple cider vinegar
1 cup soft brown sugar
½ cup grated ginger root
2 cinnamon sticks
10 cloves
1 bottle good brandy
1 cup runny honey

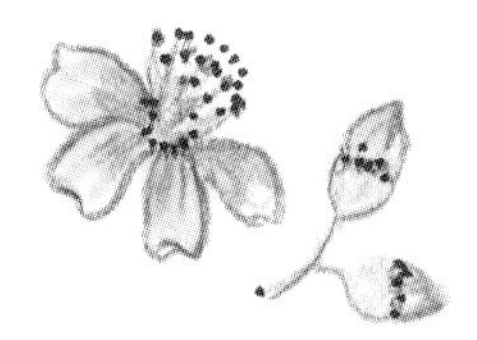

Clean and slice the crab apples, cover well and soak overnight in the apple cider vinegar, with a weight on top. The next morning sprinkle the sugar over them and leave to stand for two hours. Meanwhile add the ginger root, cinnamon and cloves to the brandy and leave to stand.

After the sugar has dissolved and mingled well with the crab apples, add the honey and stir in well. Now add the brandy and spices and pour into a wide-mouthed jar with a tight-fitting lid. Shake it up well and store in a dark cupboard all winter, giving it a daily shake and inspection. In spring, add one cup of crab apple blossoms and seal again, giving it a gentle daily shake for 14 days. Finally, strain and bottle the verjuice in a good decanter.

Serve well diluted with chilled apple juice as it is potent! Put five raisins soaked overnight in brandy into each glass. Taken as a liqueur at the end of a meal, this is a remarkable digestive, and a very little goes a long way!

Crab apple blossom sponge fingers

MAKES ABOUT 20 BISCUITS

This is an ancient spring recipe from Scotland. When the crab apples are not in bloom I use peach blossom, wisteria or even borage flowers, depending on what is flowering. They are easy biscuits to make, and keep well. I serve them with creamy desserts and ice creams, as well as for a teatime treat.

50 g castor sugar
2 eggs
1 teaspoon vanilla essence
1 teaspoon grated lemon rind
½ cup crab apple petals,
  stripped off their calyxes
50 g cake flour

Preheat the oven to 180°C. Whisk the sugar, eggs and vanilla essence until light and creamy. Mix the lemon rind and petals into the flour, then gently fold into the egg and sugar mixture with a metal spoon. Place elongated finger shapes onto a well-greased and floured baking tray, one tablespoonful at a time and spaced 3–4 cm apart. Sprinkle with a little castor sugar and bake for about seven minutes or until just browning at the edges. Remove the biscuits carefully with a spatula while still hot, and allow them to cool and firm on a wire rack. Store them in an airtight tin.

Lemon and crab apple blossom jelly

MAKES 3 JARS

This delicious jelly is a delicate version of marmalade. Serve it on toast, as a topping on steamed pudding, or as a cake filling. It is so pretty that it makes a charming gift.

1 kg fresh lemons
3 litres water
1 kg white sugar
3–4 cups loosely packed crab apple blossoms

Scrub the lemons and peel them. Shred the peel finely and simmer with half the water for 1½–2 hours. Keep the mixture covered and simmer gently. Roughly chop the lemon pulp and simmer it in another pan with the rest of the water for 1½ hours. Strain this pulp through a fine sieve and add the juice to the lemon peel mixture. Boil briskly for 10 minutes, then lower the heat and add the sugar. Stir well and simmer gently until it sets (usually about an hour). Pour a little into a saucer and let it stand. If it sets it is ready. Finally, add the crab apple blossoms and mix well. Pour into hot sterilised jars, seal while hot, and label.

Dahlia

Dahlia juarezii ● *D. rosea*

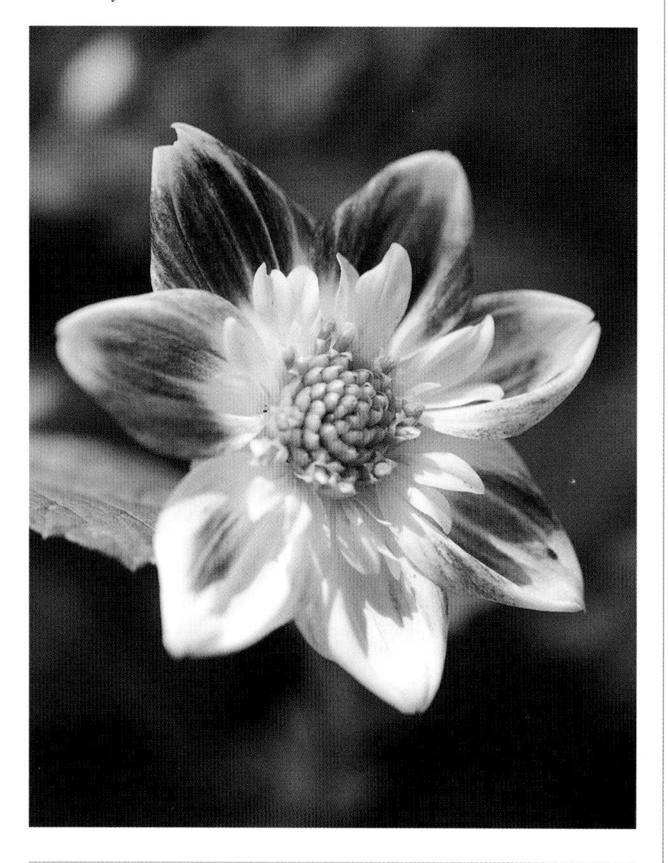

With its glorious range of colours the dahlia is spectacular in the summer border, but it is only relatively recently that it has become a garden ornamental rather than a food crop. The Mexicans used the dahlia as a food and medicine for several centuries before it was introduced to Europe in 1789 by the superintendent of the Mexico City Botanic Gardens, who sent the first seeds to botanist Cavanilles of Madrid. He named the plant *Dahlia pinnata*, in honour of botanist Dr Andreas Dahl, a pupil of the famous Swedish botanist Carolus Linnaeus.

The tubers, rather than the flowers, were eaten and are still eaten today by the Tunebo Indians in British Columbia. However, the rather pungent taste of the dahlia was not popular with the Europeans and dahlias all but disappeared there until Napoleon's wife, the Empress Josephine, became the first person in France to grow them in her world-famous gardens at Malmaison.

CULTIVATION

Dahlias come in a dazzling array of colours and make for a spectacular display in summer. Most of the single and pompon dahlias originate from *D. rosea*, while the cactus varieties originate from *D. juarezii*. They can be planted from August to November. Tubers set into richly composted soil in full sun give a display that lasts all summer long. They need little attention, other than to be cut back once they dry off in autumn, dug up and the tubers stored in early winter. They thrive with a long, slow watering twice weekly during summer.

MEDICINAL USES

Dahlia petals and the thinly sliced tubers were used by the Aztecs and later the Mexicans as an excellent skin treatment. Crushed, warmed and placed over rashes, grazes and infected scratches, the petals formed a soothing poultice that was also used over insect stings and inflamed rough areas of skin. The petals were used to make an excellent foot soak to soothe tired feet, and the same remedy was used to wash sunburned skin and rashes.

The exquisite and spectacular tree dahlia, *D. imperialis*, has 3-m-high cascades of lilac-coloured single flowers that never fail to draw the eye in their autumn glory; these flowers have been used through the centuries as a poultice. Crushed petals placed over an itchy sore spot on the skin give quick relief, and to help clear a pimple place a piece of crushed moistened petal over the spot. It will soothe and quickly bring it to a head.

Dahlia petal poultice

The exquisite tree dahlia's petals fall on the ground as the flowers mature. Gather the petals whenever you see them.

Dahlia petals
Coarse sea salt

Gently mix the petals into the sea salt, then store the mixture in a well-sealed jar or crock. To soothe aching feet or a sore back, take the salt and petal mixture, roll it into a towel that has been wrung out in hot water – about two cups – and place the poultice over the affected area. Cover and keep it warm.

Dahlia foot soak

4 cups dahlia petals
2 cups sliced dahlia tubers
4 litres water

Boil the petals and tubers in the water for 10 minutes. Leave the mixture to stand for 10 minutes, then strain and use as a wash, soaking the feet in it for a few minutes, or use the water to wash sunburned skin and rashes.

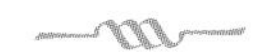

CULINARY USES

Cream cheese and dahlia dip

This Mexican spread is delicious on toast and also makes a party dip served with crudités, Melba toast or French fries. The Mexicans use chilli salsa instead of Worcestershire sauce.

250 g carton smooth cream cheese
1 cup finely grated mozzarella cheese
1 teaspoon mustard powder
1 tablespoon Worcestershire sauce or chilli salsa
2 tablespoons honey
1 teaspoon finely ground coriander seed
A little milk
½–¾ cup dahlia petals

Mix the ingredients together, adding a little milk if it is too stiff. Spoon the dip into a bowl and top with dahlia petals.

Mexican mealie and chilli dish with dahlia flowers

SERVES 4–6

Exotically different, this bright, spicy and delicious country dish varies from village to village in Mexico. Serve it in green mealie husks for a braai or a picnic.

6 mealies
1 cup onion, finely chopped
½ cup olive oil
½–1 hot fresh chilli, finely chopped
2 green peppers, finely chopped
2 cups chopped spring onions
Sea salt and black pepper to taste
Juice of 1 lemon
¾ cup mixed dahlia petals

Boil the mealies until tender, then cool them slightly and cut the kernels off the cobs. Brown the onion in the olive oil, add the chilli and green pepper, then stir in the mealie kernels and spring onions. Add the sea salt, black pepper and lemon juice. Lastly, add the dahlia petals. Serve hot in a wooden bowl and decorate with dahlia petals.

COOK'S NOTE

All the dahlia varieties are edible, although the tubers are not very palatable. While the petals are not very tasty either, they can be used as an attractive decoration, for example on rice and mealie dishes in the Mexican style.

Sundried tomato and dahlia bread

SERVES 4–6

This delicious Mexican-type bread is so quick and easy that you can make it often.

375 g white bread flour
1 teaspoon salt
3 teaspoons instant dried yeast
50 g sundried tomatoes, drained from their oil and chopped
¾ cup multi-coloured dahlia petals
5 tablespoons lukewarm olive oil
¾ cup lukewarm water

Heat the oven to 220°C. Sift the flour and salt into a large bowl. Stir in the dried yeast, sundried tomatoes and dahlia petals. Warm the olive oil in a double boiler. Make a well in the centre of the flour and pour in the warm water and oil, mixing them together well to form a soft dough. Turn the dough out onto a floured board and knead it gently for about seven minutes, turning it over and over. Grease a baking sheet and press the dough fairly flat in an oval loaf shape. Brush with olive oil and bake for about 30 minutes. It should sound hollow when you tap it and be light golden brown on top. Serve hot with butter.

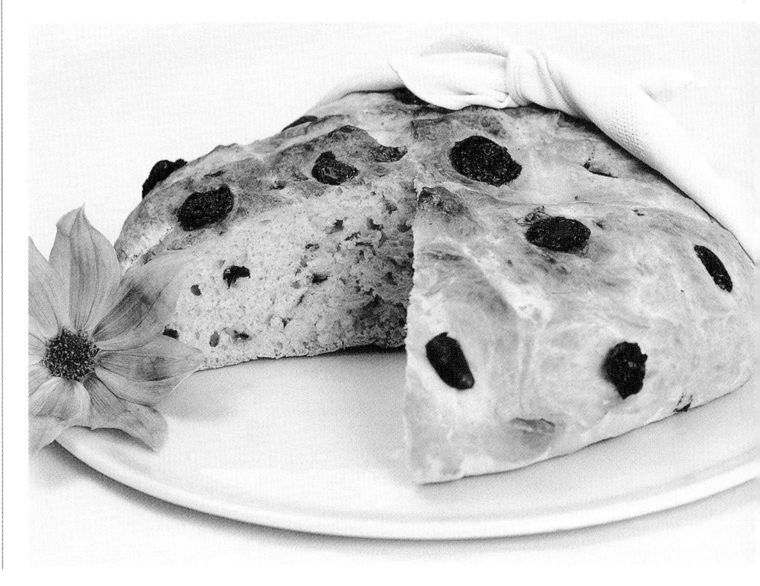

Daisy

Bellis perennis ● **Lawn daisy**

The common daisy is found in lawns and meadows all over Britain, Europe and the Mediterranean area, and has a long and colourful history as a folk remedy and medicine. Its Latin name *Bellis* comes from *bellus* meaning 'pretty', while *perennis* means 'perennial'.

Easily grown in temperate and subtropical parts of the world, it is considered one of the worst 'lawn weeds' in England. However it has long been used to treat all sorts of ailments, and it is listed in herbal writings, pharmacopoeias and ancient medicinal texts. I once read a charming description of the 'daisie' in a London museum: 'Great virtues for Daisies, which do mitigate all kinds of pains, but especially the paines of the joints, and gout, if they be stamped with new butter unsalted, and spread upon the pained place.'

I have a fond memory of learning to make a daisy chain on my first visit to England. Two elderly ladies in Sandringham's beautiful gardens in Norfolk showed me how to prick a small hole under the base of the calyx of one daisy, and push through the stem of another daisy, linking it to the next and the next, making a chain. One of the women removed the hat pin from her wide-brimmed hat to make the holes, and I completed the chain under their watchful eyes. I pressed that sweet daisy chain and have it to this day! Daisy chains originally marked the winner of a race or an event, or the doer of a good deed, and were placed upon the person's head 'in recognition of accomplishment'!

CULTIVATION

The common daisy is one of the easiest plants to grow. This pretty little low-growing perennial needs full sun and a well-dug bed with lots of compost to ensure a long flowering period. Under the heat of the African sun it is best treated as a winter annual. The hybrid daisy is readily available in nurseries during winter and spring and has the same uses as its dainty white cousin.

Plant it as a path edging or as a border plant to enjoy the thumbnail-sized daisies, as it only reaches 10–12 cm in height. Water two or three times weekly in the winter months and it will go on well into spring. Pick and dry the flowers often as the more you pick the more they produce! Plant 20 cm apart.

Today the daisy is thought to be a troublesome invader in some areas, but its ability to survive indicates its valuable medicinal constituents. Save the seed yearly and re-sow in autumn for cool-weather flowering.

Grow the daisy in-between vegetable rows such as between peas and cabbage, between lettuce and spinach, and between radishes and kohlrabi. It invigorates its companions, keeps them producing succulent leaves, and keeps slugs, snails and caterpillars away. Planted a bit closer than usual, 12–15 cm apart, they form a perfect thick barrier to deter snails.

MEDICINAL USES

Crushed daisy flowers were once used on the battlefields where they grew to staunch bleeding wounds, and as the daisy has antiseptic properties, fresh crushed flowers were associated with warfare. Salves and ointments were made by heating the fresh flowers and buds in hot lard and oil; the salve was set in small containers, making it easy to carry.

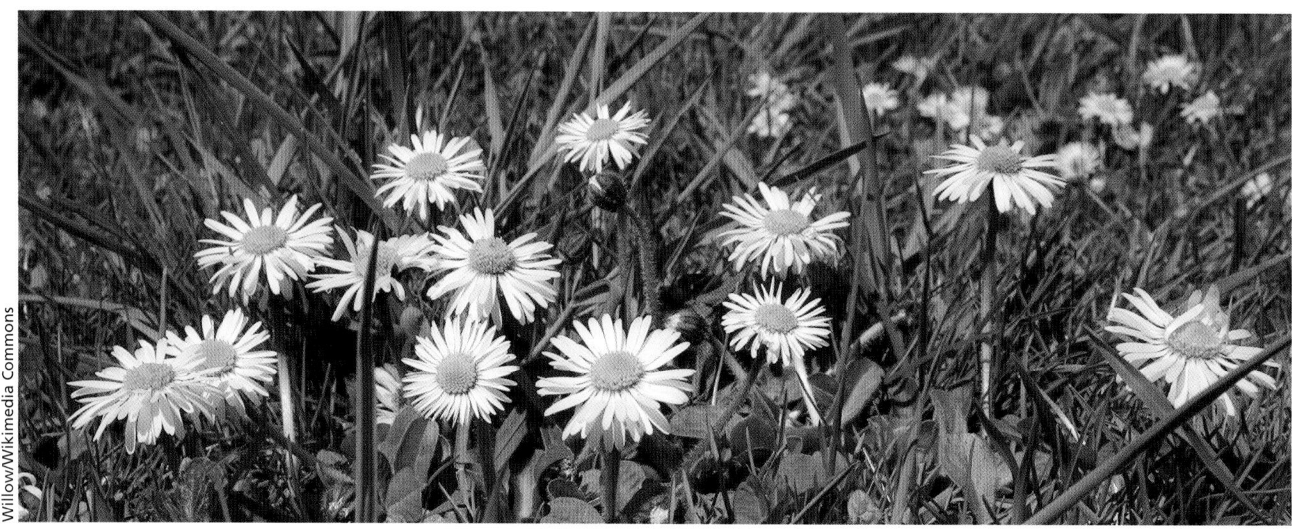

Willow/Wikimedia Commons

Saponins, essential oil, flavones, tannins and mucilage are present in varying quantities, mostly in the flowers, although the leaves contain smaller amounts. The more ornamental varieties of *Bellis perennis* daisies still contain those components.

Daisy tea can be taken to help relieve gastritis, diarrhoea, enteritis, sore throats, coughs, colds, sneezing and mucous production. Astringent and expectorant, this tea is safe for children and the elderly. To make *B. perennis* tea, pour a cup of boiling water over ¼ cup fresh flowers and one leaf. Leave the tea to stand for five minutes, stir frequently, sweeten with a touch of honey, and sip slowly for all the above ailments. A strong brew of the flowers was used in the bath to treat skin disorders, bruises, wounds and grazes.

Daisy ointment was loved by country folk and used to treat varicose veins, haemorrhoids, minor wounds, gouty joints and sore red watery eyes (rub the salve gently on the eyelids, **not** anywhere near the inside of the eye). Today *B. perennis* is a valued homeopathic remedy for deep internal bruising.

Daisy wash

Use this wash for wounds, grazes, acne and rashes.

2 cups fresh daisy leaves and flowers
1 litre water

Simmer the leaves and flowers in the water for 20 minutes, with the lid on. Allow the liquid to cool, then strain. Use as a wash or a spritz spray over the area, or as a poultice for sprained muscles, with a cloth wrung out in the warm brew.

Daisy ointment

This ointment is good for varicose veins, haemorrhoids and gouty joints. Pick the leaves and flowers in late winter and spring, when they are most prolific.

2 cups fresh daisy flowers, buds and leaves
1 cup good aqueous cream
½ cup almond oil
10 cloves
½ cup comfrey leaves, chopped

Simmer the ingredients together in a double boiler, stirring and pressing continuously for 30 minutes. Press the comfrey particularly well. Cool the mixture for 10 minutes, strain. Spoon it into sterilised glass jars, label, and store in the fridge in summer.

CULINARY USES

Daisy honey

MAKES 1 JAR

30 daisy flowers
1 jar runny honey

Submerge the flowers in the bottle of honey to infuse their delicious flavour of newly mown hay. Leave the flowers in the honey until it is finished, when you can eat the daisies. Stir a spoonful of the honey into a cup of herb tea to ease aches and pains. For a snack with the tea, put a daisy or two on a cheese sandwich – this was considered to be a good treatment for backache!

Daisy vinegar

MAKES 1 BOTTLE

Daisy vinegar was once also called daegus eage, an Anglo-Saxon word meaning the 'day's eye' (a reference to the daisy's centre with white petal 'rays' around it). The vinegar was used to flavour salads, and as a bath tonic.

50 fresh daisy flowers
1 bottle white grape vinegar

Submerge the daisies in the vinegar. Stand the bottle in the sun for 10 days, giving it a daily shake. Strain out the daisies and replace with fresh ones. Use the vinegar as a salad dressing to release stiffness and gout, or use a splash of it in the bath to ease aches and pains.

Pickled daisy buds

MAKES 1 OR 2 JARS

I once bought a small jar of pickled B. perennis *buds at a market in Spain. They were as delicious as capers, especially when served with a salad of fresh daisy leaves and flowers!*

2 cups white vinegar
1 cup honey
2 teaspoons coriander seeds
2 teaspoons mustard seeds
2 cups fresh *B. perennis* buds

Simmer the vinegar, honey and seeds together for 20 minutes, with the lid on. Pack the daisy buds into jars and pour the hot mixture over them. Seal the jars, and leave for four weeks before serving the buds with bread and cheese. Taste the Mediterranean!

Dandelion

Taraxacum officinale

This common weed with its astonishing array of health benefits is proof indeed that a weed is a plant out of place! It originated in Europe but is now widespread all over the world, its name deriving from the French *dents de lion*, meaning 'teeth of the lion', a reference to its jagged leaves. It is astonishing to think that a plant with such remarkable medicinal properties, and that was actually an official medicine in the 16th century, could have become largely forgotten, but happily it is once again the subject of a resurgence of interest and research.

Dandelion is primarily a detoxifier and a diuretic, and Arab physicians back in the 11th century recommended it as a treatment for liver and kidney ailments. In the 13th century, physicians from Myddfai in Wales named dandelion a cure-all cleanser. Those ancient physicians were amazingly accurate, as modern research has shown dandelion to be one of the most important and effective of all herbs for detoxifying the body.

CULTIVATION

I brought dandelion seeds from England 30 years ago and as it is such an undemanding and robust perennial and self-seeds, I am never without it. It is unfussy as to soil type, thrives in any sunny position, transplants easily and the rewards from the bright yellow flowers and jagged-toothed leaves are enormous.

MEDICINAL USES

Dandelion is one of the best bile stimulants known; it helps to break down gallstones, soothes chronic rheumatism, clears gout, eases painful and stiff joints, and also aids fever, constipation, insomnia, and surprisingly, hypochondria. It helps to detoxify the body after a hangover, after over-indulging or eating junk foods, and helps clear up acne and boils.

To take dandelion medicinally, eat three fresh leaves daily in a salad. The younger the leaf, the less bitter it is. Add a sprinkling of flower petals from two flowers for the beta-carotene content as well as the vitamins, minerals and amino acids the petals contain.

Dandelion flowers and young leaves in spring are considered to be a tonic, flushing toxins from the body. Spring tonic wines were made across Europe and can still be found in rural areas today.

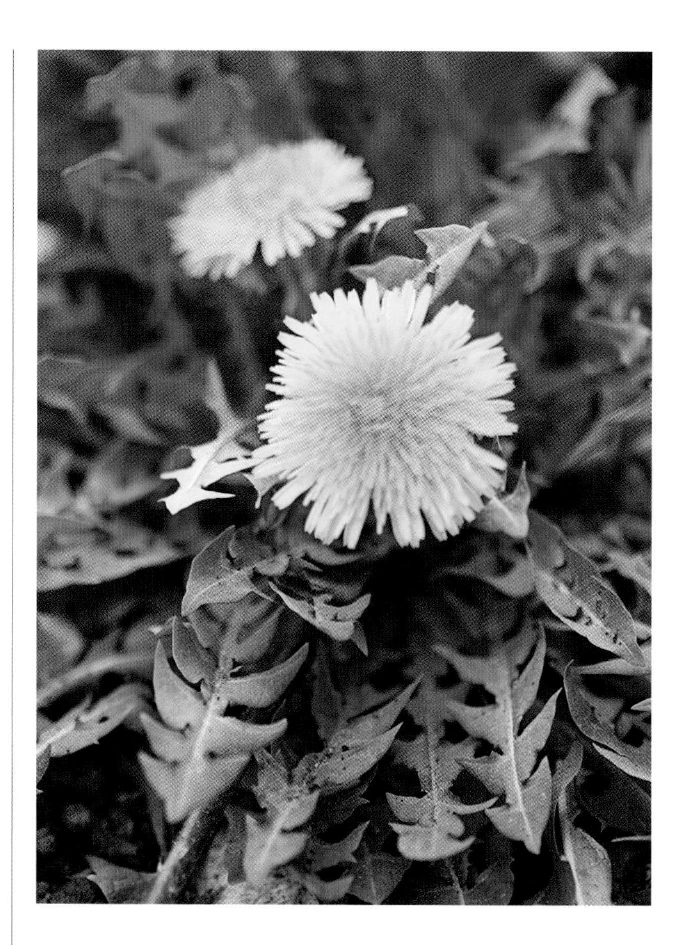

The milky latex in the stems and at the flower base is an excellent treatment for removing warts, corns and verrucas. Apply the juice frequently, at least twice a day. Repeat every day until the wart, corn or verruca subsides.

Dandelion tonic wine

This is a simple version of the traditional diuretic and digestive dandelion tonics.

2 cups dandelion flowers
2 litres water
1 cup honey
10 cloves
2 star anise
Juice of 4 lemons
1 litre good wine (optional)

Boil the flowers in the water with the honey, cloves, star anise and lemon juice. Simmer gently for 15 minutes with the lid on. Cool, strain and add the wine if desired. Refrigerate, and take a wine glass daily.

CULINARY USES

Dandelion and bacon salad

SERVES 4

This is the best known of all dandelion dishes.

4 cups fresh young dandelion leaves
2 cups dandelion flowers, calyxes removed
250 g streaky bacon
4 tablespoons olive oil
5 slices bread, cubed
Sea salt and black pepper
2 tablespoons balsamic vinegar

Tear up the dandelion leaves and mix with the flowers. Chop up the bacon and fry until crisp. Drain the bacon, and add the olive oil to the bacon fat in the pan. Fry the bread cubes in the fat and oil until golden, then remove them from the pan and drain. Mix the croutons and bacon with the dandelion leaves and flowers in a glass bowl. Sprinkle the balsamic vinegar over the salad just before serving and decorate with dandelion flowers.

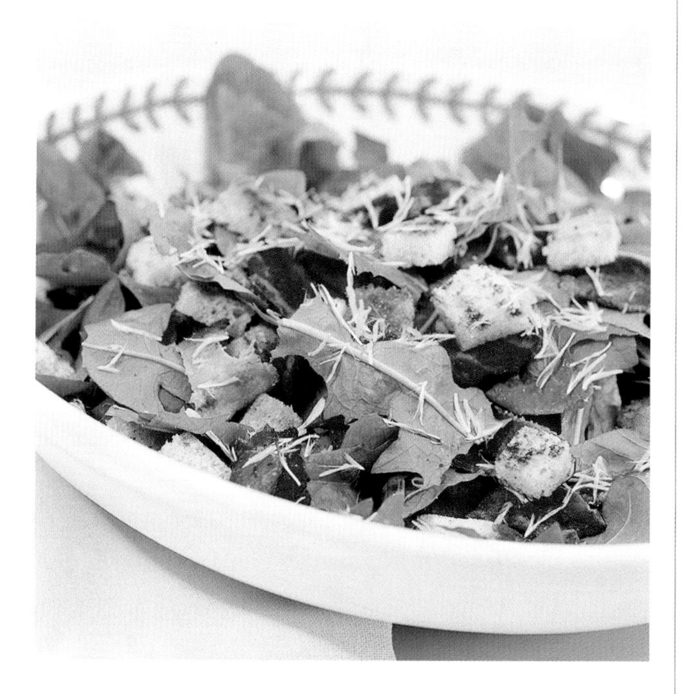

COOK'S NOTE

The dandelion's long tap root can be dried, roasted and ground to make a pleasant, healthy version of coffee, while young dandelion leaves and flowers are superb in salads and can be added to soups, stews and sauces.

Dandelion flower omelette

SERVES 1

6 dandelion flower buds
Butter
2 eggs
3 cups water
Sunflower oil
3 cups parsley
¾ cup grated cheddar cheese
Sea salt and pepper

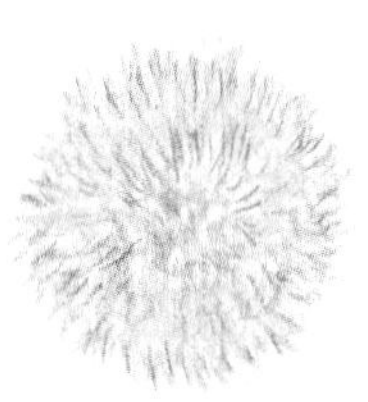

Pick flowers that are just about to open. Sauté them quickly in a little butter and set aside. Whisk the eggs with the water. Heat a little sunflower oil in a pan and pour in the egg and water mixture. Mix the sautéed dandelion flower buds with the parsley and cheese, and as the omelette sets, sprinkle this on one half of it. Add sea salt and pepper, flip the other side over to cover the cheese and flowers, and let the omelette settle for one minute. Slide it onto a hot plate and serve immediately with hot buttered toast.

Dandelion and beetroot salad

SERVES 4

This salad is both delicious and healthy. It can be served either hot or cold, and is always well received. Serve it with chicken or fish.

2 cups dandelion leaves, roughly torn
2 cups dandelion flowers
1 cup chopped celery
6 cooked beetroots,
 peeled and thinly sliced

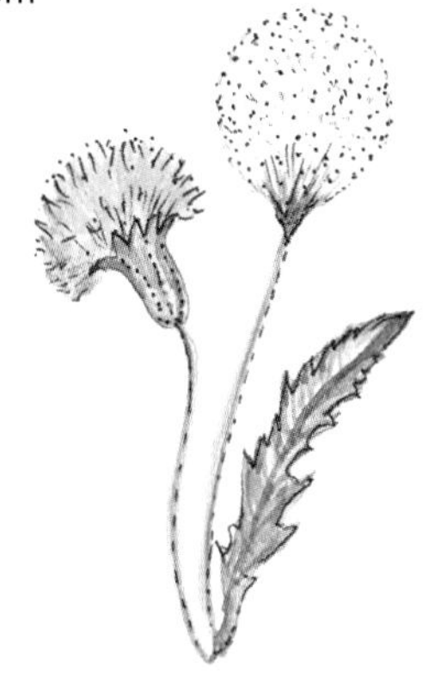

Dressing
1 cup brown grape vinegar
1 cup brown sugar
2 teaspoons mustard powder
1 teaspoon powdered coriander
½ teaspoon powdered cloves
Dandelion flowers
Chopped parsley

Mix the dandelion leaves and flowers with the celery and beetroot slices. Heat the vinegar, sugar and mustard and stir until the sugar dissolves. Add the coriander and cloves. Pour the hot dressing over the salad and serve hot sprinkled with dandelion flowers and parsley, or let it cool and serve it cold.

Day lily

Hemerocallis species

The Chinese first cultivated the day lily as a food and medicine thousands of years ago. By the 12th century it had been introduced to the New World, where it became established in the gardens of the rich. Much reverence and mystery were associated with the flower owing to its short lifespan – each exquisite flower blooms for only a day. The three petals were thought to symbolise the Trinity, and the three sepals were thought to represent yesterday, today and tomorrow, symbolising the transience and brevity of life. The flowers will last without water for a day and have been used over the centuries in religious ceremonies and to decorate shrines, fonts and places of worship in many cultures worldwide.

Pliny the Elder recommended a tea made from the dried flowers to ease the pain of childbirth. In the late 19th century, day lilies were thought to have pain-killing properties and were taken in the form of a tea to relieve rheumatism, aching joints, toothache and cramps.

CULTIVATION

Perennial, undemanding and easy, these lilies can be the backbone of a garden, or even a vegetable garden. What makes them so appealing is that they need no attention other than a deep twice-weekly watering, a few barrow-loads of compost twice a year, and occasional division. Plant them about 75 cm apart in well-dug, richly composted soil, and apart from the odd tidying up of dry leaves and stems, they can largely be left to themselves. They flower prolifically and I have counted nine or 10 blooms on a stem, opening one day after the other. You will be rewarded with a splendid display all summer long.

Day lilies take full sun and light shade equally well and adapt to all types of soil. Divide the clump every three or four years in winter by pushing two forks into it back to back and forcing them apart. Cut off the long leaves, leaving only about 10 cm, and replant in newly composted soil, watering it well. These lilies cross-pollinate easily, so within a few seasons you may find you have a new colour.

MEDICINAL USES

The earliest medicinal use of the day lily was as a tea. To make the tea, add one fresh flower to a cup of boiling water; leave it to stand for five minutes, then strain, add a touch of honey and sip slowly. The tea is a great comfort for aching muscles, strains and sprains and was often used as a lotion, with bandages soaked in the tea and bound over sprains and bruises. The brew can also be made into a mouthwash to ease toothache and mouth infections. In the past, crushed day lily petals were warmed and simply bound in place over bruises.

Day lily mouthwash

This mouthwash is used to clear oral infections and ease toothache.

1 fresh day lily flower
1 teaspoon cloves
1 cup boiling water

Pour the boiling water over the day lily flower and cloves. Swill the brew around the mouth several times during the day. Cloves are excellent as a disinfectant and as a painkiller for toothache.

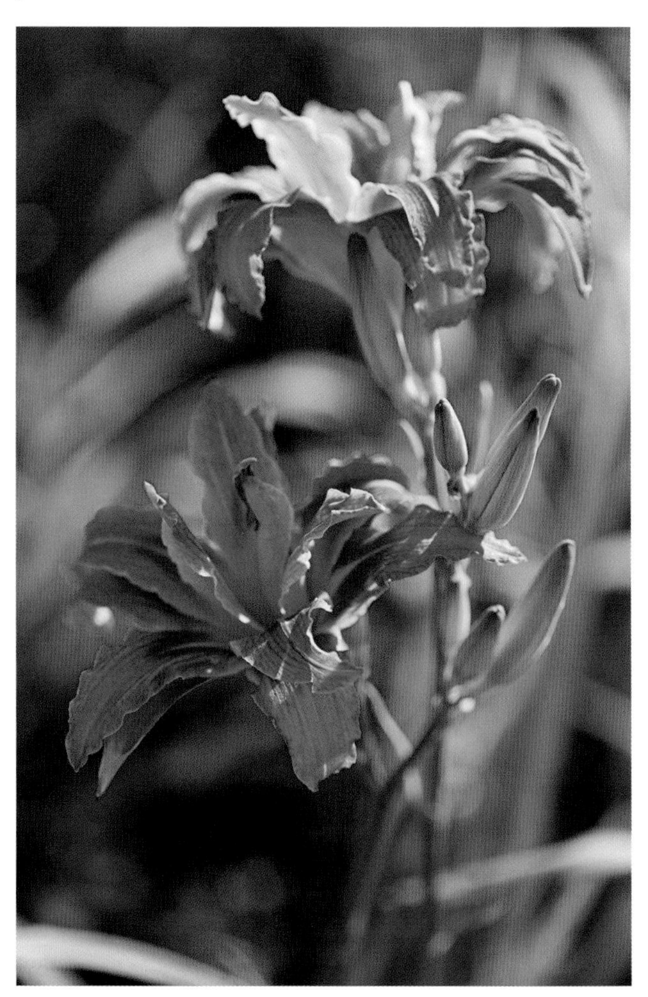

CULINARY USES

Day lily stir-fry

SERVES 4

This is a tasty, quick-and-easy supper dish that can be served in minutes and can be varied according to the ingredients you have at the time.

A little olive oil
2 onions, thinly sliced
1 packet large brown mushrooms, roughly sliced
2 green peppers, thinly sliced
8 baby marrows, cut into thin strips
10 day lily flowers and buds, thinly sliced
Juice of 1 lemon
Sea salt and black pepper to taste
½ cup chopped parsley

Heat the olive oil in a large wok or pan and add the onions. Let them brown lightly and then add the mushrooms, green peppers and baby marrows and stir-fry, turning constantly. Add the day lilies, lemon juice, sea salt and black pepper and stir well. Finally, add the parsley and serve piping hot with brown rice.

COOK'S NOTE

Cooking with day lilies is a pleasure, and their crisp, green bean-like taste enhances salads and stir-fries. The buds and flowers can be steamed or fried and complement just about any dish.

Golden day lily and yellow peach salad

SERVES 4–6

This is a golden feast for both the eye and the palate and it is my favourite summer salad. I add dandelion petals, pumpkin flowers and yellow nasturtiums for festive occasions. It is spectacular!

6 large, firm yellow peaches, coarsely grated or thinly chopped
2 cups celery, thinly chopped
2–3 yellow sweet peppers, thinly sliced
12 yellow and orange day lilies and buds
6 raw baby marrows, thinly sliced or ½ a peeled raw butternut squash, grated
4 hard-boiled eggs, chopped
1 cup grated cheddar cheese
1 cup good mayonnaise
Black pepper and sea salt to taste

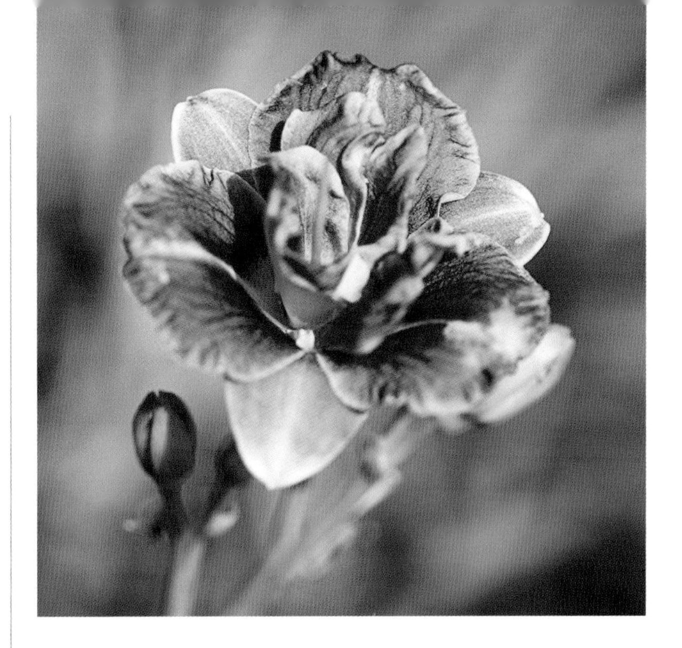

Mix the ingredients together gently and spoon into a pretty glass salad bowl. Sprinkle with a little freshly grated ginger and decorate with yellow day lilies all around the bowl.

Steamed day lilies and asparagus

SERVES 4

In spring the first asparagus comes onto the market just as the day lilies begin to flower. Pick the buds as they start to colour and steam them with the asparagus for a deliciously healthy spring treat.

4 cups day lily buds
2–3 packets asparagus

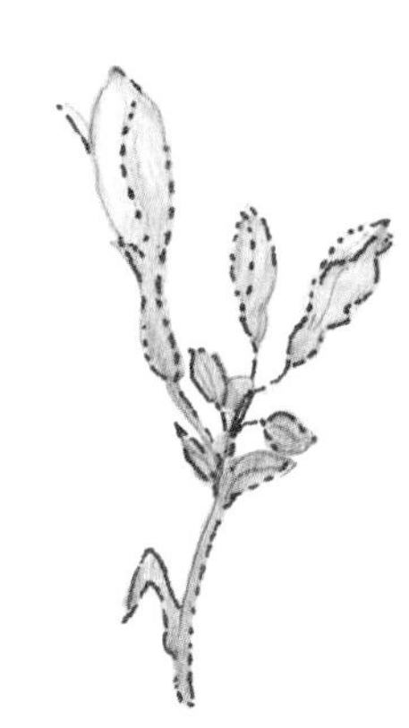

Sauce
2 eggs, beaten
2 cups full-cream milk
2 teaspoons mustard powder
1 tablespoon butter
2 tablespoons cornflour
1 teaspoon salt
Black pepper to taste
1 cup grated cheddar cheese

Place the flower buds and asparagus in a steamer and cook until they are tender. To make the sauce, whisk the eggs into the milk and mustard powder. Heat the butter and the cornflour, stirring well. Add the egg and milk mixture and stir well until it thickens. Add the salt, pepper and cheese, stirring all the time until the sauce reaches the correct consistency. Remove from the heat. Place the asparagus spears neatly on individual plates, surrounded by the day lily buds. Pour the sauce over them and decorate with day lily petals. Serve hot as a nourishing lunch dish.

Delicious monster

Monstera deliciosa • **Ceriman** • **Swiss cheese plant**

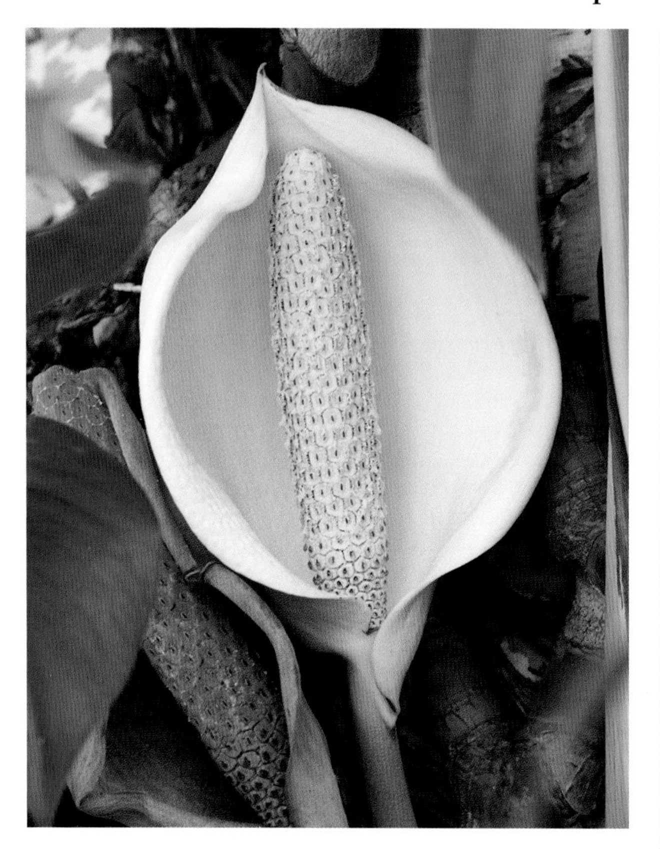

Rather surprisingly, this familiar house plant belongs to the Arum family. It originated in the jungles of Mexico and Guatemala, and is one of about 30 species of tropical climber belonging to the genus *Monstera*.

The delicious monster produces incredibly tough, woody, multi-jointed stout stems that bear huge, perforated leaves up to a metre long at intervals along the nodes. In its third year the flowering spike will appear if conditions are suitably moist. The inflorescence is a tough, creamy, arum-like flower with a bisexual spadix enclosed in a creamy white spathe. The rind that covers the spadix is covered in pale green hexagonal scales or plates, and the flower takes a year to ripen. As this happens, so the rind disintegrates and small pieces fall away, each with a succulent, exotic-tasting tip. Finally the scented, edible white pulp, which is the centre of the flower, is exposed, and it is this flower heart with its flavour of guavas, pineapple, granadilla and banana that is simply food for the gods.

CULTIVATION

The delicious monster has an extraordinary growth habit, climbing by means of masses of aerial roots. In the case of an indoor plant restricted to a pot, these roots can dangle rather untidily, but do not cut them away as the plant draws moisture from the air by means of them and they help it to survive. It continues to fruit at erratic intervals during the warm months and I have found that it does so readily if sprayed with water every week and if its aerial roots are led down into a bed of rich, moist compost that I replenish twice a year. It needs shade and protection and if it is in a greenhouse or on a verandah, it will benefit from a partner. As my grandmother used to say, they need to chat to one another so far from their jungles!

MEDICINAL USES

The spadix is the rigid core of the flower, which develops little scales. Discard the little top of each scale as there are tiny hairs of calcium oxalate on each section that can cause a burning irritation on the skin and tongue. Cut away the top and use only the ripened tips at the centre of the flower. The inner pulp and very ripe bits of the flowers are used as a treatment for skin spots, pimples, dry flaky skin on the heels and elbows and rough spots on the toes. Sticky and soothing, leave it on for as long as possible, then wash it away with tepid water to which a dash of apple cider vinegar has been added.

The soft young outer covering of the flower, the spathe, is still used in Mexico today as a comforting poultice over a sprain or bruise. Pressed open and softened in water, it makes a soothing dressing that is often used to hold other herbs in place over a wound or contusion.

The leathery little plates can be loosened off the ripe fruit and the creamy inner core rubbed onto sunburned skin.

Delicious monster spathe poultice

I was shown this very comfortable poultice for painful cracks on the heels. The spathe of the delicious monster is thought to have pain-killing properties.

1 delicious monster flower
1 tablespoon good aqueous cream
2 teaspoons almond oil
1 teaspoon rose essential oil

Cut away the inner core of the flower and discard it. Fill the spathe with the aqueous cream mixed well with almond oil and rose essential oil, smearing it into the tough spathe at the base. Now fit it over the cracked heel and gently move the spathe around the heel for a minute or two to massage the cream mixture in. Repeat this daily, using the spathe as a cup. After three days, the heel cracks should disappear. Discard the spathe and keep the heel softened and moisturised by applying the aqueous cream, almond and rose oil mixture every night.

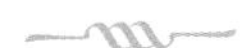

CULINARY USES

Mexican ceriman (delicious monster) drink

SERVES 4

Ripe pulp from 1 delicious monster flower,
scales removed (about ¾ cup mashed)
2 cups hot water (not boiling)
1 litre iced water
½ cup honey
1 litre granadilla or mango juice
Mint sprigs

Mash the pulp and cover with the hot water. Leave it to stand and cool, then put it through a liquidiser with a little of the iced water. Strain if preferred. Add the honey, fruit juice and mint, and chill. Serve in tall glasses with a sprig of mint. Sip slowly and relish every magical mouthful.

Delicious monster and litchi dessert

SERVES 4

This is a taste experience – since first tasting it I watch eagerly to see if my delicious monster flowers will ripen during litchi season.

2 tablespoons gelatine
1 cup warm water
1 litre litchi juice
A little sugar (optional)
4 cups litchis, peeled, stoned and sliced
1 ripe flowering delicious monster spadix,
scales carefully removed and finely mashed

Dissolve the gelatine in the warm water and stir into the litchi juice. Taste for sweetness, adding a little sugar if necessary, and stir well. Add the litchis and finally the mashed spadix. Pour into a glass bowl and set in the fridge. Serve with whipped cream.

Paradise ice-cream

SERVES 4

This unforgettable dessert is one of the quickest summer treats I know. Use either home-made or bought vanilla ice-cream.

Vanilla ice-cream
Pulp from 4 granadillas
1 cup finely crushed pineapple
1 ripe delicious monster spadix, scales removed and
finely mashed
Whipped cream

Spoon three or four balls of ice-cream into individual glass bowls. Pour a little granadilla pulp over them, and on top of that a spoonful or two of pineapple pulp mixed with the mashed delicious monster spadix. Top with a little whipped cream. This is what eating in paradise must be like!

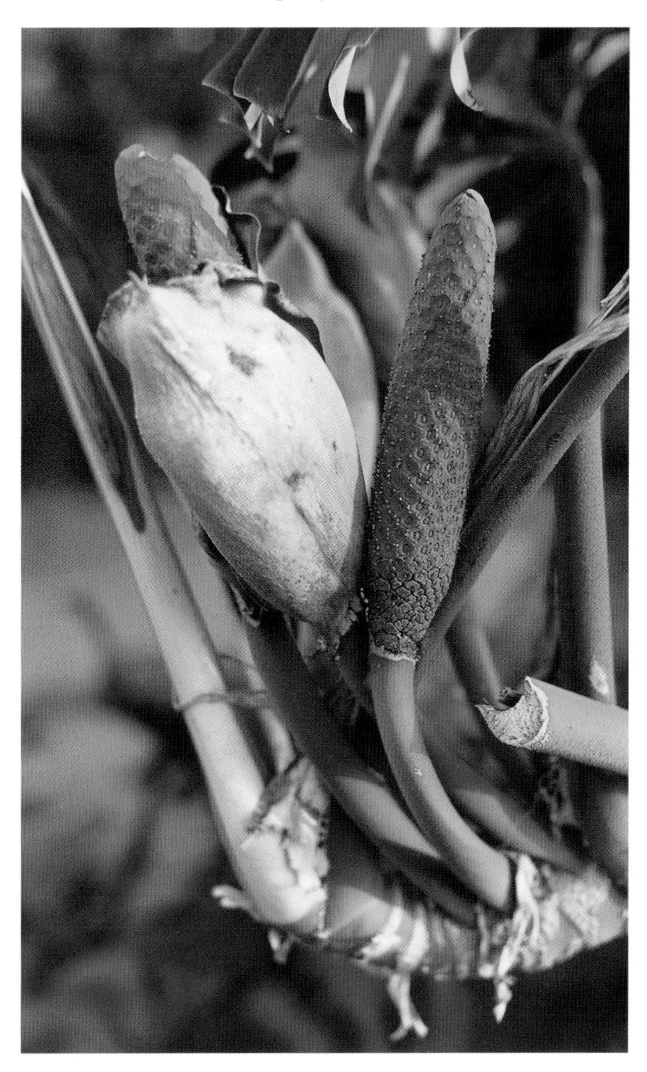

Echinacea

Echinacea purpurea ● **Purple cone flower**

Echinacea is undoubtedly one of the world's most important medicinal plants. In recent years it has drawn increasing respect from the medical profession as its ancient uses in traditional herbal medicine are being verified by scientific research. It is native to North America, and is now cultivated on a large scale worldwide.

The Sioux and the Comache Indians have used echinacea for centuries to treat the same ailments we use it for today: bronchitis, pneumonia, viral infections, acne and boils, animal and insect bites and stings, fever blisters, earache, flu, coughs and colds, sore throats and tonsillitis, skin allergies and infections, fungal infections, kidney and bladder infections, mild asthma, toothache and abscesses. It is a natural antibiotic, it boosts the immune system, and it is antifungal, anti-allergenic, anti-inflammatory and detoxifying. With all these amazing properties it is little wonder that echinacea is being researched for its ability to combat HIV – it could be set to become the plant of the new millennium.

CULTIVATION

Echinacea is an easy-to-grow perennial. It thrives in well-dug, well-composted soil, and being a prairie plant, it can do with very little water and needs little care or attention. The cushion of tough, coarse leaves gives rise to tall flowering spikes in midsummer, with bright pink, daisy-like flowers. The plant grows up to 60 cm in height, and the clumps need to be spaced 50 cm apart as they spread rapidly. The plant dies down in winter, almost disappearing from sight, and the spent flowers need to be cut. Cover with compost in spring and soak it well.

MEDICINAL USES

Echinacea is an exceptional anti-allergenic plant, and this is one of its key actions. In the case of allergic rhinitis, echinacea tea taken with three or four tablets of the biochemic tissue salt *Natrium muricatum* (available from your local pharmacy), will immediately soothe, open the nose and stop the streaming.

To make echinacea tea, pour a cup of boiling water over ¼ cup petals, leaves and root. Allow the tea to stand for five minutes, then strain and sip slowly. During an acute infection take two cups of the tea daily, and for chronic infection take one cup on alternate days. To relieve chilblains, make a cup of the tea to drink, and cool a second cup as a lotion to apply externally to sore fingers and toes. Dip pads of cotton wool into the lukewarm tea and apply to the area.

For post-viral fatigue syndrome, commonly known as ME, take a cup of echinacea tea daily and include the flower petals in the diet. Echinacea tea is being researched with favourable results as a treatment for asthma, particularly allergic asthma, and hay fever, cold sores or fever blisters caused by the *Herpes simplex* virus (see also elder flowers).

Echinacea healing cream

It is worth making your own healing creams and this easy-to-make cream has many applications.

1 cup echinacea petals and buds
1 cup comfrey flowers and buds
1 cup calendula flowers
2 cups good aqueous cream
3 teaspoons vitamin E oil
10 drops tea tree oil

Simmer the petals, flowers, buds and aqueous cream in a double boiler for 30 minutes. Strain. Add the vitamin E and tea tree oils. Mix well and pour into a sterilised jar.

CULINARY USES

Echinacea and melon fruit salad

SERVES 4–6

This pretty and healthy dessert is cool and green on a hot summer's day.

1 ripe green melon
4 kiwi fruits, peeled and sliced
3 cups green grapes, cut in half and seeds removed
4 prickly pears, peeled and sliced
1 cup echinacea petals
½ cup honey
½ cup warm water

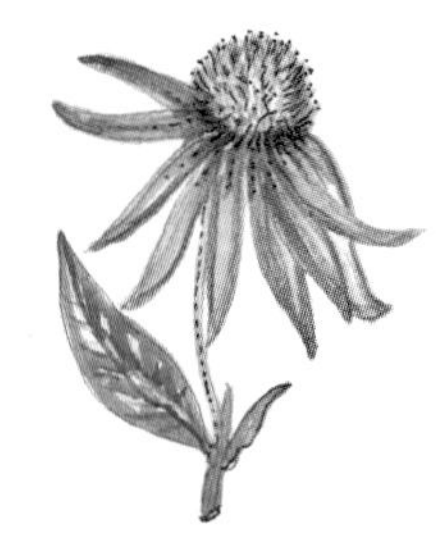

Remove the seeds from the melon and cut the flesh into squares. Mix all the fruit and the echinacea petals together in a glass bowl. Stir the honey into the warm water and pour over the salad. Allow the dessert to chill in the fridge. Decorate with fresh echinacea petals and serve with whipped cream.

American Indian savoury echinacea spread

SERVES 4

This spread makes an excellent lunch dish with sweet potatoes. Baked potatoes or even pasta can be substituted for the sweet potatoes.

4–6 large sweet potatoes
1 cinnamon stick
3 medium onions, chopped
Olive or sunflower oil
1 cup celery stalks and leaves, finely chopped
2 cups mustard greens, roughly torn
2 cups watercress sprigs or land cress leaves
1 cup echinacea petals
Sea salt and black pepper to taste
2 tablespoons honey

Boil the sweet potatoes in their skins in salted water with the cinnamon stick until cooked. Meanwhile fry the onion in the oil until it starts to brown, then add the celery stalks and leaves. Stir well. Add the mustard greens, then the watercress and echinacea petals. Stir well for about one minute and add the sea salt, black pepper and finally the honey. Split open the hot sweet potatoes and pile the echinacea spread on top. Decorate with fresh echinacea petals and a wedge of lemon.

COOK'S NOTE

Echinacea petals are fresh-tasting and tender. I only started using them in cooking a few years ago after an American Indian visitor to the Herbal Gardens described how they fry the petals with watercress, onion and mustard leaves and spread it over sweet potatoes (see recipe). I found this so interesting and delicious that it spurred me on to start experimenting.

Echinacea pane bagno

SERVES 4

Pane bagno literally means 'bathed bread'. It is a delicious salad roll, perfect as a lunchtime snack or for a picnic.

4–6 large freshly baked rolls, or 1 French loaf
1 can tuna in brine
Sea salt and black pepper
Fresh lemon juice
4 ripe tomatoes, thinly sliced
2 onions, thinly sliced

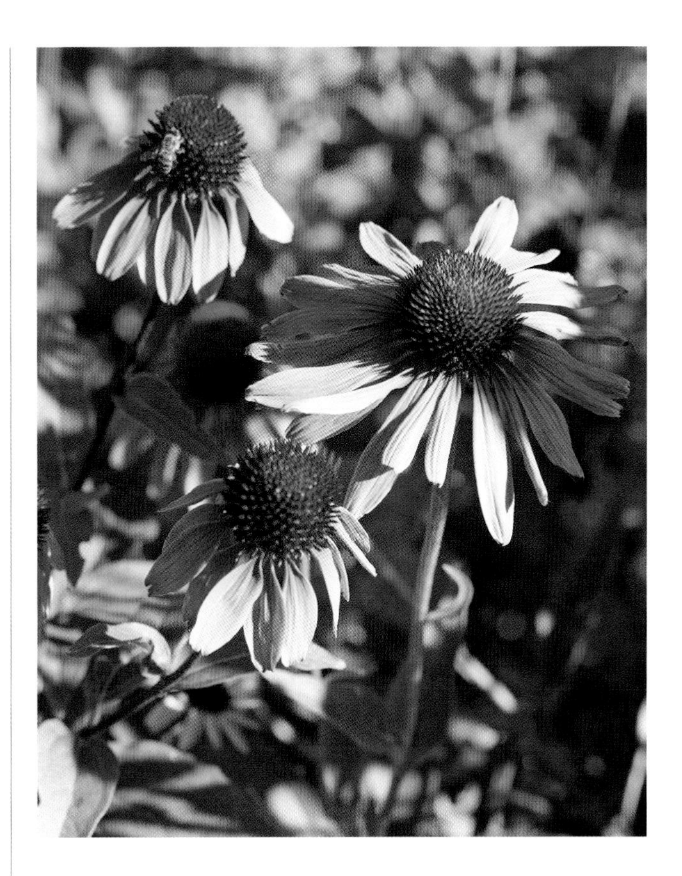

2 green peppers, thinly sliced
1 cup echinacea petals
1 cup stoned olives, chopped

Dressing
½ cup olive oil
½ cup white grape vinegar
2 teaspoons mustard powder
½ cup runny honey
Pinch sea salt and black pepper

Split the rolls or French loaf horizontally along one side, without cutting all the way through the crust. Butter both sides lightly. Mix all the dressing ingredients together in a screw-top jar and shake well. Open the bread so that it lies flat and gently dribble a little dressing along both sides. Drain the can of tuna fish and mash with a little sea salt, pepper and a squeeze of fresh lemon juice. Arrange the sliced tomatoes, onions and green peppers on the rolls, and top with the mashed tuna. Finally, sprinkle with the echinacea petals and olives. Close up the rolls or French loaf and wrap in cling wrap. Put a weight on them and leave for an hour to allow the dressing to soak in well. Just before serving, slice the rolls or loaf into manageable portions.

Elder flowers

Sambucus nigra

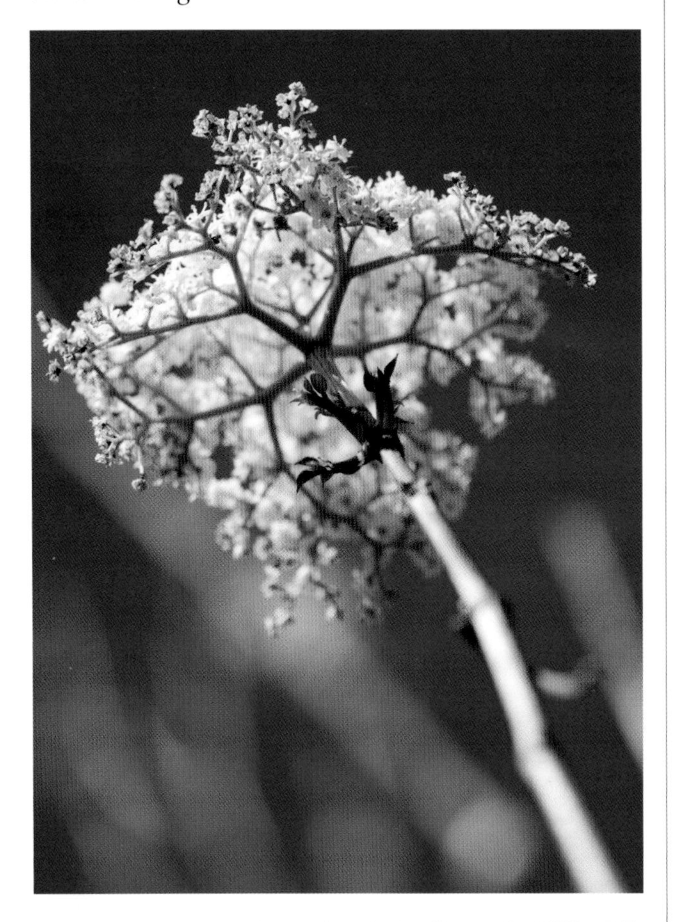

The elder is a sprawling, multi-stemmed deciduous shrub or small tree that is indigenous to Europe. It has been much revered through the centuries for its medicinal powers and it was believed to have magical protective properties. One of the most popular traditional beliefs was that it kept witches away, and in Europe elder trees were often planted close to people's homes for this reason. The purplish black berries appear after the flowers in midsummer and are particularly high in vitamins A and C; they have been made into a glorious wine or syrup for coughs, colds and bronchitis for centuries.

CULTIVATION

The elder is an undemanding shrub that requires little more than a sunny position. It will tolerate most soils but thrives in well-composted ground. Propagation is by means of cuttings in the spring, and it can be clipped back in winter to prevent it from becoming too sprawling and untidy. The elder can reach a height of about 4 m but is easily trimmed to form a hedge and can even be confined to a large tub providing that it has full sun and well-composted soil.

MEDICINAL USES

Elder is a renowned antiviral herb that helps to reduce fevers, fight flu and colds and boost the immune system. The flowers are used to tone the mucous linings of the nose and throat, helping to reduce catarrh and alleviating sinus problems, allergic rhinitis, hay fever, coughs, sore throat, postnasal drip and chronic earache. The flowers also stimulate the circulation and help to ease arthritis by encouraging sweating and urine production, which in turn remove acidity and toxic waste products from the body.

Research has found that the flowers help to break down the *Herpes simplex* virus, which is marvellous news for sufferers of fever blisters or cold sores. To rid the body of the *Herpes simplex* virus try a tea made with equal quantities of elder flowers, echinacea petals and black peppermint (*Mentha piperita nigra*). Pour a cup of boiling water over ¼ cup herbs. Allow the tea to stand for five minutes, then strain and sip. Take one cup every alternate day for two months and then thereafter once or twice a week for 4–6 months. In persistent cases, continue taking the tea twice a week for a further three or four months.

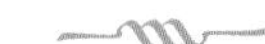

COSMETIC USES

Elder flower skin cream

Elder flowers make a wonderful healing skin cream that can be used to treat dry skin, cracked heels, and skin blemishes such as dark spots and freckles.

1 cup elder flower heads
1 cup aqueous cream
2 teaspoons vitamin E oil
4 teaspoons almond oil

Simmer the elder flower heads in the aqueous cream in a double boiler for 15 minutes with the lid on. Give the mixture an occasional stir. Strain, discard the flowers and add the vitamin E and almond oils. Mix well, and store in a sterilised jar. Apply daily to the spots and massage into rough skin. The elder flowers will soften and moisturise the skin.

Elder flower lotion

This is one of the most loved lotions in Europe. It is still used as a country cosmetic and has been well documented.

4 cups fresh elder flowers
3 strips lemon rind, thinly peeled with no pith
1 cup yarrow flowers
10 cloves, crushed
2 litres water
2 tablespoons witch hazel
10–15 drops lavender essential oil

Simmer the elder flowers, lemon rind, yarrow flowers and crushed cloves in the water for 20 minutes. Let it cool down, keeping it covered, then strain when cold. Add the witch hazel and lavender essential oil and mix briskly. Pour into sterilised spritz spray bottles and label. Use as an astringent lotion after washing the face, either spraying it on the skin or dabbing it onto the skin with a cotton wool pad. Elder flower lotion has a pore refining action and has become a traditional skin treatment for problem skin as well as for ageing skin.

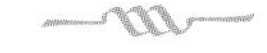

CULINARY USES

Elder flower lemonade

SERVES 8

This is an exquisite summer cordial and keeps well in the fridge.

4 cups elder flowers, pulled off their stems
Juice of 8 lemons
1 tablespoon lemon rind
3–4 cups white sugar
2 litres water

Simmer the ingredients together for 10 minutes. Add a little extra water if necessary. Cool, then strain. Pour the lemony syrup into a decanter and keep in the fridge. To serve, pour ¼ glass syrup and top up with iced water and crushed ice, or ice-cold soda water with a sprinkling of elder flowers floating on top.

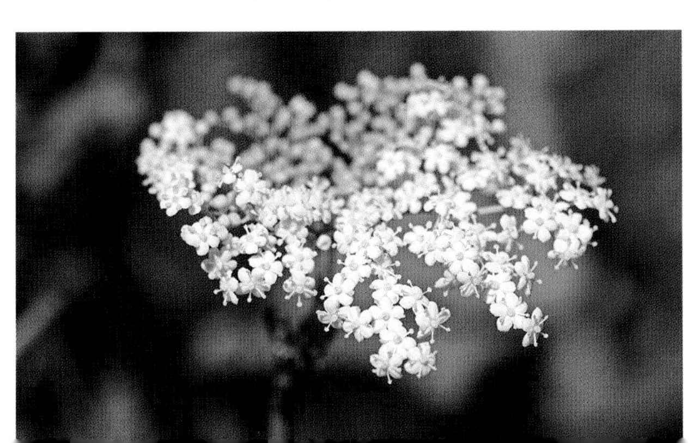

Elder flower fritters

SERVES 4

These fritters make a beautiful dessert or tea-party treat and are quick to prepare. Always make more than you think you want – they are so delectable!

12 large elder flower heads, fully open
Sunflower oil

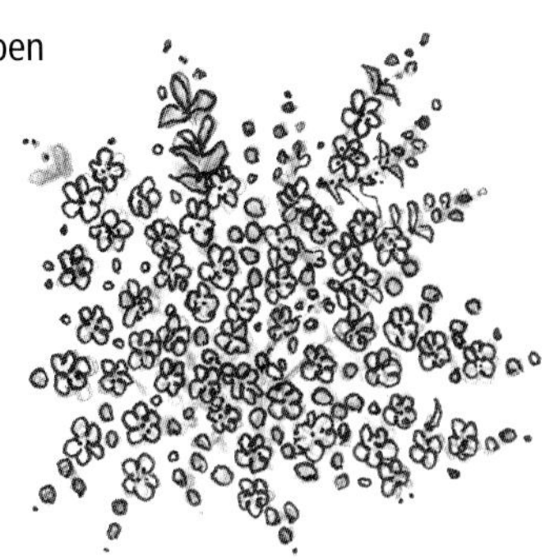

Batter
3 eggs
3 tablespoons sugar
1 teaspoon cinnamon
1 cup cake flour
1 cup milk
½ cup water

To make the batter, beat the eggs well with the sugar and cinnamon and then whisk together with the flour, milk and water to a runny consistency. Heat a little sunflower oil in a large pan. Holding each elder flower by its stalk, dip the whole flower into the batter and then immediately transfer it to the pan of hot oil. Let it cook for about two minutes or until golden brown. Transfer it to a pile of crumpled paper towel and let it drain. Place the flowers on a plate, snip off the stems, and dredge the fritters with icing sugar. Serve warm with whipped cream and sprinkle with more tiny elder flowers, stripped off their stems.

Elder flower and rhubarb dessert

SERVES 6

Elder flowers add a muscatel-like flavour to the tart rhubarb and lessen the need for so much sugar. Use this as a dessert or as a pie filling. Peaches, apples or pears can be added for a change of flavour.

12–20 long rhubarb stalks
4 cups sugar
4 cups elder flowers, stripped off their stalks
A little water

Strip the leaves off the rhubarb and cut the stems into 4 cm lengths. Place in a deep pot with the sugar, elder flowers and water and simmer gently, stirring every now and then until the rhubarb is tender and breaks up. Do not let the mixture burn. Set it aside and allow it to cool. Serve on pancakes with whipped cream or ice-cream, and decorate with more elder flowers sprinkled over the top.

Evening primrose

Oenothera biennis

The evening primrose is a hardy biennial native to North America, where it is a common weed. It has been used for centuries to treat a wide variety of ailments, and modern research is verifying these age-old uses. The Ojibwa, a North American Indian tribe, were the first to discover its medicinal properties; they used evening primrose to treat asthma and chest ailments, as a poultice and lotion for bruises and skin disorders, as a tea for fear, nervousness, panic attacks and anxiety, and for ageing women. It was brought to Europe around 1614 as a botanical curiosity and today it is recognised as one of the world's most important medicinal plants.

Leaves and flowers have long been added to soups, stews and teas, and American Indians pickled the buds in oil and salt for the winter. Simply eating one of the clear yellow flowers in the garden in the evening will set you wondering about this remarkable plant.

CULTIVATION

The evening primrose will tolerate any sort of soil and is as undemanding as any weed, merely requiring a sunny position. The leaves are arranged in rosettes in the first year and can be eaten like spinach; in the second year the leaves are arranged along the stem, and fluorescent yellow flowers that scent the night air are also produced. New flowers open every evening, only to fade and shrivel in the hot sun the following day during summer. Masses of seeds form in the capsules of the spent flowers, and it is these seeds that contain the remarkable evening primrose oil that is used for such a wide variety of ailments. The plant seeds itself prolifically all over the garden – once you have it you will find seedlings popping up everywhere. Root it out after the seed spire turns brown and scatter the seeds. The plant grows to about 1 m in height.

MEDICINAL USES

Evening primrose oil is used extensively for premenstrual tension, multiple sclerosis, as an anticoagulant and antispasmodic, and in the treatment of wounds, skin eruptions, gastric irritation such as irritable bowel syndrome, coughs, colds and menopausal hormone correction. It contains the important gamma-linolenic acid (GLA), which has been proven to lower blood pressure by preventing the clumping of platelets; it has also been shown to lower cholesterol levels and to aid weight loss. Evening primrose has also been found to be effective in the treatment of hyperactive children. To make a tea for all the above conditions, pour a cup of boiling water over ¼ cup fresh flowers and leaves. Allow the tea to stand for five minutes, then strain and sip slowly.

Evening primrose lotion for eczema

3 cups evening primrose leaves and flowers
1½ litres water

Simmer the evening primrose leaves and flowers in the water for 15 minutes. Cool, strain and apply the lotion externally, either using a spritz spray bottle or dabbing onto the skin using a cotton wool pad. Take the tea as an additional treatment.

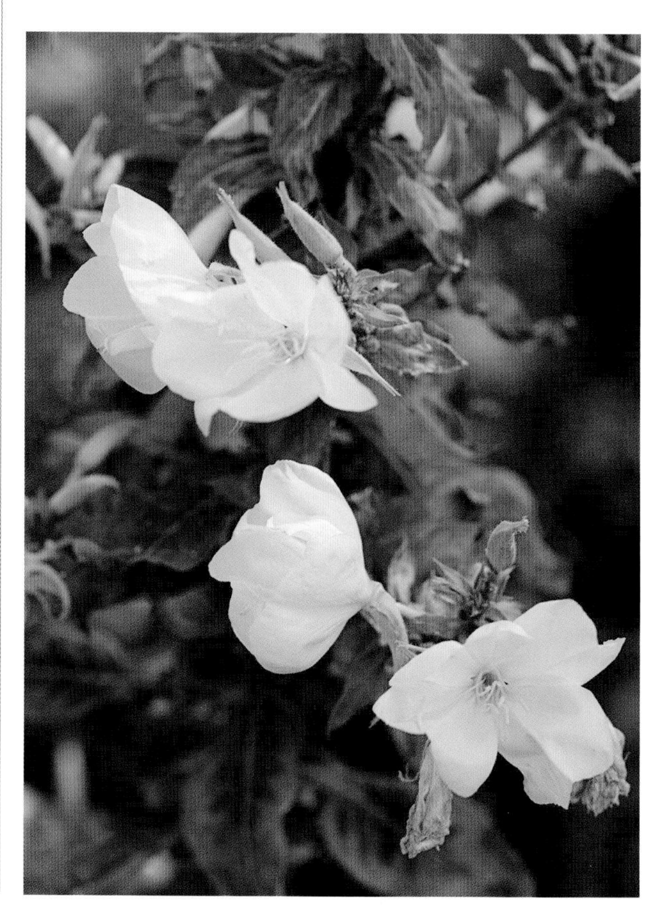

COSMETIC USES

Evening primrose oil

For very dry skin, cracked lips and dry, flaking nails, this oil will become a standby for many skin ailments.

Primrose flowers and buds
Grape seed or almond oil
30 drops lavender essential oil
3 teaspoons vitamin E oil
750 ml glass bottle

Pack the bottle with as many flowers and buds as it can hold. Fill the bottle with grape seed or almond oil and seal well. Keep it in a warm place, out of the sun, giving it a daily shake. After three days, pour everything into a double boiler and simmer it gently for 30 minutes, stirring often. Cool for 20 minutes, then strain. Add the lavender and vitamin E oils and mix well. Return the oil to the bottle or pour into smaller bottles and label. Do not expose to light; this oil must be stored in a cupboard.

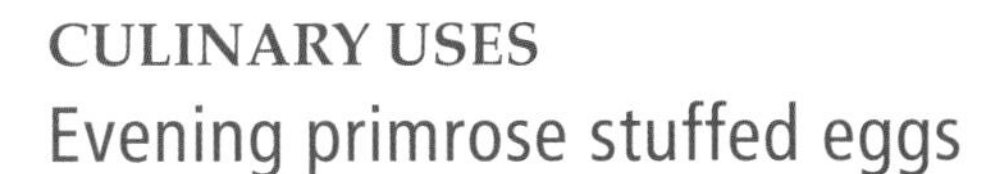

CULINARY USES

Evening primrose stuffed eggs

SERVES 6

Collect the evening primrose flowers in the early morning before they fade, and refrigerate them. This recipe is a favourite for summer picnics, and I make it often as a lunchtime snack.

1 dozen eggs
1–2 teaspoons horseradish sauce
½ cup good mayonnaise
½ cup chopped parsley
½ cup finely chopped celery
1 tablespoon Worcestershire sauce
½ cup finely grated strong cheddar cheese
Sea salt and freshly ground black pepper
1 cup roughly chopped evening primrose flowers

Boil the eggs until hard – around ten minutes – and when they are cooked, submerge them immediately in cold water. Shell the eggs, cut them in half and remove the yolks. Mash the yolks with the rest of the ingredients. Fill the hollows in the egg whites with the mixture and arrange the stuffed eggs in a flat dish on a bed of lettuce and watercress. Decorate each egg with an evening primrose petal, and serve chilled.

Evening primrose and onion scones

SERVES 6

These tasty scones are much nicer than bread rolls as an accompaniment for supper, and are quick to make.

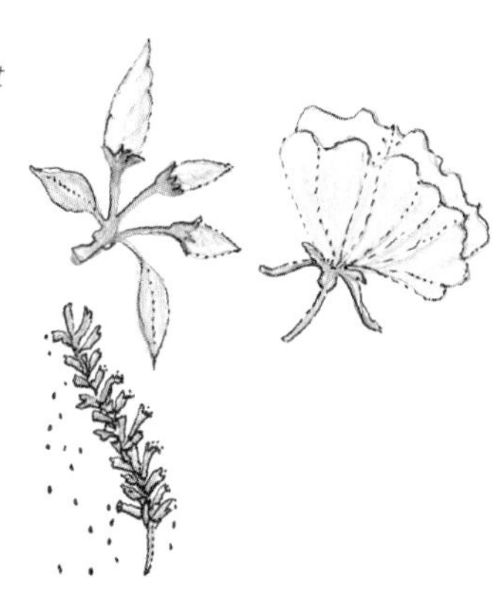

1½ cups butter, coarsely grated
2 cups cake flour
1 tablespoon baking powder
1 teaspoon salt
Pepper
3 spring onions, finely chopped
1 cup chopped evening primrose flowers
¾ cup buttermilk

Rub the butter into the flour. Add the baking powder, salt, and pepper to taste, then the spring onions and chopped evening primrose flowers. Slowly add the buttermilk and mix into a dough, adding more if it is too stiff. Turn out onto a floured board and knead briefly into a ball. Pat into an oblong about 2 cm thick and cut into neat squares about 5 cm in size. Lay these on a floured baking sheet. Brush the tops with buttermilk and bake at 180°C for about 10 minutes or until the scones start to turn golden brown on top. Serve hot with butter.

Evening primrose and pear dessert

SERVES 4–6

Make this easy dessert in autumn when there is an abundance of evening primrose flowers (the flowers last longer than one night in cooler weather).

12 pears
1 litre water
1 cup sugar
1 cup lightly chopped evening primrose petals
½ cup evening primrose buds (optional)

Core and quarter the pears and poach them lightly in the water and sugar until tender, usually about 10 minutes. Remove from the stove and allow to cool. Just before the pears are completely cool, stir in the lightly chopped evening primrose petals. Serve with whipped cream or custard, decorated with more evening primrose petals. For a slightly stronger flavour cook the pears with half a cup of evening primrose buds. Add the flowers before serving.

Feijoa

Feijoa sellowiana • **Pineapple guava** • **Brazilian guava**

This fascinating shrub is unusual in that it is a monotypic genus, which means that it is the sole representative of its genus. It was discovered in 1819 by a German explorer named Sellow, who found it growing abundantly in Brazil and named it after Don de Silva Feijoa, a San Sebastian botanist, and himself (*Feijoa sellowiana*). It was only introduced to Europe around 1890 by Edourd André, a French horticulturist who found that it thrived in his garden on the French Riviera. From there it was introduced to Australia, New Zealand and California around 1900.

Very little is known about the feijoa and there has been virtually no research done on it, which is surprising because not only is it prolific and easy to grow, but its small, green fruits that appear in abundance in late summer are exotically sweet and succulent to eat. They resemble miniature guavas, with fragrant, white, guava-flavoured flesh. Its attractive, dense grey-green foliage makes this evergreen shrub an asset in a garden of any size.

CULTIVATION

The feijoa adapts remarkably well to any soil type and temperature and can be found growing in the most unlikely spots, but it flourishes best in warm, protected, richly composted sites. It needs full sun and a deep weekly watering. When it is clipped, trained and controlled it makes a most charming topiary, a luscious espalier against strong wires on a sunny wall, a neat hedge or an attractive container plant, and can be trained over arches. Left alone, it can reach 6 m in height and spread, but pruned and controlled it is a perfect shrub for a small garden and is beautiful in all seasons. Underplant it with tansy to prevent the fruit from being stung, and hang a tin with molasses, water and fruit peels in the tree as fruit fly bait.

MEDICINAL USES

In its native Brazil, Uruguay, Paraguay and Argentina, the feijoa is used to treat certain thyroid conditions as it is rich in iodine. A tea can be made from the plant by adding a cup of boiling water to ¼ cup mixed flowers and fruit. Leave the tea to stand for five minutes, then strain and sip slowly. This same brew is used to treat dysentery and diarrhoea, but with the addition of extra flowers – two tablespoons of flowers or one tablespoon of flowers and half a tablespoon of fruit. Steep for five minutes only in boiling water, then strain and sip a little at a time. Repeat until the condition subsides.

In Paraguay, fresh crushed flowers and the ripe fruit are applied to rashes, mild burns, insect bites and stings, and itchy inflamed areas. A lotion made from the flowers can be used to soothe sunburned skin, and slices of the fruit can be used as a poultice.

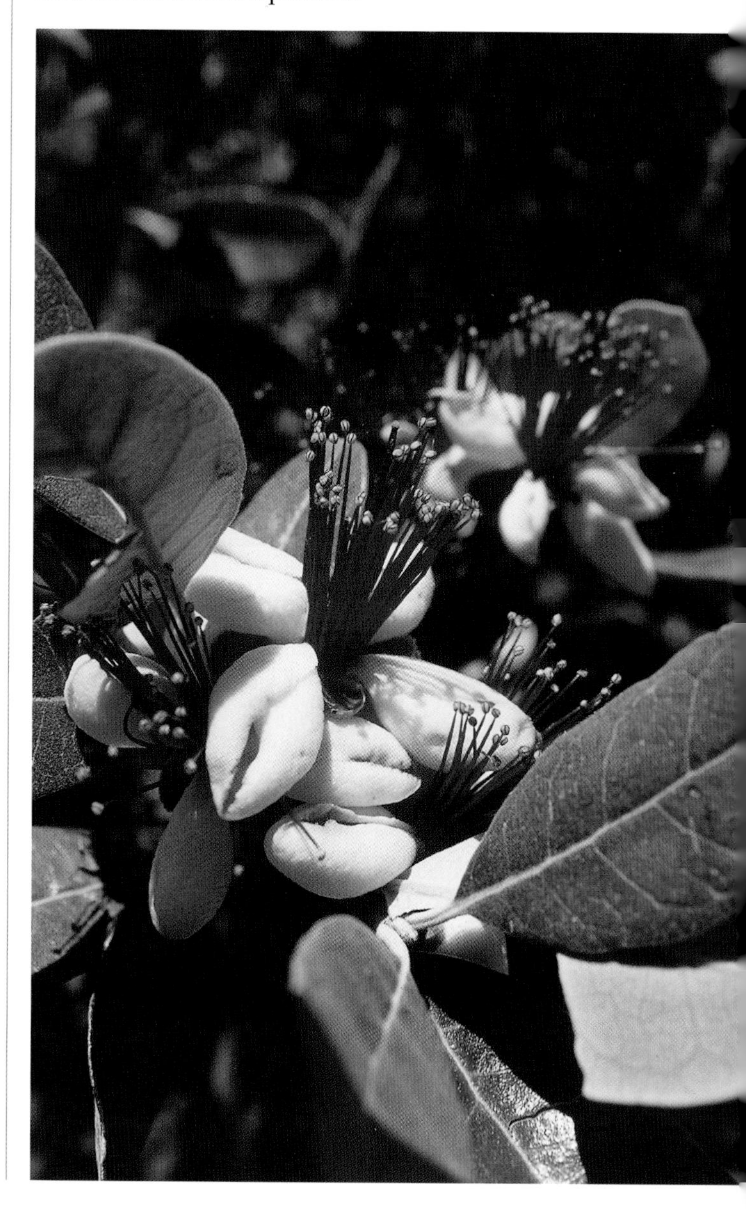

Feijoa lotion for sunburned skin

2 cups feijoa flowers
6 cloves, crushed
1 teaspoon powdered nutmeg
½ litre water
2 cups milk

Warm the flowers, crushed cloves and nutmeg in the water and milk for 20 minutes, stirring constantly. Let the lotion cool, then strain and pour into a spritz spray bottle. Spray over the sunburned area or dab on with cotton wool.

Feijoa skin cream

A modern version of a cream used in Brazil for centuries, for burns, grazes and scratches.

1 cup feijoa flowers
½ cup olive oil
1 cup acqueous cream
3 teaspoons vitamin E oil

In a double boiler, simmer together the flowers, olive oil and acqueous cream for 30 minutes, crushing the flowers well into the oil and cream. Cool for 20 minutes then strain. Add the vitamin E oil. Spoon into a sterilised jar with a well-fitting lid. Appy frequently. It can also be used for cracks at the corners of the mouth, cracked heels and nail problems. Massage well into the cuticles, especially of the toenails.

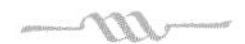

CULINARY USES

Brazilian feijoa conserve

For centuries Brazilians have used the succulent pink, curiously folded petals and red stamens of the feijoa flower to make a conserve.

4 cups feijoa flowers, calyxes removed
3–4 cups sugar
3 cups chopped ripe apricots, peaches, nectarines or plums, or a mixture
1 stick cinnamon
½ cup water

Simmer the ingredients on low heat, stirring occasionally, until the fruit is tender, about 20 minutes. Spoon into a sterilised jar and leave to cool. Serve over ice-cream, with custard and cream, or over baked custard and rice pudding. It keeps well in the fridge.

Feijoa fruit salad

SERVES 4–6

Any fruit in season can be used, but I prefer the exotic spring fruits for this light, refreshing dessert. It makes an attractive party dish.

3 cups strawberries, hulled and sliced
2 cups mulberries, stalks removed
Sugar
1 cup feijoa flowers
3 cups early peaches, peeled and sliced
1 cup granadilla juice
3 bananas, thinly sliced
1 small pineapple, peeled and coarsely grated

Sprinkle the strawberries and mulberries with sugar and leave them to stand in a warm spot to absorb the sugar for about an hour. Add the remaining ingredients, mix together, and let the fruit salad stand covered for an hour before serving to enable the juices to mingle. Dribble with a little honey and serve with whipped cream, decorated with feijoa flowers.

Buttered banana and feijoa breakfast dish

SERVES 4

This is a delicious dish for a festive brunch, or even a Sunday family breakfast.

4 thick slices tomato
4 large black mushrooms
A little cooking oil
Sea salt and black pepper to taste
Sugar
4 thick slices wholewheat toast, crusts removed
2 tablespoons butter
6 bananas, peeled and cut in half lengthways
1 cup feijoa flowers, calyxes removed
2 tablespoons chopped parsley

Fry the tomatoes slices and black mushrooms in a large pan, using a little oil. Sprinkle salt and pepper on them, plus a little sugar on the tomatoes. Cook until tender. Butter the toast, place on individual heated plates, and top with the tomato slices and mushrooms. Keep warm. Wipe the pan out and heat the butter. Add the bananas and the feijoa flowers and cook them gently in the butter for about two minutes. Arrange them around the tomato and mushroom toast and sprinkle with parsley. Serve immediately while hot, decorated with a few fresh feijoa flowers.

Fennel

Foeniculum vulgare

The ancient Greeks and Romans considered fennel to be a sacred herb and used it for slimming, much as we do today. In Anglo-Saxon times the seeds and flowers were eaten on fasting days to still hunger pangs; fennel was also used as a tonic herb, and Roman warriors took it to keep in good health when they went off to battle. Fennel was once a favourite strewing herb, especially during the Middle Ages, as its pleasant aniseed-type fragrance helped to clear the air of bad smells.

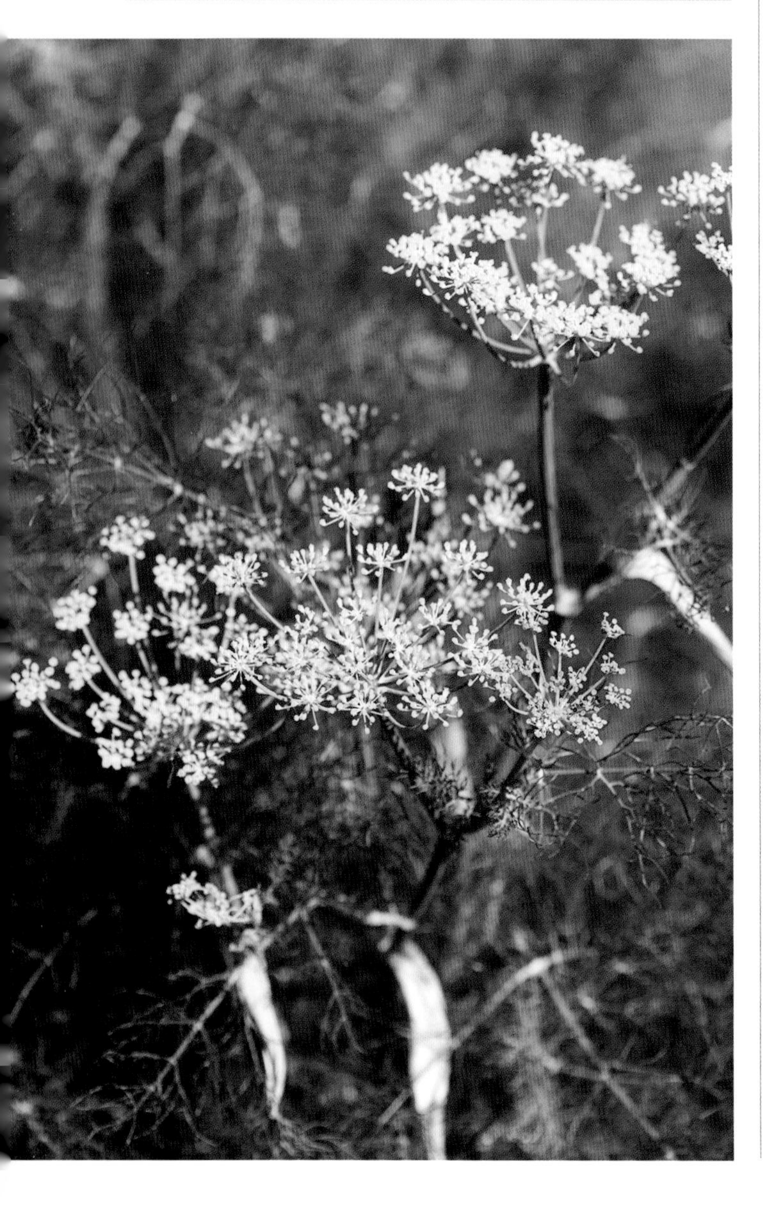

CULTIVATION

Fennel is a hardy, easy-to-grow perennial. It needs richly composted soil in full sun and a deep twice-weekly watering, and produces pretty yellow umbels of flowers that are much loved by bees and butterflies. The mature flowering stems scatter a mass of seed. Seedlings can be transplanted when they are 6 cm tall into well-dug, well-composted soil about 80 cm apart, in full sun.

MEDICINAL USES

Fennel seeds and flowers are a palatable and useful digestive remedy. Taken as a tea or chewed after a heavy meal they will alleviate flatulence, heartburn and colic, aiding the whole digestive process and easing the feeling of fullness. To make the tea, pour a cup of boiling water over ¼ cup fresh fennel leaves and flowers. Let the tea stand for five minutes, then strain. Take two cups a day during infection, followed by one cup a day thereafter for about 10 days. This tea is the world's favourite slimming drink and it is also a superb detoxifier.

Fennel is also a circulatory stimulant and anti-inflammatory, it promotes milk flow in nursing mothers, and it is a mild expectorant, and a superb diuretic.

CAUTION: Fennel is a uterine stimulant, so avoid taking too much during pregnancy. Small amounts in cooking are quite safe.

Fennel flower antacid remedy

This remedy combines three top digestive herbs, making it a most comforting antispasmodic and settling abdominal distension and bloating quickly. If you do not have flowers, use the seeds alone.

1 tablespoon fennel flowers (pulled off their stems)
1 tablespoon fennel seeds
1 tablespoon caraway flowers (pulled off their stems)
1 tablespoon caraway seeds
1 tablespoon anise flowers (pulled off their stems)
1 tablespoon aniseed

Mix the flowers and seeds together, place them in a screw-top jar and shake well. The flowers will dry naturally in the mixture if the lid is kept off. To make up the remedy, pour a cup of boiling water over one dessertspoonful of the mixture and stir well. Let it draw for five minutes, strain and sip slowly. It is quick-acting and immediately effective.

Fennel hot toddy

SERVES 1

In the 17th century this hot toddy was used in monasteries to cure everything from rheumatism and the ague, to mad dog bites and fainting fits. On a winter's night it is like a magic potion. It warms you up, lifts your spirits and chases stiffness and chills away.

1 cup boiling water
½ cup fennel flowers
4 cloves
1 teaspoon crushed cinnamon (not powdered cinnamon)
Juice of 2 lemons
1 tablespoon honey
Dash of good brandy

Pour the boiling water over the fennel, cloves and cinnamon. Let the mixture stand for five minutes, keeping it covered to retain its warmth, or place it in a pot on the stove on low heat for five minutes. Strain, and add the lemon juice, honey and brandy. Sip slowly – and watch your mood change radically!

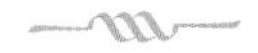

COSMETIC USES

Fennel has been used since ancient times to make a facial steam for cleansing oily skin and clearing spots, blackheads and acne.

Fennel facial steam

1½ litres boiling water
2 cups fennel leaves and flowers

Pour the boiling water over the fennel leaves and flowers. Make a towel tent over the head, and lean over the steaming bowl for a few minutes. Rinse in tepid water to which a dash of apple cider vinegar has been added. Pat dry. Do this once a week to help clear problem skin.

CULINARY USES

Fennel flower slimmer's salad

SERVES 4

This is one of my favourite salads and all of us, even those not anxious to slim, should eat it once a week or fortnight to keep the body clear of toxins. Should you be coming down with flu or a cold, add extra lemon juice and sprinkle a little cayenne pepper over the salad. This often stops the infection in its tracks.

1 butter lettuce, roughly torn
1½ cups chopped celery, leaves included
1½ cups alfalfa sprouts or fresh young lucerne leaves
1½ cups fennel leaves and flowers, roughly chopped
1½ cups peeled chopped cucumber
1½ cups finely grated carrot
½ cup chopped parsley
Juice of 1 lemon

Mix the ingredients together in a large bowl, and pour the lemon juice over the salad. Decorate with fennel flowers. Do not add salt or pepper.

COOK'S NOTE

Fennel flowers, nipped off their stems and fried, make a delicious addition to the salad or sprinkled over a soup. Fry the flowers quickly in a hot pan with a touch of olive oil and sprinkle with salt and paprika.

Fennel flower soup

SERVES 4–6

Another superb detoxifying dish, this soup is a good anti-inflammatory as well as being rich in vitamins and minerals. It is also excellent for bringing down high blood pressure.

3 cups finely chopped leeks
1 tablespoon sunflower oil
2 cups chopped fennel stalks, leaves and flowers
1 cup pearl barley, soaked overnight
2 cups finely chopped celery
1½ cups finely grated turnip
1½ cups finely grated carrot
1 cup split peas
½ cup grated fresh ginger
Juice of 1 lemon
Sea salt to taste
A little cayenne pepper
1½ litres water or vegetable stock

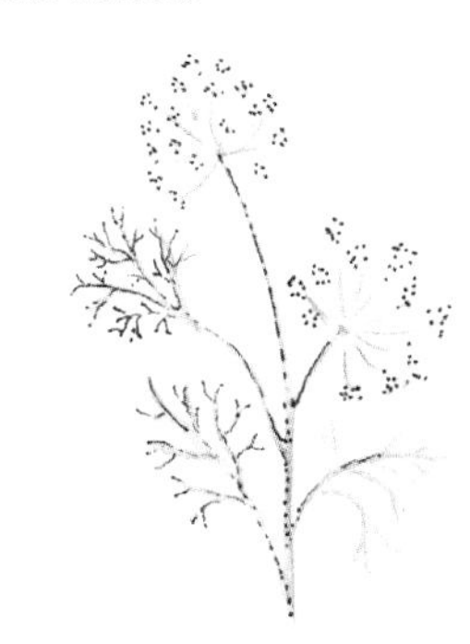

Lightly brown the leeks in the sunflower oil. Add the remaining ingredients and simmer for about one hour. Add a little extra water if necessary.

COOK'S NOTE

The leeks browned in the oil give a good flavour to the fennel flower soup. For those on a fat-free diet, omit the oil. Finely chopped fennel leaves are delicious in fish dishes and on green beans.

Fig

Ficus carica

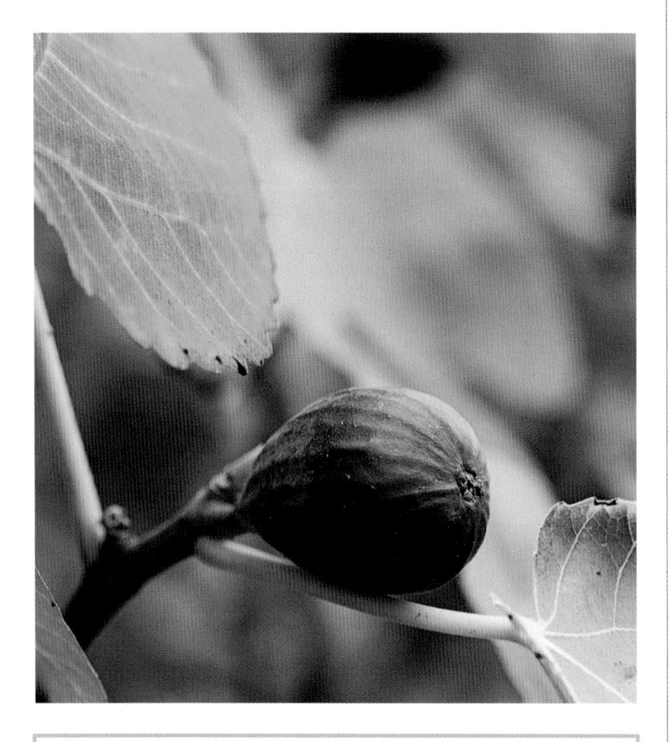

The fig really is a flower with a swollen calyx, with the stamens and petals all inside! Small wasps act as pollinators, entering the 'flower' through the hole at the base, known as the ostiole. This structure is unique to the *Ficus* genus.

From its early Mediterranean beginnings, this much-loved fruit has spread throughout the world as one of the oldest food crops, a medicinal remedy, and a prized garden feature.

Figs probably originated in Syria, and have been cultivated across Mesopotamia and Egypt since 4000 BC. The Phoenicians took the fig into China and India. It was one of the plants grown in the Hanging Gardens of Babylon, and the dried fruits were traded on the great trade routes. Figs were a major crop in ancient Greece and Pliny the Elder (AD 23–79) described 29 cultivars thriving at that time.

Drawings of the fig were found in the Gizeh pyramid and in the archives of great antiquity. Many of the ancient varieties still exist today, and the Kadota fig remains a favourite. We grow several varieties at the Herbal Centre gardens and make jams, preserved whole figs, jellies and dried figs the way the ancient growers did.

CULTIVATION

Dig a wide deep hole in full sun, and fill it with a really huge amount of rich compost. Set a wide pipe at an angle into the hole so that a hosepipe can be inserted to get water down to the roots in a long, slow, deep watering, twice-weekly.

Propagation is from cuttings taken in the dead of winter, at the first stirrings of spring. I have learned that twigs with four nodes on them are best so that two nodes can go underground for good rooting to occur. Keep the deep pot or bag constantly moist and shaded until the first buds appear.

Lavender and rosemary are great companions, and with elderberries and lemon verbena nearby, no unwanted insects come near the figs. Remove overripe figs as fruit flies and fruit beetles will descend upon them. Give each fig tree a barrow of compost two or three times yearly, and make a huge sturdy dam around each tree so that you can flood it with water twice-weekly.

MEDICINAL USES

Ancient medical texts referred to the fig fruit as 'fig flowers' or 'flowers of fig'. The fruit was used as a constipation remedy, and a valuable alcoholic drink for toning the digestive system was made from thinly sliced figs and honey, left to ferment. This potent brew was prized in Turkey, Spain and Italy.

'Syrup of figs' is an ancient gentle laxative. Most chemists stocked it during my childhood and my grandmother made her own. No-one suffered from constipation, flatulence, colic or indigestion with a dose of this marvellous medicine!

Fresh figs are excellent as a natural laxative. Four fresh or dried figs eaten daily first thing in the morning will move sluggish bowels. Soak dried figs in warm water overnight and enjoy them with a cup of herb tea – mint tea is a favourite! In many countries, two dried figs softened in water overnight have formed part of the diet for centuries – bladder, bowel, kidney, stomach and even weight problems are eased and corrected by this.

Figs build bones, so for osteoporosis be sure to grow a fig tree in your garden as the fruit are abundant in vitamins A, C and E, as well as many minerals like calcium, potassium and phosphorus, and to a lesser extent iron, copper and manganese.

Fig twigs stripped of their leaves and pressed into flour bins will keep weevils away, and the milky sap dries up warts (the sap is released when a leaf is picked). Drip the sap onto the wart at least three times a day.

Syrup of figs for digestive upsets and constipation

10 thinly sliced figs, skin intact
1 cup honey

Simmer the figs and honey in a double boiler. Stir frequently for 30 minutes, warming the syrup thoroughly. Strain, pour into a sterilised bottle and label. Take one dessertspoonful daily for digestive upsets and constipation. The syrup is safe for children – two teaspoons is usually the right dosage.

CULINARY USES

Fig ice-cream

SERVES 4–6

16–20 ripe figs, peeled and chopped
4 cups plain Bulgarian yogurt
1–2 cups whipped cream
Sprinkling of nutmeg and cinnamon

Peel the figs and chop roughly. Stir in the yogurt and cream. Add the nutmeg and cinnamon and mix well. Taste, and if it is not sweet enough add a little runny honey, tasting as you go. Pour into freezing trays and place in the freezer. Check every 15 minutes and stir gently. Freeze solid. Serve with a sprinkling of chopped almonds or pecan nuts in individual glass bowls.

Quick fig jam

Ripe figs
Soft brown sugar
Stevia syrup (1 cup stevia leaves and flowers)

Cut ripe figs into quarters and weigh them. Toss them in a large heavy-bottomed pot. Weigh half the amount of soft brown sugar, and add it to the stevia syrup. To make the syrup, boil one cup of lightly chopped stevia leaves and flowers in one litre of water for 20 minutes. Allow the syrup to cool, and strain. Taste the syrup and add to the fig mixture a cup at a time, until you get the desired taste you feel is most delicious. Simmer the jam, stirring frequently, until the figs are translucent and a drop or two of the sugar mixture sets on a cold saucer. Spoon into sterilised glass jars right to the top, screw on the sterilised lids and label.

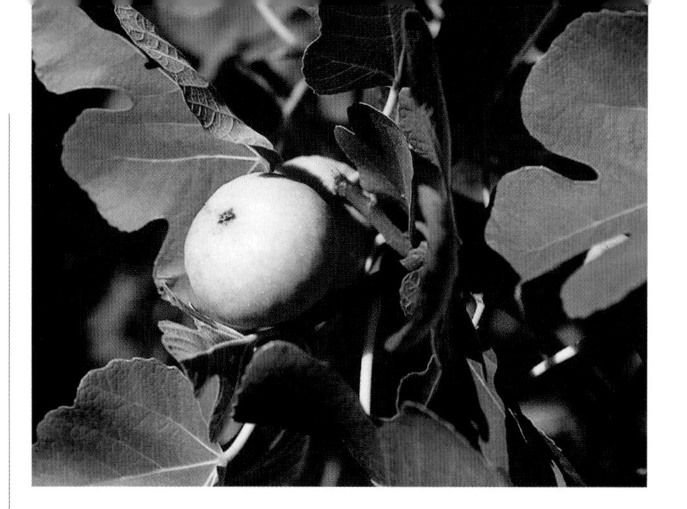

COOK'S NOTE
Dry ripe sliced figs in the summer sun on stainless steel trays or in a dryer. They make a delicious dried condiment. Chop the dried figs and serve with ice cream.

Fig savoury salad

SERVES 4–6

This is a real party platter and one that even the pickiest eater will enjoy! Use black figs as they hold their shape beautifully.

2 butter lettuces, leaves separated
Slices of mozzarella cheese, enough for each half fig
12 black figs, cut in half
Pickled sweet chillies or cucumbers
Twists of thinly sliced cold beef or strips of chicken breasts
Squeeze of lemon juice
Black pepper

Lay the butter lettuce leaves out like little boats on a large platter. Place a slice of mozzarella cheese in each one, topped with half a fig, cut side up. Place a pickled chilli or pickled cucumber on top of the fig, and tuck a slice of rolled-up cold beef or sliced chicken breast around it. Add a squeeze of lemon juice. Grind black pepper over the salad and serve as a first course or as a snack with drinks on a summer evening. Simple and simply delicious!

COOK'S NOTE
For breakfast try fresh or honey-baked figs with homemade Bulgarian yoghurt or fresh cream, sprinkled with pecan nuts or macadamias. It is absolutely irresistible! Figs are even used to flavour coffee, and *fiquette*, a type of liqueur made with ripe figs and juniper berries, remains a popular choice overseas.

Fruit sage

Salvia dorisiana ● **Giant woolly sage**

There are hundreds of species belonging to the genus *Salvia*, but very little has been written about this spectacular variety with its huge, shocking pink flowers, large leaves and unmistakable fruity scent and flavour. A cousin to *S. elegans* and *S. officinalis*, it endeared itself to gardeners in centuries past, but as more and more hybrids have become available it has sadly been all but forgotten. There is little evidence of its uses in ancient herbals other than as a strewing herb, and because of its fruity fragrance it is sometimes confused with pineapple sage, with its masses of tiny red flowers. If it were not for one little cutting brought into South Africa with a few other botanical specimens for research, fruit sage would not be available here today, and I hasten to resurrect it, as from the tiny cutting in the Herbal Centre trial gardens it has become queen of the winter garden and a favourite in the nursery. It grows 1½–2 m in height and width, with great sprays of fragrant, thumb-length, brilliant pink flowers. Sunbirds adore the flowers for their fruity nectar.

CULTIVATION

Grow fruit sage in full sun in a large, compost-filled hole. It needs protection during very cold winters and should be pruned back neatly after the early spring flowering period is over. It needs space but can also be potted into large tubs and clipped and trained. On a hot patio the huge velvety leaves are a wonderfully handy insect repellent. Rub the leaves onto chair legs, table tops and benches to keep flies and mosquitoes away. Your guests will be intrigued by the fruity scent.

MEDICINAL USES

The genus name *Salvia* derives from the Latin *salvere*, meaning 'to save', and the name is apt as all species have amazing medicinal properties. Among other things, sage is a valuable digestive aid, a herbal remedy for both animals and humans, and burning sage will clear toxins, bad air and odours.

A tea made from the flowers is an excellent digestive that eases a feeling of fullness, slight nausea, colic and flatulence, and helps you relax. To make fruit sage tea, pour a cup of boiling water over ¼ cup flowers. Leave the tea to stand for five minutes, then strain and sip slowly. It is a most useful relaxing herb and a bunch of leaves and flowers tied up and tossed into the bath will do more to help you unwind than anything else I know. The soothing oils seem to ease aching muscles and rashes and dry, itchy skin. A leaf placed in one's shoe on a long walk will ease tiredness and soothe blisters, and crushed flowers placed over an insect bite and bound in place will take away the redness and itch.

Fruit sage poultice for bruises and strains

Fruit sage leaves
Hot water

Place the fruit sage leaves in hot water for a few seconds, then pat them dry and place them immediately over a bruise, a pulled muscle or a strain, or a tired, aching joint. The poultice will soothe and relax the area.

Fruit sage and almond oil rub for bruises

1 cup fruit sage flowers
3 fruit sage leaves
1 cup almond oil

Simmer the flowers and leaves in almond oil for 30 minutes, stirring frequently. Cool and strain. Pour the oil into a dark bottle and label. Warm the oil before use by standing the bottle in a bowl of hot water. Massage oil gently into the bruised area.

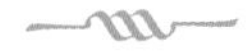

CULINARY USES

Fruit sage dessert whip

SERVES 4–6

2 large eggs, separated
300 ml thick cream
6 tablespoons white sugar
3 tablespoons gelatine
4 tablespoons hot water
300 ml plain yoghurt
Pulp of 4 granadillas
½ cup fruit sage flowers, calyxes removed

In three separate bowls, whip the egg whites; the cream; and the yolks and sugar. Dissolve the gelatine in the hot water and allow it to cool (stand the bowl in iced water).

Add the cooled gelatine quickly to the egg yolks, and then add the yoghurt and granadilla pulp, whisking evenly all the time. Now add the cream and fold in the egg whites. Pour into a glass dish and place the fruit sage flowers in a pretty pattern over the top of the dessert. Chill until set. Decorate with a little spray of fresh flowers as you take it to the table.

COOK'S NOTE

Fruit sage flowers have a sweet, fruity taste. Sprinkle them onto salads and scatter them over desserts and into fruit drinks or use them as an attractive garnish. Remove the calyxes before serving.

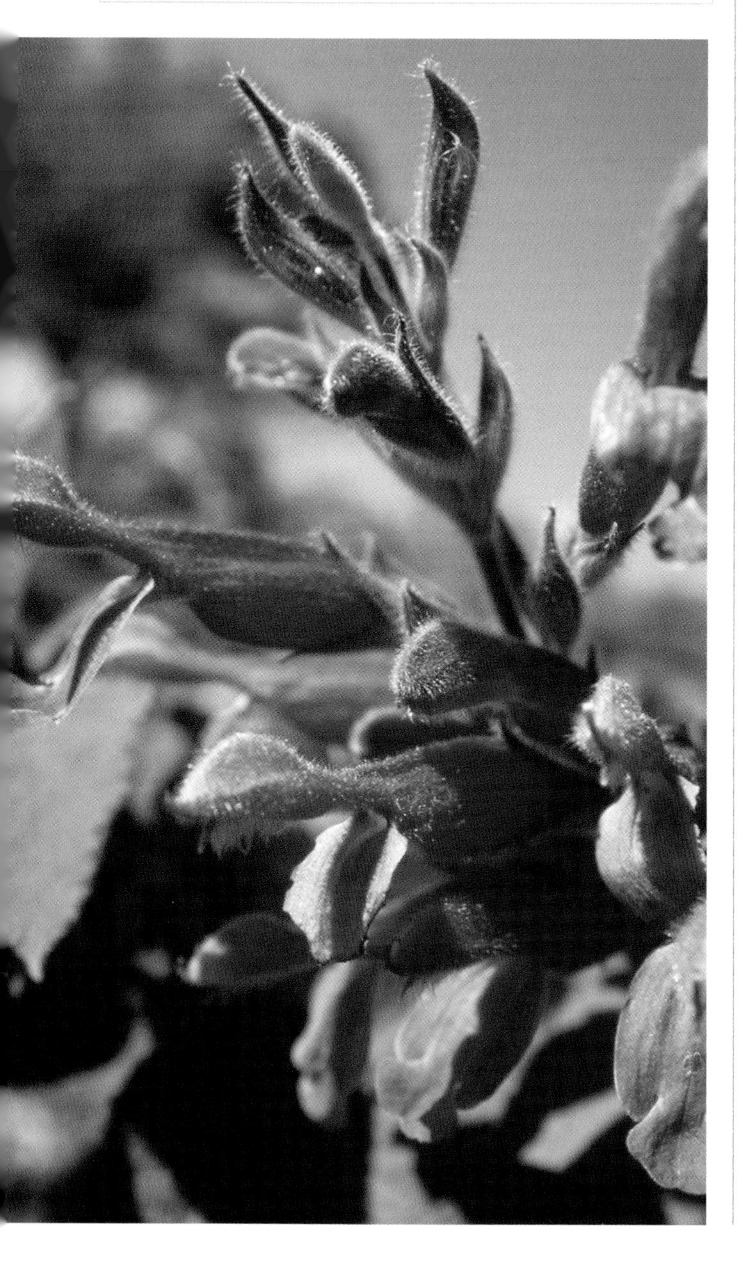

Baby carrots with fruit sage and honey

SERVES 4–6

Large carrots can also be used for this delicious dish but cut them into fine rounds. Serve as a vegetable dish with roast meat or roast chicken.

36 baby carrots, well washed
4–5 tablespoons butter
¾ cup honey
1 teaspoon salt
½ cup sesame seeds
1 tablespoon freshly grated ginger root
Juice of 1 lemon
2 tablespoons chopped fruit sage flowers, calyxes removed

Boil the carrots until tender (use just enough water to cover them). Melt the butter and add all the ingredients except the carrots. Sauté while stir-frying continuously; keep turning the seeds and fruit sage in the butter. Drain the carrots in a sieve until dry and add them to the butter and honey mixture, turning them until they are well coated and just starting to brown. Transfer to a serving dish, and spoon the remaining butter and honey mixture over the carrots. Serve hot.

Roast pork and fruit sage

SERVES 6

This dish is superb for a Sunday dinner and it is equally delicious served cold.

2½–3 kg leg of pork
1 large sheet of tin foil
½ cup honey mixed with 2 teaspoons mustard powder
Sea salt and black pepper to taste
1 cup chopped celery stalks and leaves
½ cup fruit sage flowers chopped, calyxes removed
2 onions, peeled and thinly sliced
2 apples, peeled and thinly sliced

Preheat the oven to 180°C. Trim the pork of excess fat and place on a double layer of tin foil. Spread the honey and mustard mixture over the pork. Sprinkle with salt and pepper, then lay the celery and fruit sage on the roast and cover with the onion rings and apples, and sprinkle with a little more salt and pepper. Wrap up the tin foil tightly so that all the juices are retained. Place in a large baking tray and roast until tender, about an hour and 10 minutes. Serve with roast potatoes, roast onions and vegetables, and decorate with fruit sage flowers. The flowers give an exotic taste to the pork!

Fuchsia

Fuchsia species • *F. corymbiflora* • *F. denticulata* • *F. racemosa*

The fuchsia is native to central and southern America and parts of New Zealand. In 1690 a French missionary priest, Charles Plumice, discovered a fuchsia in Mexico and sent it back to France, naming it after the celebrated Bavarian botanist Leonard Fuchs (1501–1566). Nearly all traces of the plant were lost for the next century, but a few specimens were taken to Kew by a Captain Firth. Years later, in 1793, an avid gardener, James Lee, spotted a flowering fuchsia on a windowsill in London and begged a cutting from the woman who lived there, who had received it from her sailor son. Lee raised the first plant from that cutting, took more cuttings, and established a small nursery that marked not only the beginnings of his fortune, but a new fashion in potted plants.

CULTIVATION

Cuttings can be taken easily and need little attention, simply keep them moist and shaded in boxes filled with sand. Once planted out in semi-shade or full shade, they will give years of pleasure and ask little in return other than a deep watering twice-weekly, or daily if they are in tubs or hanging baskets, and a dressing of peat and wood ash (not coal ash) over their roots in winter. Plants should be pruned back in spring, and can take quite vigorous pruning if they are well established, but they do need winter protection.

MEDICINAL USES

No proper research has been done on the fuchsia's medicinal and culinary values, but in South America the crushed petals and juice from the berries have long been used to treat skin ailments, freckles, small blisters and rashes. The flowers of the New Zealand tree fuchsia (*Fuchsia arborescens*) are eaten and used crushed on bites, scratches and grazes, the pinky juice relieving itching and redness. They are also used in bathing water to soothe inflamed blisters and sunburn.

In rural parts of Scotland, *F. magellanica* flowers are crushed and wrapped around corns or callouses on the feet and kept inside the shoe all day. Fresh flowers can be reapplied at night, held in place with a bandage, and by the next morning the painful corn is something of the past.

A superb fuchsia jelly can be made to relieve sore throats and tonsillitis, to soothe the early stages of a cold, and to strengthen the voice.

Healing fuchsia jelly

This jelly is useful for treating sore throats, tonsillitis, mouth ulcers and gum ailments.

1 cup fuchsia flowers
1 cup fuchsia berries
½–1 cup honey
1 cinnamon stick
Juice of 1 lemon
2 cups water
1 apple, peeled and chopped
2 tablespoons gelatine

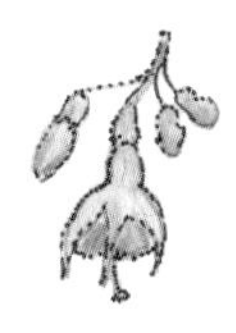

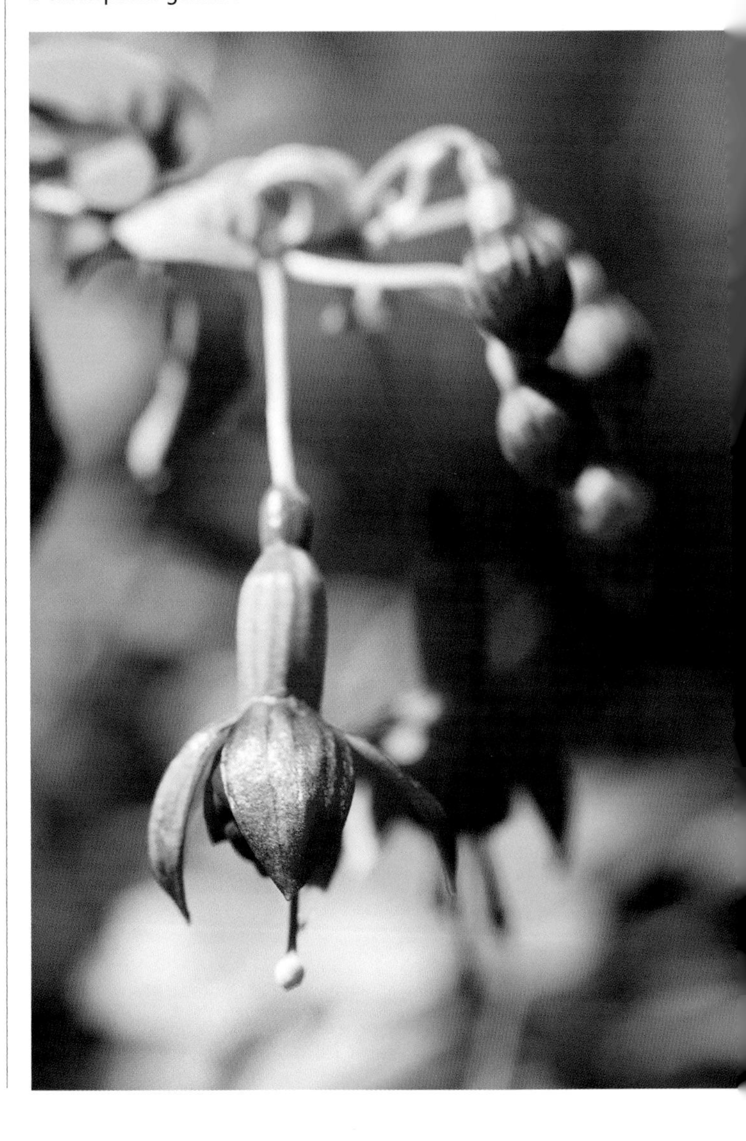

Simmer the flowers and berries with the honey, cinnamon stick, lemon juice, water and apple for 10 minutes. Cool and strain, then add the gelatine dissolved in a little hot water. Allow to set in the fridge. Take a tablespoonful at a time and hold it in the mouth for as long as possible to derive maximum benefit.

CULINARY USES

Cold chicken and fuchsia salad

SERVES 4

This is a superb lunch or picnic dish, and it can be varied with salads in season such as avocados and winter lettuces.

1½ cups good mayonnaise
4 cups diced cooked cold potato
Sea salt and black pepper to taste
1 cooked cold chicken, cut into slices and bite-sized pieces
1 pineapple, peeled and cut into small wedges
3 cups torn fresh spinach leaves
2 cups chopped celery
Juice of 1 lemon
1 cup fuchsia flowers
2 spring onions
4 hard-boiled eggs, shelled and quartered
1 butter lettuce

Mix the mayonnaise into the potatoes, and season. Mix in the other ingredients, except for the fuchsia flowers, spring onions, hard-boiled eggs and lettuce. Line a bowl with the lettuce leaves and pile the mixture into the lettuce-lined bowl and decorate with the eggs, spring onions and fuchsia flowers. Serve chilled, with crusty brown bread.

Fuchsia ice-cream topping

SERVES 4–6

Use this as a topping for ice-cream, rice pudding, sago pudding, mashed bananas or even oats porridge. It is so pretty that served with cream it quickly makes a party piece. For the fresh fruit, use peaches, nectarines, strawberries, mangoes, mulberries or a combination thereof. Select small fuchsia flowers so that you can keep them whole.

3 cups fresh fruit, peeled and cut up
Sugar to taste (about 1 cup)
½ cup water
½ cup desiccated coconut
1 cup small fuchsia flowers

Simmer the fruit, sugar, water and coconut gently in a double boiler, stirring often, until tender and syrupy. Cool. Add the fuchsia flowers and pour the topping over the ice-cream or pudding. Decorate with more fresh fuchsia flowers. For a beautiful summertime party dish, layer ice-cream and the topping and fresh fuchsia flowers in individual tall glasses. Serve decorated with a mint leaf or two and a fresh fuchsia flower, and eat with long spoons.

COOK'S NOTE

I tasted fuchsia petals in a beautiful red pomegranate drink in a London restaurant many years ago – long before pomegranate became the important health food we know today. The whole flower was cut in half, covered with castor sugar and brushed with a pinch of nutmeg. This exquisite flower, decorated in this manner and propped on the edge of the glass completely won me over. It was a delectable combination.

Fuchsia and potato mash

SERVES 4

That familiar comfort food, the mashed potato, can become a party dish if one livens it up with the addition of a few brightly coloured fuchsia petals and a sprinkling of parmesan cheese and aromatic spices.

6 large or 8 medium potatoes
1 tablespoon butter, cut into small pieces
¾ cup hot milk
Sea salt and black pepper
2 teaspoons crushed coriander
1 teaspoon powdered nutmeg
1 teaspoon powdered allspice (pimento berries)
¾ cup fuchsia petals
Parmesan cheese
Chopped parsley
Fuchsia flowers

Peel the potatoes and boil until soft. Drain off the water and mash immediately. Add the butter, hot milk, sea salt and black pepper to taste. Mash until light and fluffy, adding more hot milk if necessary. Fork in the coriander, nutmeg and allspice, and finally, add the fuchsia petals. Pile into a glass serving dish. Keep hot, and just before serving top with a light sprinkling of parmesan cheese and decorate with chopped parsley and fuchsia flowers.

Gardenia

Gardenia jasminoides

The exquisite gardenia, with its waxy white, heavily fragrant flowers and glossy green leaves is native to China, where it has been revered for its medicinal, cosmetic and fragrant properties for over 2 000 years. The Chinese add fresh flowers to the bath, and tie them in muslin with a handful or two of salt to use as a scrub to soften and cleanse the skin. In past centuries, gardenias were cultivated for the empresses of Japan to wear in their hair, for corsages, and for use in the bath. In the cooler months they were cultivated in tubs in greenhouses to ensure their bounty of flowers.

Gardenia flowers are still used in cooking in many rural areas today, and can be added to sugar, drinks, fruit salads, desserts and syrups. To scent tea in the ancient Chinese way, tuck a fresh gardenia flower into a tin of loose tea leaves, close the tin securely and leave it for four or five days, or until the flower dries, while it imparts its heavy, beautiful fragrance to the tea leaves. Flowers tucked into raw rice, oats or sago will impart the same sweet, heady scent.

CULTIVATION

The gardenia is beautiful enough to be a focal point in a frost-free garden, demanding little more than a large hole filled with good alkaline leaf mould or lime-free compost well mixed with peat. It prefers a partially shady spot but will also thrive in full sun, providing it has a bit of afternoon shade. A deep weekly watering is all that is required, and dead-heading of its spring to late autumn flowers. It will do well in a large tub, where it can be kept trimmed into a ball shape. In open ground gardenias will reach a height of up to 2 m and about 1–1.5 m in width, and they benefit from an occasional dressing of peat to keep the leaves from turning yellow.

Propagation is by soft-wood cuttings in spring and hard-wood cuttings in late summer. They provide a mass of blooms, and cut flowers floating in a shallow glass bowl will scent a room for days.

MEDICINAL USES

In traditional Chinese medicine a soothing lotion was made to wash sores, grazes and insect bites. Drink a little of this infusion to relieve flu, to lower a temperature, and to cleanse the liver. Interestingly, ancient Chinese drawings depict the gardenia root, fruit and flowers being used to treat snakebite.

In Indonesia, where the gardenia is grown extensively, the leaves and flowers are made into a tea. To make the tea, add ¼ cup chopped leaves and flowers to a cup of boiling water, leave to stand for five minutes, then strain. This can be taken to ease tight, asthmatic breathing, lower a fever, calm heart palpitations, lower high blood pressure and to ease stress, fear and anxiety. Take half a cup in the morning and half a cup in the evening. Sipped slowly, the warm tea sweetened with a little honey is comforting and relaxing.

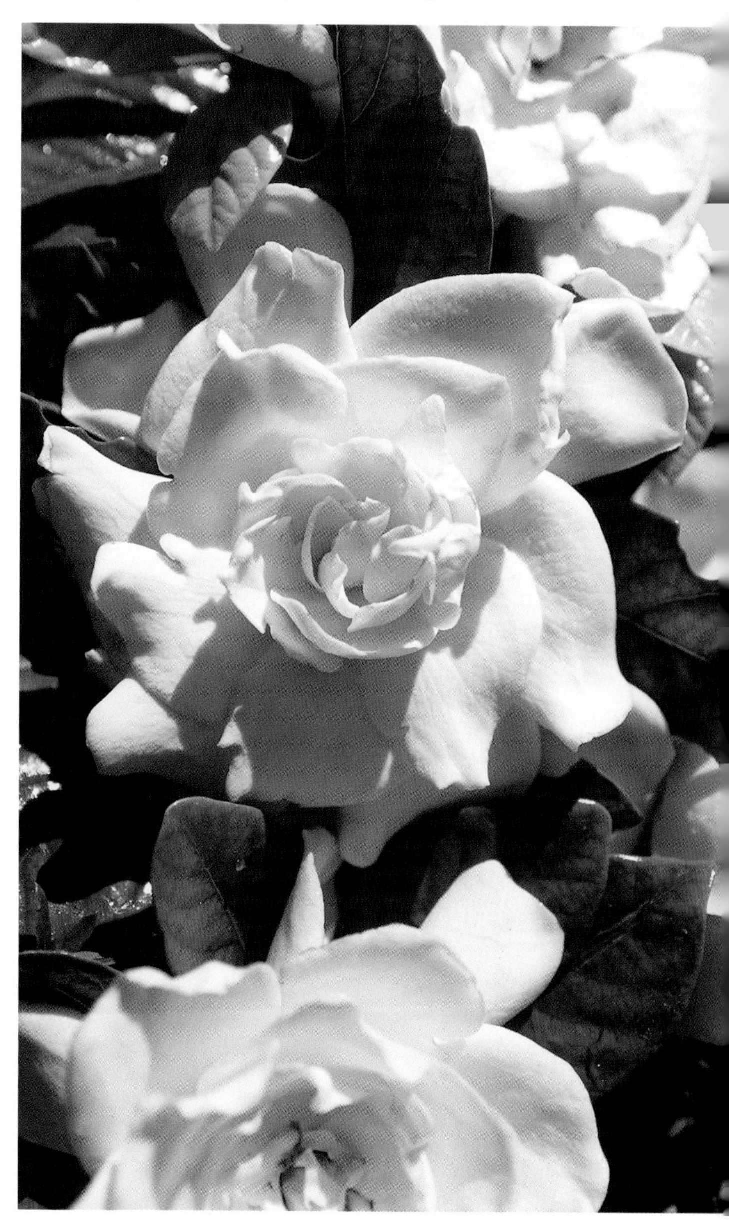

Gardenia lotion

This lotion is soothing on grazes, sores and insect bites.

2 cups mixed gardenia flowers, leaves and roots
2 litres water

Boil the ingredients together for 15 minutes, with the lid on. Cool the mixture a little, strain, and use as a wash on the skin conditions described.

Gardenia flower wash

Use this wash for red inflamed skin, sunburn, windburn and itchy rashes.

1 cup chopped gardenia petals
1 cup aqueous cream
½ cup rosewater

In a double boiler, simmer the petals in aqueous cream and rosewater for 20 minutes. Cool, strain and spoon into a jar. Use a scoopful to wash the affected area. It is immediately soothing. It can also be used on blisters on the feet, over chafed areas and for facial skin problems. Keep the wash on the side of the bath and use for all sore, red spots.

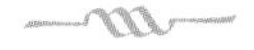

CULINARY USES

Gardenia chocolate mousse

SERVES 6–8

This decadent mousse is food for the gods, and so easy to make.

250 g dark chocolate
4 eggs, separated
2 tablespoons soft butter (at room temperature)
4 tablespoons castor sugar
3 tablespoons dark rum
1 cup cream
4 tablespoons thinly sliced gardenia petals

Break the chocolate into pieces and melt in a double boiler. Whisk the egg whites until stiff. Whisk the butter and sugar together until creamy, then add the beaten egg yolks and rum. Whisk the cream until stiff. Gently combine all together, and finally add the gardenia petals. Pour into a pretty glass bowl and refrigerate. When you are ready to serve, decorate with a sprinkling of gardenia petals and a whole flower in the centre.

Gardenia milkshake

SERVES 1

Energising and nourishing, this exotic milkshake is a meal in a glass and very refreshing on a hot day. Children love to drink it with a straw.

1 glass milk
1 ripe banana
1 egg, well beaten
1 tablespoon honey
6 gardenia petals
1 teaspoon cinnamon

Blend all the ingredients (except for the cinnamon) in a liquidiser. Pour into a glass and sprinkle cinnamon over the frothy top. Drink immediately and feel your energy levels rise!

Gardenia and litchi fruit salad

SERVES 6

This is one of the most exquisite desserts I know, and it is perfect for a special occasion. The litchis are essential to the recipe, but the other fruits can be varied according to what is available or in season, such as mango slices, peaches, grapes, watermelon, kiwi fruit or green melons. Tinned litchis can be substituted for fresh ones.

4 cups peeled, stoned litchis
3 cups mango or peach slices, or other fruit
5–6 tablespoons grape juice
1 tablespoon grated ginger
2 tablespoons castor sugar (or 1 tablespoon honey)
3 gardenia flowers, petals separated
and calyxes discarded
1 cup whipped cream

Arrange the fruit in individual glass dishes with a dash of grape juice. Mix the ginger and castor sugar (or honey) together and sprinkle a little over the fruit. Keep chilled. Just before serving, chop the gardenia petals, sprinkle over the fruit, and top with the whipped cream.

COOK'S NOTE

It is essential to handle gardenia petals with the greatest of care as they turn brown very easily; it is important to prepare and add them just before serving. Sprinkle the petals with lemon juice to prevent them from discolouring.

Garland chrysanthemum

Chrysanthemum coronarium • **Chop suey greens** • **Edible chrysanthemum**

This attractive, bright and easily grown annual is popular in oriental cuisine, and has only recently been introduced to the rest of the world. It has been grown for centuries in gardens all over the East, and in China particularly, for use in stir-fries and teas and for its marvellous medicinal properties. The ancient Chinese used this chrysanthemum as a blood tonic, to help clear toxins from the body and to assist the functioning of the kidneys and bladder. It is a gentle diuretic and also a deodoriser.

The leaves are used extensively in cooking as a chop suey green and big bunches of the pungent, crisp feathery leaves are now sold in markets all over the world. The bright yellow petals are crushed into butter, fat, batters and sauces to lend colour and flavour. Finely chopped raw leaves and flowers sprinkled over stir-fries and rice dishes add a rich, full taste and help to clear the body of toxins, an important benefit if one has eaten food that is too rich or spicy.

CULTIVATION

The garland chrysanthemum likes well-dug, richly composted soil in full sun and a lot of water – a deep soaking at least twice-weekly. It does not do well in the heat of midsummer and is best grown as a winter or cool-weather crop. It will survive frost and cold winds, but does best in a protected area, where it will reach 1 m in height and even in width, with a glorious show of bright yellow daisy-like flowers that go on and on until the heat makes them bolt. Picking of leaves and flowers benefits the plant. Sow fresh seed in trays every February for winter planting and transplant the seedlings once they are big enough to handle. Shade and protect the small plants in the beginning and do not let them dry out.

MEDICINAL USES

A tea made from the leaves and flowers is a gentle diuretic that helps with cystitis and water retention. To make the tea, pour a cup of boiling water over ¼ cup flowers and leaves. Leave the tea to stand for five minutes, strain and drink. One cup a day is sufficient, but in the case of swollen feet, add fennel flowers and leaves and celery leaves, and drink two or three cups through the day.

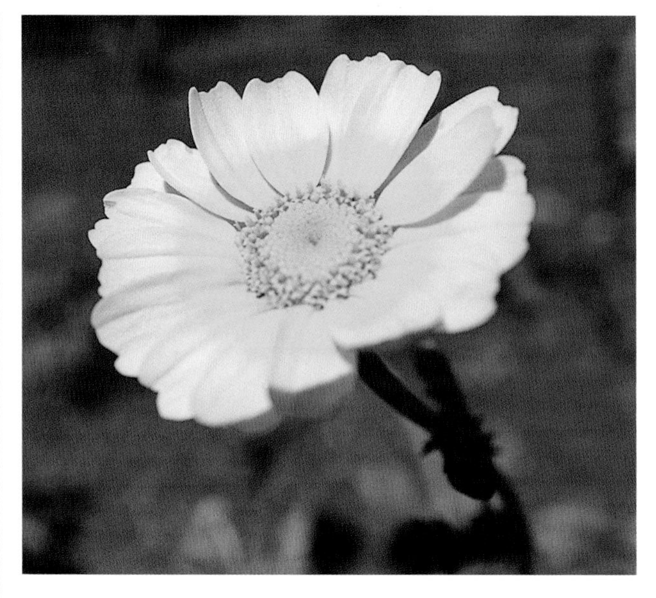

As a tonic herb the garland chrysanthemum is much loved in China as it is rich in minerals, amino acids and vitamins A, D and E. A thin soup can be made as a spring tonic and blood and kidney purifier, and to clear up a lingering cold and clear the chest of mucous.

Garland chrysanthemum tonic broth

Take this broth to purify the blood and kidneys.

1 cup chopped garland chrysanthemum flowering tops
1 cup finely chopped celery
1 cup finely chopped parsley
3–4 cups water

Simmer the ingredients together for 30 minutes to make a thin tonic soup. Take one cup of broth, warmed, two or three times a day. It is quite pleasant. Flavoured with a dash of lemon juice, sea salt and cayenne pepper, this soup will also clear up a lingering cold and clear the chest of mucous.

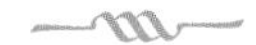

COSMETIC USES

Garland chrysanthemum lotion is excellent for oily, spotty skin, and fresh crushed flower petals, moistened in hot water, can be applied to spots and pimples.

Garland chrysanthemum lotion

This lotion is used to treat oily, spotty skin.

1 cup garland chrysanthemum flowers and a few leaves
1 cup bran
2 cups water

Boil the flowers, leaves and bran in the water for 20 minutes. Allow the lotion to cool, strain, and use it as a rinse after washing the face. Alternatively, use the lotion unstrained as a massage mask over the face to clear oiliness. It leaves the skin feeling soft, refreshed and refined.

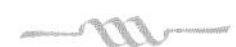

CULINARY USES

Garland chrysanthemum croutons

SERVES 4

Serve sprinkled over a light vegetable soup or as a snack with drinks, or mix into rice and serve with soy sauce.

Sea salt and pepper
2 teaspoons mustard powder
4 thick slices brown bread
¾ cup sunflower oil
1 large onion, cut into rings
2 cups garland chrysanthemum flowers, cut into quarters

Sprinkle salt, pepper and mustard powder over the bread and cut the slices into small squares. Heat the oil in a pan, and gently fry the bread with the onion rings and garland chrysanthemum flowers until they all start to turn golden, turning often. It is easier if you do this in small batches rather than in one go. When the croutons start to crisp, lift them out and drain on crumpled paper towel.

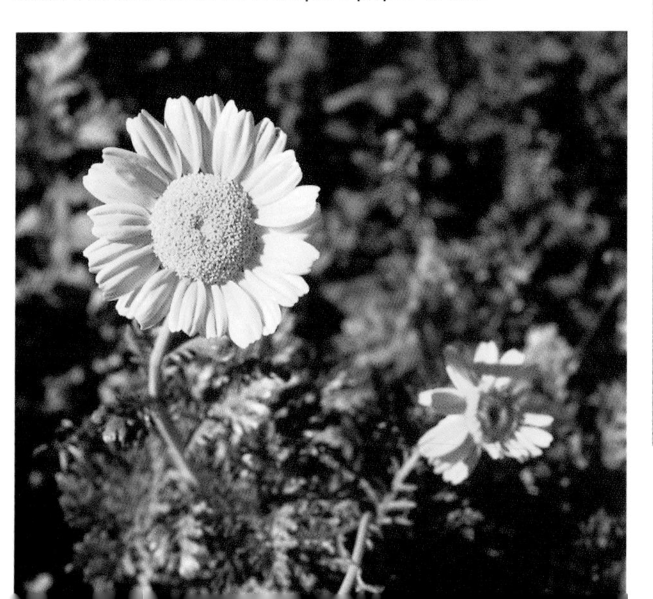

Garland chrysanthemum stir-fry

SERVES 4

The spicy taste of these easy-to-grow flowers gives this basic stir-fry a different taste. Add seasonal ingredients to ring the changes.

1 cup finely chopped onions
Sunflower oil
1 cup thinly shredded carrots
3 cups thinly shredded cabbage
½ cup thinly shredded ginger root
1 cup garland chrysanthemum petals
1 cup garland chrysanthemum leaves
Juice of 1 lemon
Sea salt and black pepper to taste
Dash of soy sauce

Fry the onions in oil until they start to brown. Add the carrots and cabbage and stir-fry briskly. Add the other ingredients and keep stirring until the vegetables are tender but still crisp. Do not overcook. Serve piping hot with rice.

Garland chrysanthemum and apple dessert

SERVES 4

This dessert is delicious on a winter's night and it is quick and easy to make. Serve with custard or cream for a party dish.

6 apples, peeled and cored
2 litres water
1 cup honey

Topping
1 cup garland chrysanthemum flowers, quartered
½ cup butter
1 teaspoon cinnamon powder
1 teaspoon allspice powder
½ cup soft brown sugar
¾ cup pecan nuts, finely chopped
1 cup sunflower seeds

Cook the apples and honey in the water for 15 minutes. To make the topping, gently fry the garland chrysanthemums in the butter, add the spices and stir-fry well. Add the sugar, pecan nuts and sunflower seeds and cook for two minutes. Spoon the cooked apples into a glass dish, sprinkle with the spicy topping and keep hot in the oven. Serve hot with whipped cream or custard, decorated with a sprinkling of garland chrysanthemum petals.

Gladiolus

Gladiolus hybrids

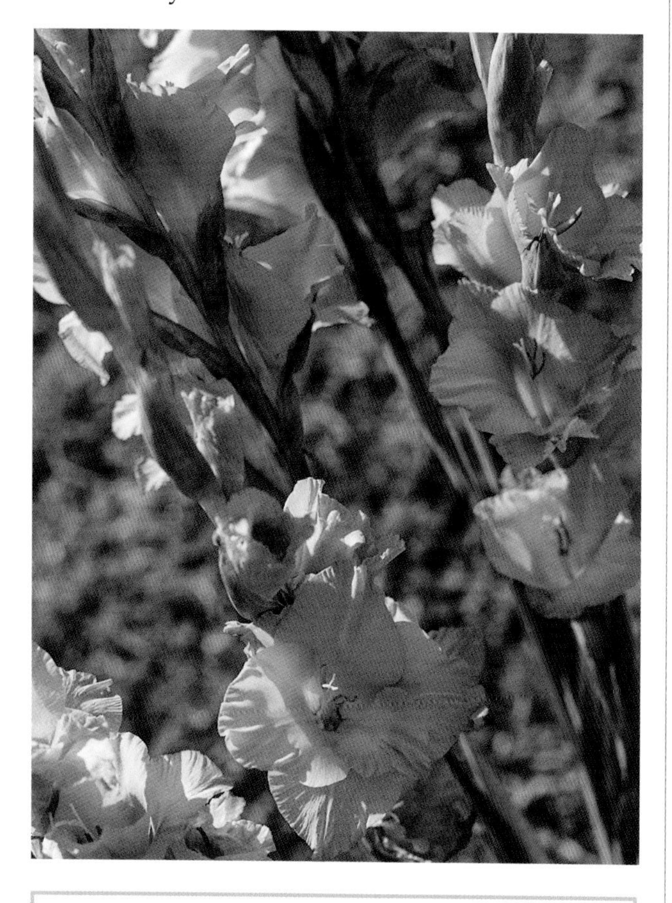

The huge variety of gladioli cultivated today are believed to have descended from the bright orange parrot flower, *Gladiolus dalenii* (formerly *G. natalensis*), which is indigenous to South Africa and was taken to England in the early 1700s. In 1904 one of the engineers responsible for building the bridge that spans the Zambezi River at the Victoria Falls, Sir Frederic Fox, found the pretty *G. primulinus* growing wild in the perpetual spray of the falls and took it to the Royal Horticultural Society in England. From there, Unwins of Cambridge, a long-established seed firm, developed new hybrids using those original corms.

CULTIVATION

I became intrigued by this easy-to-grow plant in the early 1960s, when my mother-in-law grew an acre or two of breathtaking hybrids for the local florists in Rustenburg. I learned how they were packed for transporting – tied onto river reeds in fan shapes so as not to bruise the exquisite opening blooms – and I also learned that one needs to spray for thrips in order to protect the buds. In my world that was not acceptable, so, with the help of a patient farmhand, I began cultivating organically grown gladioli far from her area.

Gladiolus corms need to be planted in spring in deep, richly composted furrows in full sun. The corms must be spaced 30 cm apart, and water needs to flood over them. A long, slow, twice-weekly watering – not just a trickle from a hosepipe – will increase stem length and number of florets. Gladioli need sunlight to form buds. They are not frost-resistant: in cold areas the corms must be lifted in late autumn, stored in straw during winter in a closed shed – no wind or draught on the corms – and then replanted in spring. Large corms should be planted 10–13 cm deep, and smaller ones 7 cm deep, exactly.

In the 1960s gladioli were the favoured cut flower, but today they are seldom seen. In my herb garden I grow the wild orange gladiolus for medicinal purposes and find that it multiplies quickly and easily. Space them 25 cm apart and stake if the flowering spike becomes too heavy.

MEDICINAL USES

Both the corms and flowers of *Gladiolus dalenii* have been used as food and medicine by several African tribes, and several smaller varieties of corms have been roasted in coals and used as a poultice for drawing out boils and abscesses. Throughout the centuries, a drink made by boiling the corms of some gladiolus varieties has been taken by those who overindulged in alcohol. As gladiolus corms can be easily confused with other plants, care must be taken in selecting the right corm. Traditionally, the Zulu and Sotho people have used the corms of wild gladioli, ground down to a fine meal, to treat dysentery, diarrhoea and stomach upsets, and farmers in KwaZulu-Natal make an infusion of the corms and lower portion of the leaves for coughs and colds. Use one dessertspoonful of corms (peeled and finely chopped) and leaves to a cup of boiling water, leave to stand 5–6 minutes, strain and drink.

Gardening in the summer heat, we soon learned that a crushed gladiolus flower would soothe a blister or heal a scratch from the secateurs. Zulu flower-pickers showed us how to crush and squeeze the petals into a tight ball, which they rubbed over their fingernails to strengthen them and prevent them from breaking (the dark red flowers give the nails a beguiling pink tinge!). Gladiolus petals placed in a jar of water and left in the sun for a few hours make a soothing wash for hot, tired feet.

Gladiolus flower lotion for sores

12 gladiolus flowers, chopped
4 cups water
1 piece of bulrush stem and root, the size of a forefinger

Simmer the chopped flowers in water, stirring frequently. Crush the bulrush stem and root and add to the pot. Simmer for 30 minutes. Allow to cool, then strain and use for small cuts, grazes, burns, red chafe marks and mosquito bites.

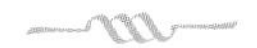

CULINARY USES

Stuffed gladiolus flowers

SERVES 8

This summer starter is real party fare. Choose fully open flowers and remove the sheath of calyx.

2 cups mashed, drained tuna in brine
¾ cup good mayonnaise
⅓ cup sesame seeds
½ cup finely chopped celery
½ cup finely chopped green pepper
Juice of 1 lemon
Sea salt and black pepper to taste
2–4 flowers per guest

Mix the tuna, mayonnaise and the rest of the ingredients well. Spoon teaspoonfuls into each open flower and pat into shape. Arrange the flowers in a circle on a bed of lettuce on a serving platter. Serve chilled with wedges of lemon.

Gladiolus and bean stew

SERVES 6–8

I first tried this tasty stew in the Eastern Cape over 30 years ago. The elderly farm worker who gave me the recipe told me that his grandmother cultivated wild gladioli around their grass hut especially for this purpose. Use any organically grown gladiolus flower. The beans have to be soaked overnight beforehand.

500 g haricot beans
500 g large butter beans
4 large onions, finely chopped
A little sunflower oil
6 large tomatoes, skinned and chopped
1 finely chopped chilli, seeds removed
1 tablespoon crushed coriander seeds
1 cup brown sugar
1 cup brown grape vinegar
1 litre hot water
3–4 cups gladiolus flowers, roughly chopped
1 cup celery leaves
A little parsley

Soak the haricot beans and butter beans in a generous amount of water overnight. The next morning sauté the onions in the oil, then add the tomatoes, chilli, coriander seeds, sugar, vinegar and water. Rinse and drain the beans, and add them. Simmer gently with the lid on, adding more water from time to time and stirring well frequently. When the beans are tender, add the gladiolus flowers, celery leaves and parsley. Simmer for five more minutes. Serve the bean stew piping hot with *stywe* pap, polenta or brown rice.

Gladiolus and avocado open sandwich

SERVES 4–6

This recipe is so quick and easy, and always popular. Open sandwiches can be varied according to ingredients available, but this combination remains a favourite and is spectacularly beautiful.

8 slices dark rye or pumpernickel bread
Horseradish sauce
8 thin slices ham
Cucumber slices
8–10 gladioli flowers, calyxes removed and petals separated
2 avocados, mashed with salt, pepper and lemon juice
1 cup grated mozzarella cheese
1 butter lettuce
Cherry tomatoes
Chopped parsley

Spread the bread with butter, followed by a thin layer of horseradish sauce. Lay the ham on the bread. Place the cucumber slices on top of the ham; then lay the gladiolus petals on top of the cucumber so that the petals form a frill around the edge of the bread. Pile on the mashed avocado, and top with the mozzarella cheese. Arrange the sandwiches on top of lettuce leaves on individual plates with cherry tomatoes. Sprinkle with parsley.

Goldenrod

Solidago virgaurea ● *S. canadensis*

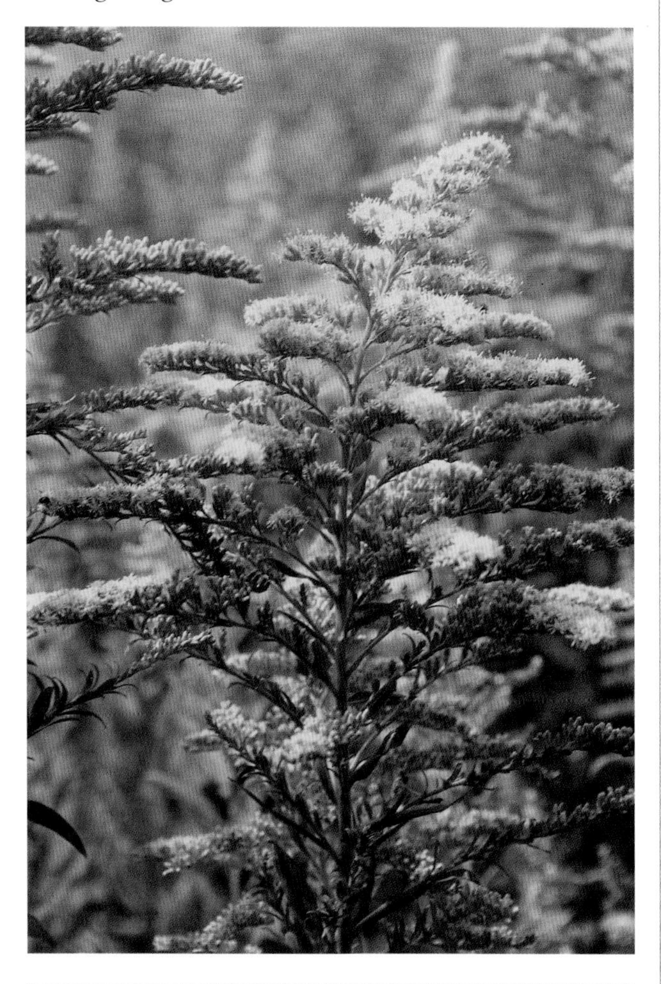

Most species of goldenrod are native to North America and were reputedly spread around the world by soldiers and gypsies. The plant has been used medicinally since ancient times and is cultivated today for herbal and homeopathic remedies. The North American species, *Solidago canadensis*, was brought over to Britain in 1648 by John Tradescant. The European and Asian species, *S. virgaurea*, also known as Aaron's rod, was once called 'wound weed' because it reputedly had wonderful healing properties. Goldenrod's generic name, *Solidago*, comes from the Latin *solido*, meaning 'to join or make whole'. Today many cultivars have been hybridised from those original species. Both these species are the best for medicinal purposes.

CULTIVATION

S. virgaurea, the European variety, is a clump-forming perennial with long, slender-toothed leaves and multi-branched stems about 75 cm long, with tiny yellow flowers that brighten the autumn border. A waste-ground weed, it will grow in any soil as long as it is in full sun. All it needs is a barrow of compost every spring, a deep weekly watering, and literally no other attention; however, cut back the spent flowering spires in winter and divide the clump occasionally.

S. canadensis is the tall flowering variety and forms a spectacular clump. Its flowering spires reach over 1.5 m in height; like *S. virgaurea*, it requires a deep weekly watering, full sun and a good amount of compost each spring.

MEDICINAL USES

It is the flowers of the goldenrod plant that have medicinal value; the flowers can be dried on brown paper in the shade and stored in airtight jars for winter use. They have diuretic, antiseptic and anti-inflammatory properties, and are an important anti-oxidant. They are effective in relieving urinary tract ailments, from cystitis to more serious conditions such as kidney stones and nephritis. They also help to relieve backache caused by kidney conditions, and they ease arthritis. Goldenrod's saponins act specifically against the *Candida* fungus, which causes oral and vaginal thrush, and it is a valuable herb for chronic sinusitis and nasal catarrh. It has a mild yet thorough action and is helpful in treating gastroenteritis and diarrhoea in both adults and children. Recent research has found that goldenrod reduces hot flushes significantly during menopause. With this amazing array of healing properties we should all be growing goldenrod!

As a general tonic and as a treatment for any of the above ailments, goldenrod health tea is wonderfully soothing. For acute conditions, take up to three cups through the day, while for chronic conditions take no more than one cup daily. Make the tea fresh every time. The honey and cayenne pepper can be left out if preferred.

Goldenrod health tea

SERVES 1

1 cup boiling water
3 cups flowering goldenrod sprigs
2 cloves
1 mint leaf
Honey to taste
Tiny pinch cayenne pepper

Pour the boiling water over the goldenrod flowers and mash well with a teaspoon. Add all the other ingredients and stir well. After five minutes, strain and sip slowly.

Goldenrod douche

2 cups goldenrod flowering heads,
  or 1½ cups dried flowers
2 litres water
½ cup apple cider vinegar

Simmer the goldenrod in the water for 15 minutes. Allow the mixture to cool for 10 minutes, strain out the flowers, and add the apple cider vinegar. Use the full quantity as a douche, and repeat the process on the next two nights to clear the infection. This brew can also be used frequently as a wash or lotion.

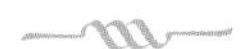

CULINARY USES

Goldenrod and celery health drink

MAKES 3 GLASSES

This is a superb drink for any bladder or kidney ailment, and for cystitis I know no better drink. It is also excellent as a general health builder and detoxifier. It can also be served chilled with freshly squeezed orange juice. As with any herbal remedy, remember to discuss it with your doctor first.

2 cups barley water
2 cups boiling water
1 cup goldenrod flowers
½ cup chopped parsley
1 cup chopped celery
Juice of 1 lemon

Make the barley water by boiling a cup of pearl barley in two litres of water for 40 minutes. Keep topping up and simmer gently with the lid on, then strain.

Pour the boiling water over the goldenrod flowers, parsley and celery. Leave the mixture to stand for five minutes, then put through a liquidiser. Strain, and add the barley water and lemon juice. Drink slowly, either warm or cold. During acute infections, such as an acute cystitis attack, drink three times a day and add extra water.

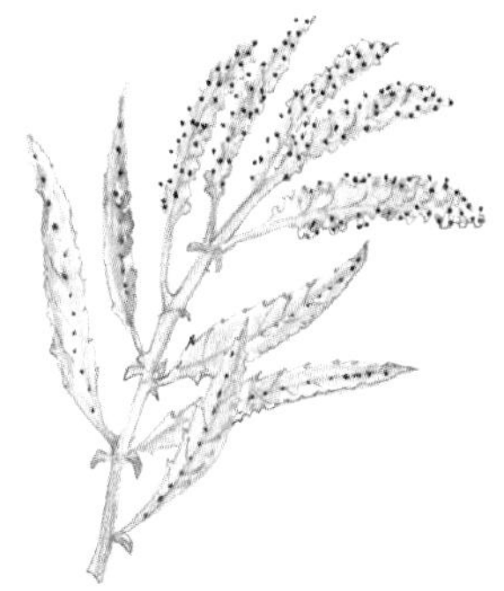

Goldenrod soup

SERVES 6–8

This old American Indian recipe is not only delicious, but health-building too. I make it every autumn when the goldenrod is in flower.

2 cups chopped onion
A little olive oil
2 cups chopped celery
3 cups green mealies, cut off the cob
2 cups grated sweet potato, skin left on
2 cups grated butternut or pumpkin
2 cups chopped green pepper
2 cups peeled, chopped tomato
2 cups goldenrod flowers, pulled off their stems
Juice of 2 lemons
Sea salt and cayenne pepper to taste
2½ litres water

Lightly brown the onion in a little olive oil, then add the celery and stir-fry briefly. Add all the other ingredients, and stir well. Cover and simmer until tender. For a change you can add two cups of mushrooms or two cups of leeks, or replace the water with chicken stock. Serve the soup hot with crusty brown bread. It keeps well in the fridge.

Goldenrod and apple chews

MAKES 15–20

Much loved by children, these round 'chews' are a sugar-free health treat.

1 kg cooking apples
1 cup unsweetened apple juice
1 teaspoon powdered cinnamon
¾ cup chopped stoned dates
½ cup chopped goldenrod flowers and buds
¾ cup chopped pecan nuts

Peel and slice the apples and place them in a heavy-bottomed pot. Add all the remaining ingredients, except for the pecan nuts, and simmer gently over a low heat for three or four hours. Stir frequently and let it melt together to form a thick dough. Scrape the dough into a shallow bowl and leave it to cool, then roll the dough into balls and coat them with the chopped pecan nuts so that they do not stick together. Twist each ball into a small piece of greaseproof paper, ready for the lunchboxes.

Granadilla flower

Passiflora edulis ● *Passiflora* species ● **Passion flower**

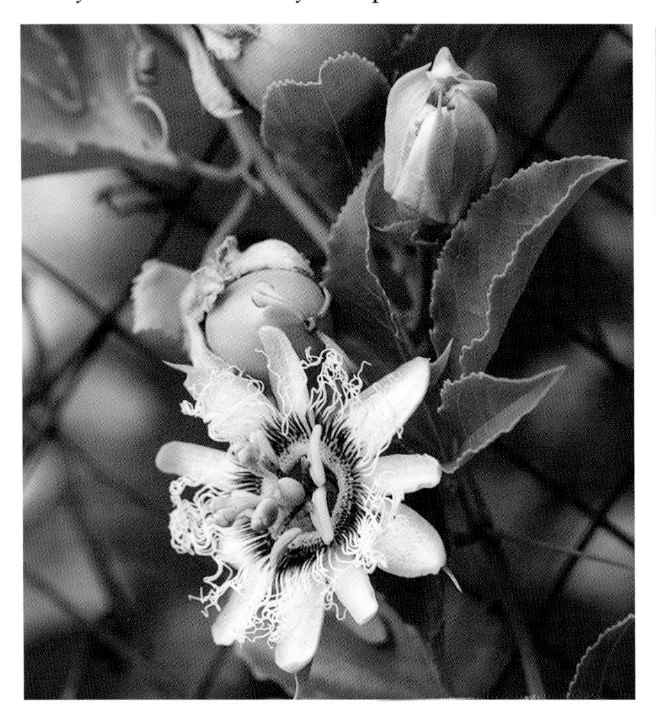

CULTIVATION

The vine needs full sun, a deep, richly composted hole, and a fence or support to grow up. It needs to be protected from winter frost and I usually replace my vines every four or five years. Keep vines lightly tied up and trimmed, apply a seaweed foliar feed every six months, and water deeply twice a week, and you will be rewarded with an abundance of flowers and fruit.

MEDICINAL USES

It is fascinating to know that the fruit, leaves and flowers of the granadilla have been used through the centuries to calm nervousness, to soothe, tranquillise and quieten, and to allay fears and anxiety. For those suffering from insomnia and panic attacks, this plant may prove to be particularly useful. There are about 400 different granadilla species and a number of them have a similar sedative action. *Passiflora incarnata* and *P. quadrangularis* have been found to contain serotonin, one of the main chemical messengers within the brain. To make a calming tea, pour a cup of boiling water over one granadilla flower (calyx and stem removed). Leave the tea to stand for five minutes, then strain and sweeten with a touch of honey. The delicious fruit is also a digestive aid.

Native to America and first recorded in Europe around 1699, the granadilla flower is also known as the passion flower, and is traditionally associated with Christ's Passion. Spanish monks first noted its symbolism, but it was a botanist and physician in the 16th century, Monardes (after whom bergamot, *Monarda didyma*, is named), who first recorded in writing the symbolic interpretation of the flower.

The pillar or column at the centre of the flower was said to represent the cross, with the three stamens inside the column suggesting the Holy Trinity. The five anthers under the stamens were thought to indicate Christ's five wounds when nailed to the cross. Beneath the three stigmas is a small, swollen seed vessel, said to denote the sponge soaked in vinegar that was held up to Christ's mouth. The three stigmas were thought to represent the three nails that pierced his hands and feet, and the calyx was said to represent the halo. The corona of fine tendrils is usually purple; this was believed to depict the crown of thorns stained with Christ's blood, and the 10 petals surrounding the flower were said to indicate 10 of the 12 disciples (excluding Peter who denied him and Judas who betrayed him). The digitate leaves were thought to suggest the hands of the persecutors, and the long green tendrils along the stem the whips that lashed him. The colour purple was thought to symbolise the robe thrown over Christ in mockery, and white the purity of Christ's love.

Calming granadilla syrup

1½ cups boiling water
2 granadilla flowers, green calyx removed
Pulp of 4 ripe granadillas
2 teaspoons honey

Pour the boiling water over the granadilla flowers. Add the fruit pulp, stir well and steep for five minutes. Strain and add the honey. Pour half a cup of the brew at a time and sip slowly. Children enjoy this warm tea, and it settles, calms and unwinds them after a rushed and busy day. Keep excess in the fridge – it will last a day or two – and warm half a cup when needed. I use a small stainless steel double boiler pot to warm special drinks like this.

Hot granadilla insomnia remedy

Monks in the Mediterranean area grew granadilla for treating stress and insomnia, and became known for the 'passiflora remedy', recording it in their pharmacopoeias. 'Passiflora' became a valuable remedy and is still used as a distress remedy all over the world, thanks to those early recordings. Make it fresh every night.

1 granadilla flower, chopped, calyx removed
½ cup unsweetened fresh granadilla juice
¾ cup boiling water
1 teaspoon honey
2 cloves, crushed

Simmer all the ingredients in a double boiler for 15 minutes, stirring frequently. Let it stand for five minutes to cool, then strain it and sip it slowly just before going to bed.

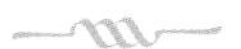

CULINARY USES

Passion flower nectar

SERVES 4–6

At the end of a hot day there is nothing nicer than this relaxing, exotic fruit drink.

1–3 teaspoons honey
1 cup granadilla pulp
2 cups granadilla juice
1 cup granadilla flowers, roughly broken
3 cups chopped watermelon, seeds removed

Put all the ingredients into a liquidiser and blend for two minutes. Pour immediately into glasses with crushed ice, and add a dash of soda or iced water if desired. Top each glass with a luscious granadilla flower and let your guests savour its delicate fragrance.

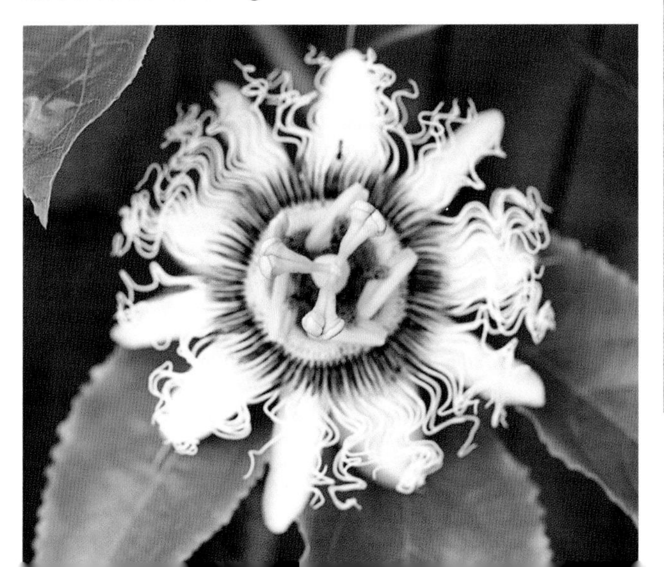

Passion flower cake topping

Bake your favourite sponge cake in a large cake tin or pyrex dish and use this incredible topping instead of icing. The sides of the dish need to be high to hold the topping while it sets.

4 bananas, thinly sliced
1½ cups granadilla pulp
½ cup sugar
2 tablespoons gelatine
1 carton smooth cream cheese
1 cup granadilla flowers

Gently poach the bananas in the granadilla pulp and sugar. Remove from heat and allow the mixture to cool. Mix the gelatine in a little warm water and add to the banana and granadilla mixture. Mix well. Fold in the cream cheese. Discard the calyxes from the granadilla flowers, strip off the petals, chop them up and mix in. Pour the topping over the cake and place in the fridge to set. It should take about an hour. Serve decorated with whipped cream and fresh granadilla flowers.

Passion flower tropical fruit salad

SERVES 6

Make this in midsummer with all the exotic fruits available. Change the fruits according to what is in season.

½ cup sugar (optional)
1–1½ cups granadilla pulp
2 cups papino, cut into cubes
2 cups peeled, cubed mango
2 cups peeled litchis, cut in half
1 cup kiwi fruit, peeled and sliced
1 cup granadilla flowers, cut into quarters, calyxes discarded

Mix about half a cup of sugar into the granadilla pulp if it is too tart. Mix all the cut fruit together gently and place in a glass bowl. Pour the granadilla pulp over the fruit salad. Sprinkle with the granadilla flowers and place a whole flower in the centre. Pipe rosettes of whipped cream around the sides of the bowl, and serve with extra whipped cream or with ice-cream. Wait for the applause!

COOK'S NOTE

The most delicious way of serving granadilla is to use the fruit and flowers together. The monks warmed the flowers in honey and served them with goat's milk yoghurt, with the pulp of the fruit poured over the top.

Hawthorn

Crataegus oxyacantha • *C. monogyna*

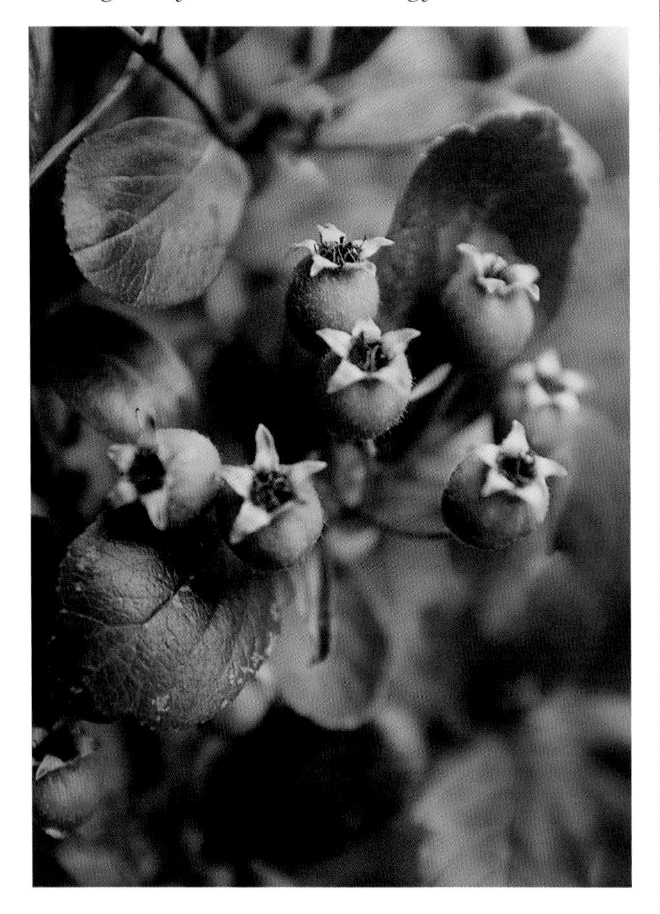

In the Middle Ages hawthorn was a symbol of hope. It is an ancient herb, indigenous to the British Isles and Europe, where it still grows in hedgerows today. It makes a charming tree, spectacular with its heady white blossoms in spring, its glossy green leaves in summer, and its brilliant red berries in autumn and early winter.

Medicinally, only two species, *Crataegus oxyacantha* and *C. monogyna*, may be used. Many hawthorn species with red berries are for sale in nurseries, so it is important to get the correct species if you are planning to use them in a home remedy.

CULTIVATION

Hawthorn is slow-growing; it will reach about 8 m in height if left unchecked, or it can be pruned and trained to form a superb hedge or boundary, or trimmed as a specimen tree. All hawthorns do best in cold areas, withstanding icy winters, frost and even snow, but they are also able to adapt to hot areas. In Europe a new hawthorn called *C. azarolus*, or 'azarole', has been hybridised, the fruit of which is more appetising and makes a good jam.

MEDICINAL USES

Hawthorn is used principally for circulatory and heart ailments such as angina, heart strain and coronary disease as it has antispasmodic and sedative properties and it is an effective vasodilator. It normalises both high and low blood pressure by regulating the action of the heart. Excellent for stress and heart tension, it helps hearts weakened by age, and is also helpful for nervous heart problems, irregular heartbeat and arteriosclerosis. Historically it has also been used to help remove kidney and bladder stones, for treating diarrhoea, and as a diuretic. The bark has been used to treat malaria and other fevers, and although the tiny red berries are not very appetising, they are perfectly palatable, and like the flowers, they are important for heart ailments and circulation.

Crushed hawthorn flowers and buds or crushed hawthorn berries are excellent in a cream for poor circulation and chilblains. Hawthorn flower tea is marvellous to help you unwind, to ease tension and anxiety, and to help lower high blood pressure. To make the tea, pour a cup of boiling water over one tablespoon of fresh hawthorn flowers plus one or two hawthorn leaves. Allow the tea to stand for five minutes and strain. Sweeten with honey if desired, and sip slowly.

Hawthorn flower de-stressing drink

This precious drink remains one of the original favourites going back to medieval times. The flavoured honey can be made in spring, when the plant is in flower.

Clusters of hawthorn flowers
1 jar of runny honey (citrus works particularly well)
¼ cup crushed hawthorn berries
Boiling water

Press the flowers into the honey jar using a long spoon. It will keep for many months, so make several jars. In late summer and autumn, fill a quarter of a cup with the crushed berries. Fill the cup with boiling water and sweeten with the hawthorn flower honey. Stir well and sip slowly. Preserve the hawthorn berries in the same way as the flowers.

Hawthorn cream

Use this cream for chilblains and poor circulation.

1 cup hawthorn flowers, buds or fruit
1 cup aqueous cream
10 drops rose geranium oil
2 teaspoons vitamin E oil

Simmer the hawthorn and aqueous cream in a double boiler for 20 minutes. Strain and add the rose geranium oil and vitamin E oil. Store in a sterilised jar and use as a massage cream on hands and feet after a hot bath.

Sage and hawthorn flower tea for menstrual problems

SERVES 1

1 cup boiling water
¼ cup fresh mixed sage and hawthorn buds and flowers, plus 1 or 2 leaves of each plant

Pour the boiling water over the flowers. Leave the tea to stand for five minutes, stir well, strain and sip slowly. It will ease bloating and premenstrual tension, regulate oestrogen flow, ease menstrual and menopause problems, and slow down a racing heart.

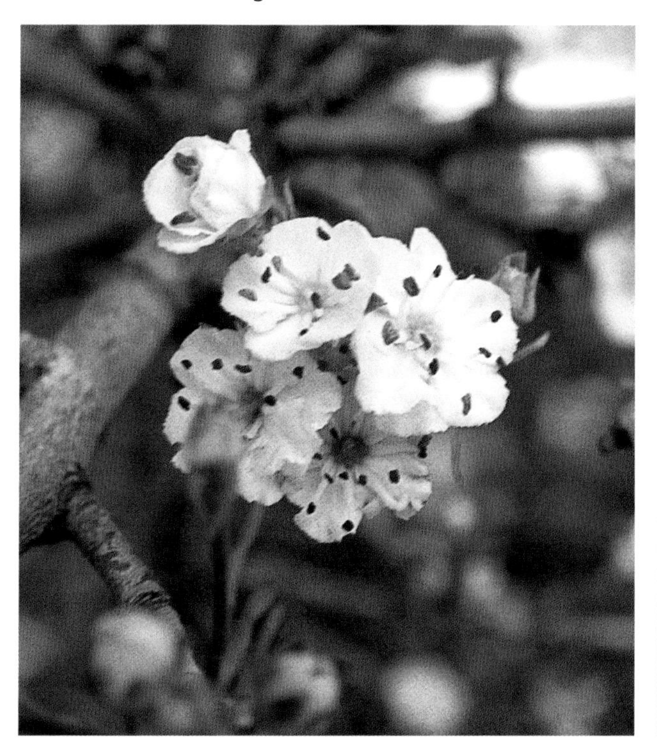

CULINARY USES

Hawthorn pancakes with lemon curd

SERVES 4–6

This is a delicious teatime treat and so quick to make in spring when the flowers are abundant.

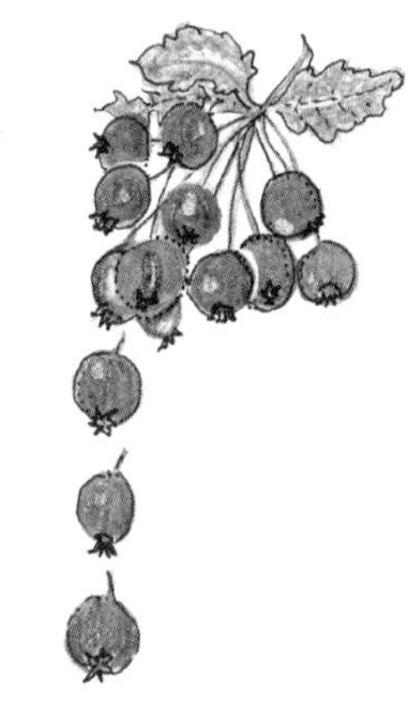

Sunflower oil
1 egg
1 cup milk
2 cups cake flour
A little water
½ teaspoon sea salt
1 cup hawthorn buds and flowers, pinched off their stems
Lemon curd

Heat a little oil in a large flat pan. Whisk the egg into the milk. Whisk the flour into the egg and milk mixture with a little water to make a runny consistency. Add the sea salt and the hawthorn buds and flowers. Drop a spoonful or two of the batter at a time into the pan and tilt it so that the batter is thinly spread. As soon as the pancake bubbles, flip it over. When it is done, slide it onto a plate. Spread with lemon curd, roll it up and keep it hot. Add a little cream when serving and decorate with fresh hawthorn flowers.

Chicken and hawthorn flower stir-fry

SERVES 4

This is a delicious supper dish that takes so little time and effort to prepare; I make it when the spring blossoms are at their best. The chicken breasts are easiest to slice when semi-frozen. You can substitute thin slices of beef or mutton for the chicken.

3 skinless chicken breast fillets, thinly sliced
2 leeks, thinly sliced
2 cups thinly sliced button mushrooms
1 cup thinly sliced celery
1 peeled, grated apple
1 cup hawthorn buds and flowers, stripped off their stalks
A little olive oil
Sea salt and black pepper
Fresh lemon juice to taste

Brown the chicken and leeks, then add the remaining ingredients, stirring continuously. Once the chicken is done, spoon the stir-fry onto a bed of brown rice, decorate the plate with fresh hawthorn blossoms all around, and serve hot.

Hollyhock

Alcea rosea

The common hollyhock is native to China and was taken to Europe in the 16th century, where it became a much-loved cottage garden plant. Known as 'holyoke' or 'beyond-sea rose', it was grown far and wide for its medicinal properties, as a dye, as well as for its edible flowers. Monks in Europe used the darker red petals of the spectacular flowers to colour wine and medicines, and the flowers were added to batters, soups and stews as a health-giving, soothing tonic.

CULTIVATION

The hollyhock is easy to grow, and seeds are available in nurseries and in seed catalogues worldwide. All that is required for a spire of breathtaking flowers is a well-dug, richly composted spot in full sun. Sow the seeds directly into the ground where they are to grow, 75 cm apart, and keep them moist and shaded. Hollyhock has a long tap root and does not like to be transplanted, but very small plants can be relocated quickly, provided that they are immediately submerged in water once they are removed and then kept moist and shaded in their new positions for a week or two. The hollyhock is supposedly a biennial, but I find that it mostly does better as an annual. In warm areas the tall flowering spire is quick to mature, and during midsummer it makes an eye-catching display in the border.

MEDICINAL USES

The hollyhock has a soothing effect on the mucous membranes and is useful for treating coughs, colds and bronchitis. Hollyhock species have been used since 300 BC to treat earache due to chronic catarrh, and hay fever with catarrh and allergic rhinitis. Hollyhock counters excess stomach acid, peptic ulcer pain and soothes and eases gastritis, irritable bowel syndrome, diverticulitis, colic and even diarrhoea.

A warm, comforting tea made from hollyhock flowers will ease cystitis and frequent urination. The leaves and root are also used, and its close cousins, the marshmallow, *Althaea officinalis*, and the common *Malva sylvestris*, are used in the same way. To make hollyhock tea, pour a cup of boiling water over one hollyhock flower. Leave the tea to stand for five minutes, strain, sweeten with honey and add a squeeze of lemon juice. Sip one cup daily as a treatment for all the above conditions. In the 16th and 17th centuries hollyhock tea was popular for easing irregular menstruation, for spongy gums (used as a gargle and as a tea), and to dissolve 'coagulated blood from falls, blows and knocks'.

As a lotion used for washing and as a douche, hollyhock has a soothing effect on tender, inflamed skin, and it will soothe rashes, boils and even abscesses.

Hollyhock lotion for inflamed skin and boils

4–6 hollyhock flowers
2 litres water
½ cup apple cider vinegar

Boil the flowers in the water for 10 minutes, strain and add the apple cider vinegar. Use as a wash or douche to soothe tender skin, abscesses, rashes and boils. A warm poultice can be made by soaking a towel in the brew and placing it over the boil or abscess. Repeat twice a day.

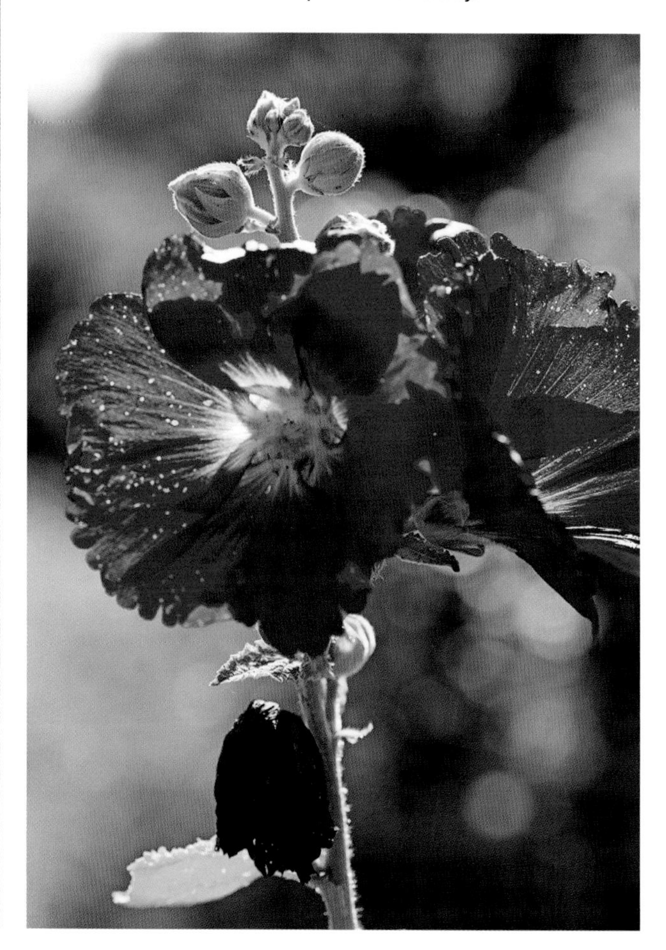

CULINARY USES

Hollyhock summer fruit salad pancake

SERVES 4–6

1 ripe orange-fleshed melon (spanspek) or green melon, cut into cubes
1 pineapple, thinly sliced and cut into cubes
2 cups grapes, seeded
2–3 cups mango, peeled and cubed
2 bananas, thinly sliced
Juice and pulp of 6 granadillas
Petals from 6 hollyhock flowers, calyxes discarded

Pancake batter
2 cups flour
1 cup milk
1 cup water
2 beaten eggs
Pinch salt

Mix all the fruit together and set aside. Whisk the pancake ingredients together well. Heat a little oil in a large pan, pour in about half a cup of batter and tilt the pan to spread it thinly. Flip each pancake over to cook the other side. Place the pancakes on individual plates, top with spoonfuls of the fruit salad, decorate with whole hollyhock flowers and serve dusted with icing sugar and whipped cream.

Hollyhock scones

MAKES 10 SCONES

This is a quick recipe and a favourite Sunday afternoon treat.

2 cups cake flour
Pinch salt
1 tablespoon baking powder
5 tablespoons butter, coarsely grated
4 tablespoons sugar
½ cup milk
2 eggs
½ cup granadilla pulp
6 hollyhock flowers

Sift the flour, salt and baking powder into a large bowl. Rub in the butter until the mixture resembles fine bread crumbs. Dissolve the sugar in the milk. Whisk the eggs into the milk and sugar until creamy, add the granadilla pulp and whisk well. Add to the flour mixture and mix lightly to form a ball. Turn onto a floured board and pat out to 2 cm height. Cut round shapes with a pastry cutter.

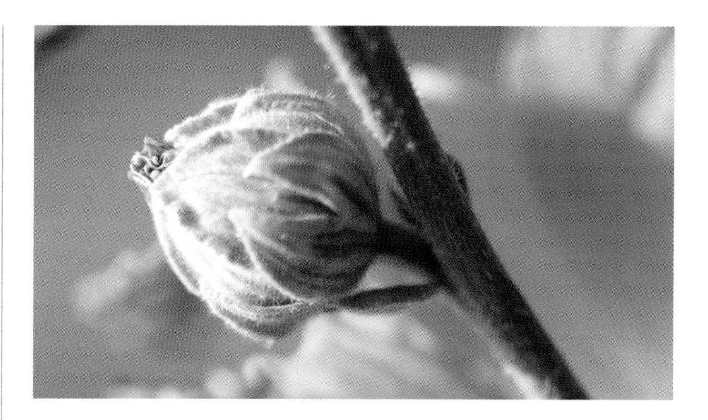

Place on a floured baking sheet and bake at 180°C for about 10 minutes or until the scones begin to turn golden. Cool slightly. Split the scones, spread with butter and a hollyhock flower (remove the calyx) or a few petals. Dust with icing sugar and decorate the plate with hollyhock flowers. You can spread the scones with strawberry jam or honey before topping with the hollyhock petals.

COOK'S NOTE

Hollyhock flowers are delicious added to green salads and fruit salads, whisked into drinks and used to decorate puddings. Cooked in syrup, they make a delicious sauce over rice and sago pudding.

Hollyhock and green bean salad

SERVES 4–6

4 cups young green beans
1 large onion

Dressing
1 cup plain Bulgarian yoghurt
½ cup fresh lemon juice
½ cup honey
½ cup chopped spring onions
2 teaspoons mustard
Hollyhock flowers
Chopped parsley

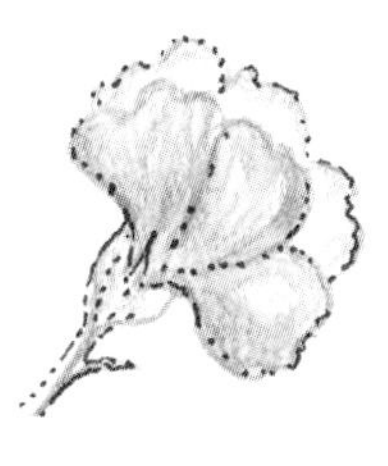

Top and tail the beans and simmer in salted water until tender. Strain and cool. Slice an extra-large onion into fairly thick rings. Place a handful of beans through each onion ring and place on individual plates – the bean bundles should look as though they are neatly tied by the onion. Liquidise the dressing ingredients and pour over the beans. Place two hollyhock flowers over each end of the beans. Sprinkle with parsley and serve chilled with cold chicken or cold meat.

Honeysuckle

Lonicera species • **Woodbine**

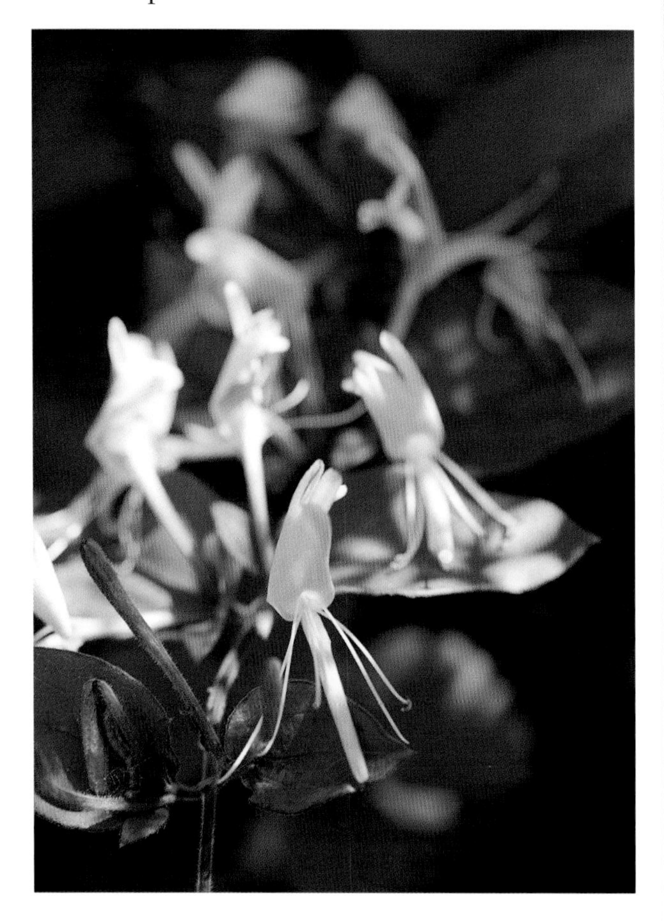

Also known as woodbine, honeysuckle is a perennial evergreen climber, native mainly to Europe and the Caucasus, but some species are also found wild in North Africa, North America and western Asia. There are many kinds of honeysuckle, all of which are exquisitely fragrant, and all with similar medicinal properties. The genus was named in the 16th century by a German physician, Lonicer, who strongly advocated its medicinal properties, but monks in Europe had been using honeysuckle for centuries to treat chest ailments, hay fever and homesickness. The most commonly used species are *Lonicera caprifolium*; the pink flowering, more bushy *L. periclymenum*; and in old gardens the winter-flowering, sweet *L. fragrantissima*, a shrubby plant that has tight, stalkless clusters of creamy white flowers on bare branches.

CULTIVATION

I grow honeysuckle over fences and arches and place shaded benches nearby, where one can sit and enjoy the glorious scent. It goes on undemandingly year after year, scenting the hot summer days and nights with its heady fragrance. An arch of honeysuckle over a gate was an old tradition in rural gardens as a blessing for all who entered. Easy to grow, all it needs is a deep, well-composted hole, a good strong support and a deep weekly watering. I tie and wind in the tendrils continuously and every winter tidy up the thick growth. New plants can be propagated by merely pulling up rooted runners and replanting them, keeping them moist until they root well. Honeysuckle is tolerant of adverse conditions, and will thrive in spite of heat, drought, bitter winter winds and even neglect.

MEDICINAL USES

Honeysuckle flowers have emollient, expectorant and antispasmodic properties, and crushed and pounded in a gentle cream, they make a soothing, pain-relieving treatment for swollen, aching haemorrhoids. Made into a lotion, honeysuckle quickly soothes skin inflammations, aches and dry rashes.

For a heart tonic, and to help relieve asthma, hay fever and rheumatism, an ancient remedy was to take a cup of honeysuckle tea and eat honeysuckle flowers once a day for a period of 10 days. To make the tea, pour a cup of boiling water over ¼ cup fresh flowers. Allow the tea to stand for five minutes, then strain, sweeten with honey and sip slowly.

Recent research has found honeysuckle flowers, and to an extent the leaves, to be outstanding in the treatment of colitis. I have made honeysuckle syrup for many years and keep it as a standby for coughs, chills, sore throats, runny noses, tight chests and exhaustion. It is an old-fashioned remedy but works as well today as it did in our grandmothers' day.

Honeysuckle cream for haemorrhoids

1 cup honeysuckle flowers
½ cup pennywort leaves (*Centella asiatica*)
1 cup aqueous cream
1 teaspoon vitamin E oil

Simmer the honeysuckle flowers and pennywort leaves in the aqueous cream in a double boiler for 20 minutes, stirring frequently. Stand for 15 minutes to cool, then strain. Discard the pennywort leaves and add the vitamin E oil. Mix well, then spoon it into a sterilised jar with a well-fitting lid.

Honeysuckle lotion for sunburn, dry rashes and eczema

2 cups flowering honeysuckle sprigs, leaves included
2 litres water

Boil the flowering sprigs in the water for 20 minutes. Cool and strain. Use as a splash, lotion or as a spray in a spritz bottle for skin inflammations, sunburn, rashes and eczema.

Honeysuckle cough syrup

2 cups honeysuckle flowers and buds
2 teaspoons aniseed
1 tablespoon fresh lemon thyme sprigs
Juice of two lemons
2 teaspoons lemon zest
about ½ cup honey
½ cup stevia flowers
500 ml water

Simmer the ingredients gently for 15 minutes with the lid on. Remove from the heat and allow the mixture to cool. Strain, and discard the herbs. Pour into a bottle with a tight-fitting lid and keep in the fridge. Take one tablespoon of the syrup in about ¾ cup hot water twice a day, the second dose preferably just before going to bed.

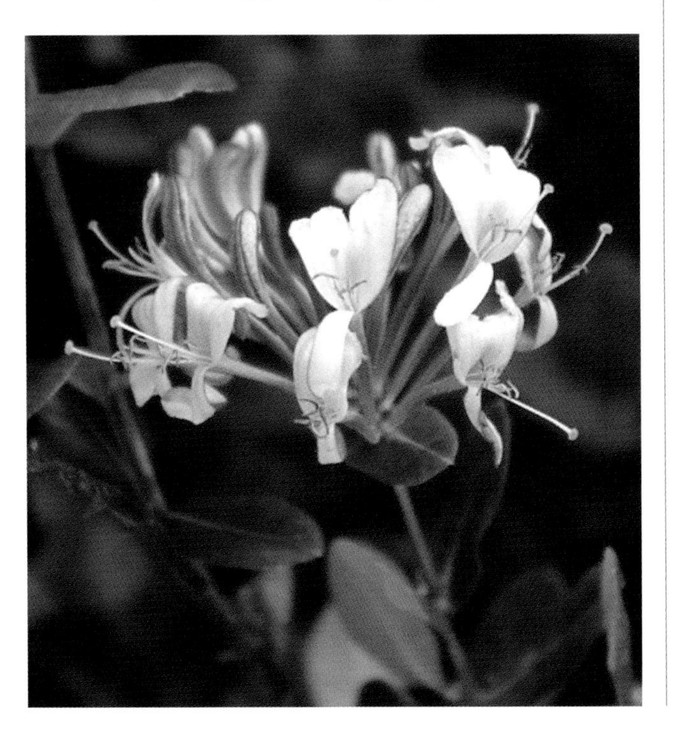

CULINARY USES

Honeysuckle energy drink

SERVES 1

This is an excellent exam-time drink that will give energy and a sense of wellbeing. It is also nourishing for invalids and for those who are overworked and overtired. Make it fresh every time and do not let it stand.

1 egg
1 tablespoon honey
1 tablespoon sunflower seeds
1 banana
1 cup milk
1 tablespoon chopped almonds
½ cup honeysuckle flowers

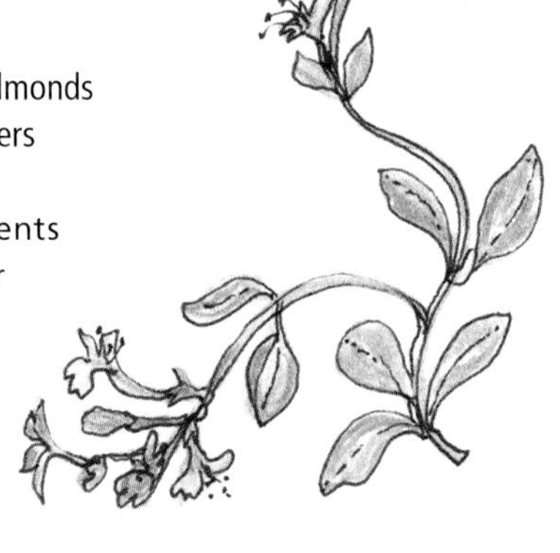

Whisk all the ingredients together in a blender for three minutes. Pour into a glass and drink immediately, sipping slowly.

Honeysuckle fruit salad

SERVES 4–6

1 pawpaw peeled, seeded and diced
Juice of 2 oranges
4 ripe guavas, peeled and grated
2 ripe bananas, peeled and diced
2 cups sultana grapes, seeds removed
2 Golden Delicious apples,
  peeled and grated
1 cup honeysuckle flowers

Mix all the ingredients together in a glass bowl. Dribble a little honey over the fruit salad and sprinkle with honeysuckle flowers. Serve chilled with custard, whipped cream or ice-cream.

> COOK'S NOTE
> **Grow honeysuckle near the kitchen and pick the flowers for salads, fruit salads and stir-fries. The buds can be used in pickles with onions and cucumbers. Honeysuckle can even be used in milky desserts. Honeysuckle is a versatile plant.**

Hyssop

Hyssopus officinalis

Native to southern Europe, hyssop is a lovely, free-growing perennial that is a tough yet persistent roadside weed, particularly in the Balkans and Turkey. It loves sunny places and does well in poor, barren soil, preferring roadsides to the garden! The beautiful blue flowers are borne in late summer and are much loved by bees and butterflies.

Once considered nature's cure-all, hyssop has been a revered herb since the earliest times. It was used by the ancient Greeks for purifying temples and for the cleansing of lepers. It is mentioned in the Bible: 'Cleanse me with hyssop and I shall be clean' (Psalm 51 v. 7). Over the centuries people have thought that this reference could have been to oreganum, marjoram or winter savory, but it is now believed that it probably refers to the same hyssop we know today, as modern research has found that the mould that produces penicillin grows on hyssop leaves. This could have acted as antibiotic protection for lepers when they were bathed in hyssop.

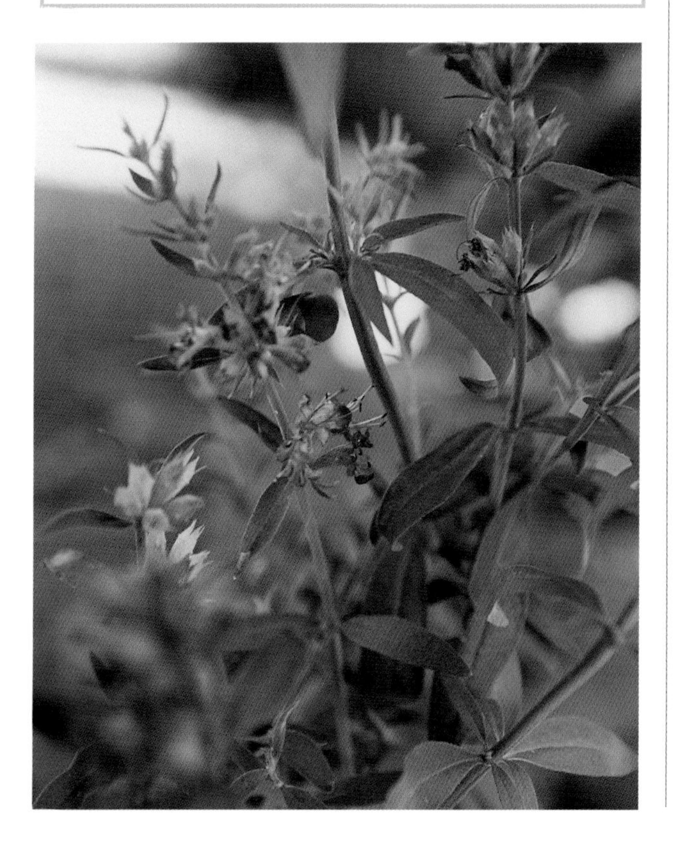

CULTIVATION

I do not find hyssop particularly easy to grow, as my hot mountainside garden is too taxing for it, but it does do well if it likes the spot. It is a short-lived perennial, and full sun, lightly dug soil and not too much attention or water seem to be all that it requires. You will be rewarded with 30-cm-high flowering spikes and an equal spread. Cut off the spent flowers from time to time. New cultivars in Britain range from white through to pale blue and pink flowering spikes, and all seem to have similar properties. Propagation is by seed and by means of small cuttings taken from around the base of the plant. In the hot area where I live, I find that it does best with afternoon shade. Hyssop will thrive in the cooler areas of the country with a yearly dressing of compost as it takes light frost and cold winds well.

MEDICINAL USES

The diverse uses of hyssop have earned it a rightful place in folk medicine through the ages; these uses have been verified by modern research. It was prescribed in ancient times for asthma, stomachache, nasal catarrh and pleurisy. Today it has been found to relax peripheral blood vessels and to have significant antiviral properties, particularly with the *Herpes simplex* virus. It is expectorant, anticatarrhal, anti-inflammatory and antispasmodic. It eases chest colds and asthma, clears bronchitis and urinary tract inflammation and is used with figs for constipation. To make hyssop tea, pour a cup of boiling water over ¼ cup flowering sprigs. Let the tea stand for five minutes, then strain. Sweeten with a little honey if desired, and sip slowly.

CAUTION: Do not take hyssop during pregnancy or nervous irritability, as strong doses can induce muscular spasms.

Hyssop cough syrup

1 cup hyssop flowering sprigs
6 cloves, crushed
Juice of 2 lemons
2 teaspoons finely grated lemon rind
2 cups boiling water
½ cup honey

Simmer the hyssop sprigs, cloves, lemon juice and lemon rind in the water for 15 minutes, stirring frequently. Cool for 10 minutes. Strain. Add the honey and mix well. Children love this cough mixture. Give two teaspoons at least eight times during the course of the day.

Hyssop and fig constipation remedy

1 cup sliced fresh or dried figs
(peeled if they are fresh)
1 cup hyssop flowering sprigs
2 cups water

Simmer the fig slices and hyssop flowering sprigs in water in a double boiler for 20 minutes. Cool. Strain it through a coarse sieve or remove the flowers and mash finely. Take two teaspoons with hyssop tea first thing in the morning, and again late morning if necessary.

To make an excellent lotion for cuts, scrapes, grazes and bruises, boil up a handful or two of hyssop flowers and flowering sprigs with an equal quantity of water for 20 minutes. Allow it to cool and then strain it.

CULINARY USES

Hyssop meal-in-one chicken dish

SERVES 4–6

This is a popular, easy-to-make chicken dish that I make on top of the stove in a large cast iron pot. It keeps well and reheats well. The hyssop imparts a delicious, fresh flavour that combines nicely with all the vegetables. To ring the changes, add sliced mushrooms, sliced aubergine and sliced tomatoes.

1 large chicken, cut into pieces or 1 pack chicken pieces
2 large onions, peeled and sliced
Olive oil
2 green peppers, sliced
3 green mealies, cut off the cob
4 large potatoes, peeled and cubed
2 cups peeled, diced carrots
½ cup hyssop flowers
Salt and pepper to taste
Juice of 1 lemon
1 litre chicken stock

Brown the chicken pieces and onion in the oil. Add all the other ingredients and stir, adding the chicken stock last. Simmer with the lid on for about 30–40 minutes, stirring every now and then, or until the chicken is tender. Just before serving, thicken the sauce with a little cornflour mixed with water if desired. Serve with brown rice or crusty bread.

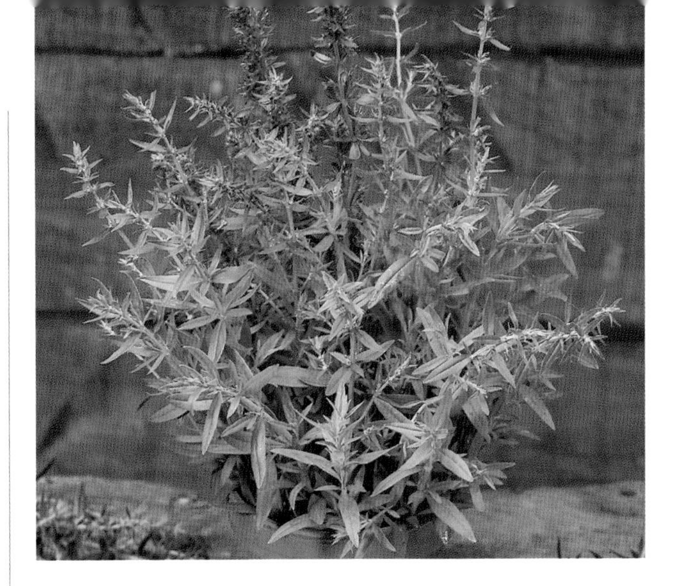

Green hyssop salad

SERVES 4

This salad cleans the palate and is so refreshing that I serve it with any rich meat dish.

3 cups torn or thinly shredded lettuce
2 cups watercress
2 cups chopped celery
1 cup thinly sliced cucumber
½ cup hyssop flowers, pulled off their calyxes
Juice of 1 lemon
Chopped parsley

Toss the lettuce, watercress, celery, cucumber and hyssop flowers together lightly. Sprinkle the lemon juice over the salad and add a little chopped parsley.

Poached nectarines and hyssop

SERVES 4

This is a delicious dessert and very quick and easy to make.

1½ cups castor sugar
2½ cups water
4 large or 8 small nectarines, pricked all over with a fork
½ cup hyssop flowers, calyxes removed

Choose a pot large enough to hold all the nectarines. Boil the sugar and water for five minutes before lowering in the nectarines and hyssop flowers. Turn down the heat, cover the pot, and let the nectarines simmer for about four minutes. Remove from the stove and cool. Carefully remove the nectarines and place them in a glass bowl. Pour a little of the syrup over them and decorate with fresh hyssop flowers. Serve with whipped cream, custard or vanilla ice-cream.

Jasmine

Jasminum officinale • *Jasminum multipartitum*

This exquisite plant, with its sweetly scented, star-shaped flowers, was first introduced to Britain and then Europe via the ancient trade routes from the East in about 1548. The Chinese first used the flowers as a flavouring in tea centuries ago, and later in perfumery.

There are about 300 *Jasminum* species throughout the tropical and subtropical regions of the world. The beautiful Arabian jasmine, *J. sambac*, native to south-east Asia, is also added to ordinary tea and used in Buddhist ceremonies. It flowers all year round and remains a valuable food flavourant. *J. multipartitum* is indigenous to South Africa and its flowers are used in traditional medicine.

All the jasmines grown today have some medicinal, fragrant or culinary use. *J. officinale* is the best species for the perfume industry and for medicinal use.

CULTIVATION

It is only recently that the summer-flowering medicinal jasmine, *J. officinale*, has become available to gardeners in the southern hemisphere, and its more fragile, trainable growth makes it a popular plant for fences and columns, and for pruning and clipping into bushes. It has the additional advantage of flowering all through the summer. Just three flowers in a room will impart a marvellous scent that is soothing, calming and uplifting.

Growing your own jasmine is so easy that no garden should be without it. All the jasmines take full sun to partial shade and require no more than a good twice-weekly watering and a dressing of compost twice a year. Tidying and pruning off the spent flowers is essential to prevent new growth from climbing over the old wood, forming untidy nests.

MEDICINAL USES

Jasmine oil is used to lift depression and ease stress, and has a calming and soothing effect. Ancient Indian and Chinese doctors, herbalists and religious sects used jasmine as a sedative to treat a number of ailments and as a muscle relaxant, usually in the form of a tea or added to oil as a massage for stiffness and soreness. Later, jasmine infusions were added to the bath to release tension and to oils and creams to soothe dry and sensitive skins.

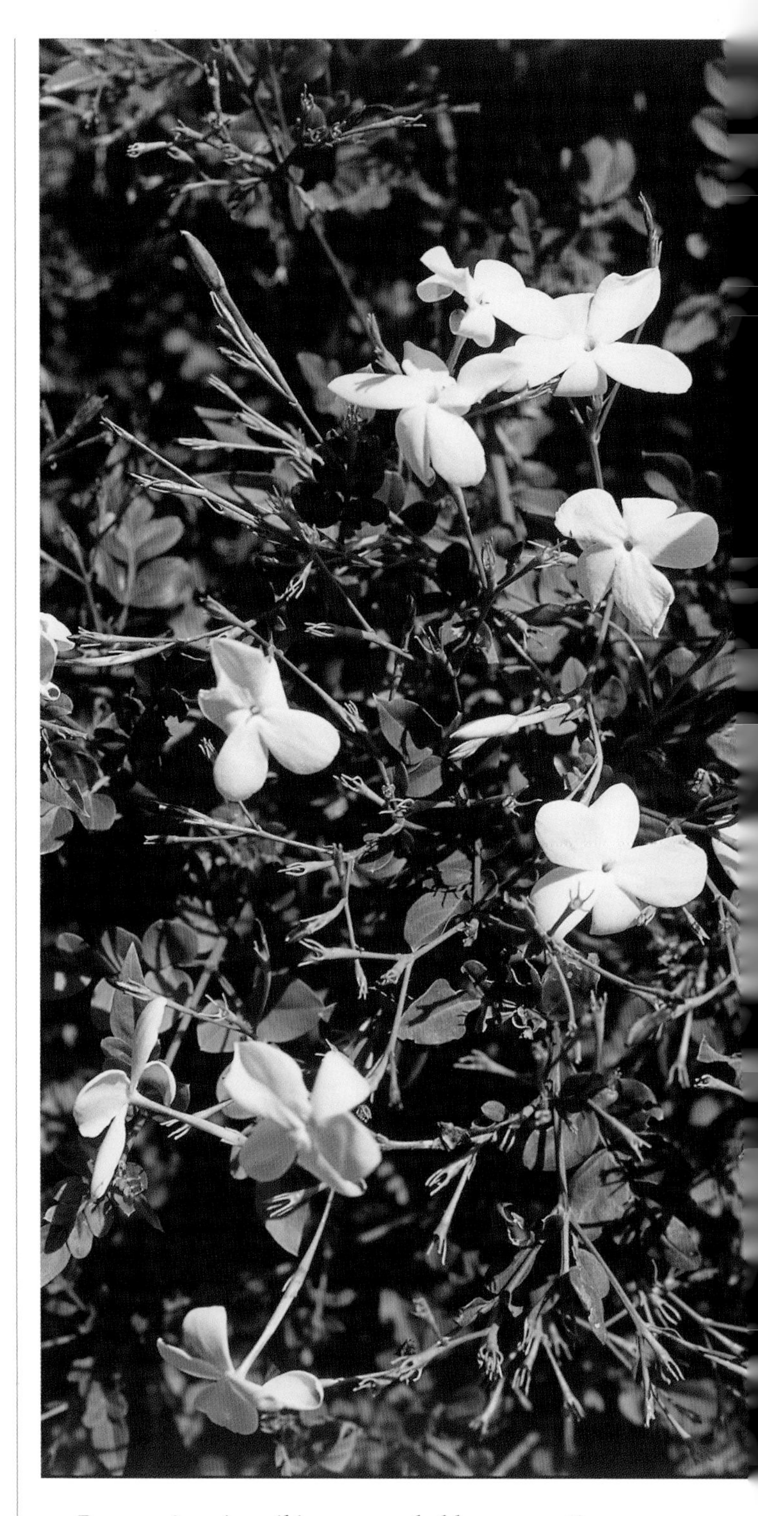

Because jasmine oil is so remarkable as an anti-depressant and for anxiety-related sexual problems in both men and women, it is superb as an aromatherapy massage oil. A few crushed jasmine flowers rubbed on the temples will ease a tight throbbing headache.

CAUTION: Avoid jasmine oil during pregnancy as it is a uterine stimulant.

Jasmine massage oil

An effective treatment for relieving tension, jasmine massage oil can become quite the panacea, and it needs to be made carefully!

1 cup almond oil
2 cups freshly picked jasmine flowers

Put the almond oil and jasmine flowers in a double boiler with the lid on. Simmer gently for an hour, stirring frequently. The oil needs to penetrate the soft waxiness of the flowers, so stirring the flowers together with the oil is vitally important. After an hour, strain using a new sieve. Set the flowers aside and bottle the fragrant oil in a sterilised, dark glass bottle with a well-fitting screw-top lid. To test the strength of the oil, spread a drop or two onto the skin on the inside of the wrist and gently rub it in. If it becomes uncomfortable, itchy or raises a red spot, wash it off immediately with warm water and milk. If the oil is too strong, dilute it with more almond oil or add a tablespoon of the jasmine-infused oil to half a cup of good aqueous cream. Test again until it is comfortable.

Store the jasmine flowers in a screw-top glass jar to use in the bath, just a few at a time. They will be fragrant and rich in oil and will make for a relaxing bath experience. True jasmine essential oil is considered the most precious oil in the world and it is the most expensive of the essential oils!

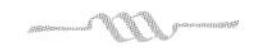

CULINARY USES

Jasmine cordial

Jasmine flowers have been used in cooking for centuries. I was intrigued to find recipes in ancient herbals using the flowers in delicious cordials and syrups. These are refreshing and fragrant, and as a bonus they soothe anxiety and calm restless children. Use only J. officinale *for this.*

1 cup honey
2 cups jasmine flowers, pulled from their calyxes
Juice of 1 lemon
1 teaspoon lemon zest, finely grated
1 teaspoon freshly grated nutmeg
1 litre water

Simmer all the ingredients together for 15 minutes in a double boiler. Remove from heat and allow the mixture to cool. Strain, discard the flowers and bottle the syrup. Take one tablespoon of syrup in a glass of chilled water with crushed ice and sip slowly. As a nightcap, take one tablespoon of syrup in a cup of hot water, stir well and sip slowly.

Jasmine tea

Use J. officinale, J. sambac *(Arabian jasmine) or our own indigenous jasmine,* J. multipartitum. *Use a tin or glass container rather than plastic.*

2 cups fresh jasmine flowers, pulled out of their calyxes
250 g loose Ceylon or green tea
1 airtight cake tin or large glass jar with a good lid

Mix the flowers into the tea leaves in the tin or glass jar, covering the flowers completely with the tea leaves. Seal and leave undisturbed for five days. Open and check that the fragrance is as strong as you would like it, adding more fresh jasmine flowers if necessary. By now the flowers should be almost dry. Spoon the tea and the jasmine flowers into smaller tins or bottles with lids that seal well, to lock in the fragrance. To make the tea, place 1–3 teaspoons of the mixture in a tea pot, cover with about two cups of boiling water and let it draw. Use a tea strainer and serve either black with lemon or add a little milk.

Jasmine and strawberry dessert

SERVES 4

This is one of the most attractive and enchanting desserts I know. Serve it on hot summer nights under the stars with the scent of jasmine in the air, to a group of appreciative friends.

3–4 cups fresh strawberries
Castor sugar
1 cup jasmine flowers, pulled out of their calyxes
2 tablespoons Tia Maria or your favourite liqueur
4 cups soft vanilla ice-cream
1 cup whipped cream

Hull the strawberries and cut them into thin slices. Sprinkle them with castor sugar and leave to stand at room temperature for at least an hour before serving. Meanwhile, marinade the jasmine flowers in the liqueur. When ready to serve, spoon a layer of strawberries into individual glass bowls, followed by a layer of ice-cream and a layer of marinated jasmine flowers, then repeat the layers, finishing with a layer of flowers. Top with whipped cream and decorate with whole strawberries and fresh jasmine flowers.

Judas tree

Cercis siliquastrum ● *C. canadensis* ●
Red bud tree

The Judas tree is a small, attractive tree that originates in Asia and the Mediterranean regions, so named because legend has it that Judas hanged himself from a tree of this species.

Tough, resilient, drought-resistant and even to a large extent frost-resistant, it used to be a garden favourite and was commonly available in nurseries, but sadly it seems to have gone out of fashion. Its pinky-mauve, almost magenta-coloured pea-shaped flowers are strikingly beautiful in spring, when the bare branches are covered in masses of brilliant blossoms, which withstand the early spring winds. The tough camel's foot-type leaves give dense shade in summer.

Cercis canadensis or red bud tree, a North American native, is its close relative. Both grow to about 5–8 m in height and form attractive, wide, shrubby trees that make superb focal points in a small garden as their growth habits are gently twisted and contorted to form a mass of fascinating branches.

CULTIVATION

To plant a Judas tree, all that is required is a deep, well-watered hole filled with compost, in a sunny position. Sink the plant into the hole without disturbing the roots. Water the sapling well once a week, making sure that it has a big 'dam' around it to hold both compost and water. Do not plant anything close to its trunk. It needs no pruning.

MEDICINAL USES

Once used to treat anaemia and lack of energy, the Judas tree was an important ingredient in the convalescent's diet, as well as during periods of overwork and stress, or for students writing exams. It has been used through the centuries to treat kidney stones, respiratory ailments and swollen feet during pregnancy. It is a gentle diuretic and will clear a runny nose and ease a tight chest and laboured breathing. The flowers are rich in carotene, high in vitamins and minerals and have been found to help dissolve fatty deposits in the blood and liver when combined with parsley.

To make Judas flower health tea for all the above conditions, pour a cup of boiling water over ¼ cup fresh flowers. Allow the tea to stand for five minutes, and strain. Sweeten with a little honey and add a squeeze of lemon juice. The flowers can also be used to make a soothing cream to help heal skin rashes, infected sores and fungal conditions.

The American Indians used the red bud to treat ailments ranging from toothache and bladder infections, to spotty skin and split toe nails, using crushed flowers as a poultice or lotion and adding them to teas.

Judas tree flower cream

This cream is very useful for treating rashes, infected sores, fungal conditions and swollen feet.

1 cup Judas tree flowers
1 cup good aqueous cream
3 teaspoons vitamin E oil
2 teaspoons tea tree essential oil

Boil the flowers and aqueous cream in a double boiler for 20 minutes. Strain through a fine sieve. Discard the flowers and add the vitamin E and tea tree oils to the cream. Stir well and spoon into a sterilised jar. Massage into affected areas and into swollen, tired feet, especially during pregnancy.

COSMETIC USES

During my years of lecturing beauty school students, this oil became a favourite because of its exceptional skin softening properties. A mere ½–1 teaspoon is all that is needed in the bath.

Judas tree bath oil

2 cups fresh Judas tree flowers and buds
½ cup grape seed oil
½ cup good olive oil
2 tablespoons almond oil
20 drops rose essential oil

Simmer all the ingredients except the rose oil together in a double boiler for 20 minutes, stirring frequently. Allow to cool for 10 minutes, then strain into a glass bowl. Whisk in the rose oil and immediately pour the bath oil into a sterilised dark glass bottle with a well-fitting lid. Add ½–1 teaspoon to the bath, under hot running water to disperse it. This oil is excellent for dry skin in winter.

To make a good body lotion, whisk together two teaspoons of this oil, a cup of aqueous cream and a cup of distilled water. Pour it into a jar with a well-fitting lid. Massage gently into dry skin, especially on the legs and feet.

CULINARY USES

Judas tree pickle

MAKES 2–3 JARS

This old recipe was popular long before commercial pickles became available. Use them on sandwiches and with cold meats and cheeses.

2 cups water
3 cups brown grape vinegar
2 cups brown sugar
½ cup mixed coriander seeds, peppercorns and caraway seed
2 cups small young cucumbers, thinly sliced
4 cups pickling onions, peeled and sliced in half
2 cups sliced green pepper
2 cups Judas tree flowers

Boil the water, vinegar and sugar together with the spices for 10 minutes. Meanwhile, pack bottles with the vegetables and flowers. Ensure that the bottles have well-fitting lids. Pour the vinegar and sugar mixture over the vegetables and flowers until each bottle is full. Seal immediately while hot. Wipe down the bottles and label. Leave to mature for at least two weeks.

Judas tree stir-fry

SERVES 4

This makes a delicious quick supper dish. Vegetables in season can be added to ring the changes.

A little olive oil
2 thinly sliced onions
4 potatoes, peeled and thinly sliced
2 cups thinly sliced mushrooms
2 cups Judas tree flowers
Juice of 1 lemon
½ cup chopped chives or spring onions
Sea salt and black pepper to taste
½ cup parsley

Heat the oil in a frying pan or wok and brown the onions lightly. Add all the other ingredients except the parsley. Stir-fry quickly. Serve piping hot sprinkled with parsley and decorated with Judas tree flowers.

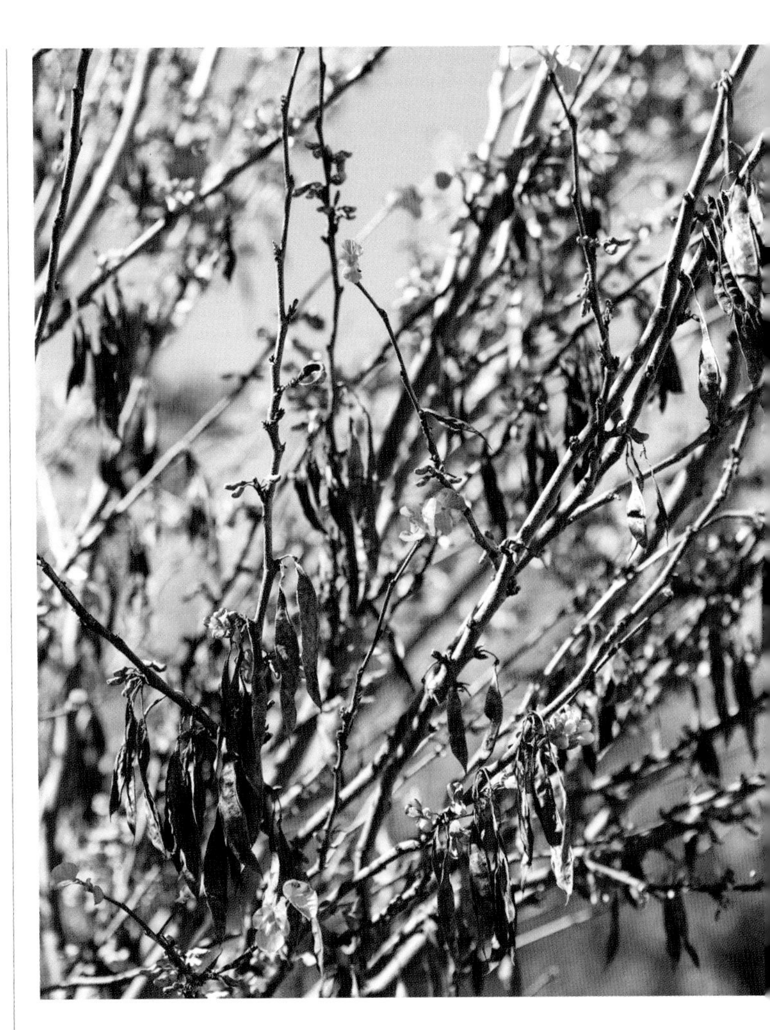

Judas tree flower and mulberry jelly

SERVES 4–6

The Judas tree flowers when mulberries are ripe, so this makes a delicious springtime dessert.

1 cup white sugar
2 cups mulberries, stalks removed
2 cups water
1½ tablespoons gelatine mixed into ½ cup warm water
1 cup Judas tree flowers
1 cup cream

Put the sugar, mulberries and water together in a pot and bring to the boil. Simmer for 10 minutes. Allow to cool, then blend in a liquidiser. Add the dissolved gelatine. Pour into a bowl, add the Judas tree flowers and stir well. Refrigerate to set. Meanwhile, whisk the cream until it stands in peaks, and refrigerate. Before serving, spread the cream over the surface of the jelly and decorate with a sprinkling of Judas tree flowers.

Korean mint

Agastache rugosa

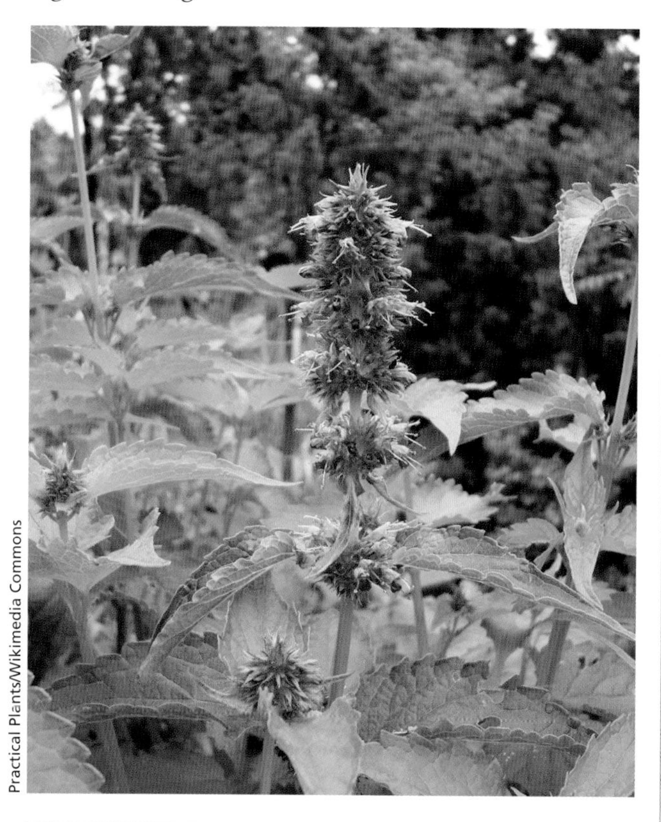

Practical Plants/Wikimedia Commons

This free-flowering perennial is native to Korea, parts of China, Laos and areas of Russia, growing wild on mountain slopes and along roadsides. Cultivated as a medicinal plant in China, its name, *Huo Xiang*, was first mentioned in the ancient Chinese pharmacopoeias as far back as AD 500. Today it is still used as a warming, stimulating herb in Chinese medicine, and scientific studies all over the East prove it to be quite exceptional for treating viral infections, ringworm, fungal infections, digestive disorders, morning sickness, nausea, vomiting and abdominal bloating. It has become a favoured garden plant and is now grown all over the world.

CULTIVATION

Growing Korean mint is easy as all it needs is full sun, well-dug, well-composted soil and a deep twice-weekly watering. It is tall and hardy, growing to about 50 cm in height, with a mass of fragrant mauve plumes about 2–4 cm long, much loved by bees and butterflies. Cut back the tall flowering stems when they start to look untidy at the end of summer but remember that the more you pick the more they grow; I find that I can pick the long sprays three or four times during the summer and new fresh stems quickly appear. Propagation is from rooted cuttings taken from the base of the perennial clump during autumn. If these are kept warm and protected throughout the winter, by late spring you will be able to plant out quite a show.

MEDICINAL USES

A lotion made from the leaves and flowers is used in Chinese medicine to treat ringworm and fungal infections. The Chinese also made a paste of boiled Korean mint leaves and flowers, mashed with a neutral cream, such as aqueous cream or petroleum jelly. This was spread on a cloth, placed over the fungal infection, and held in position with a bandage. Today Korean mint cream remedies are made for athlete's foot or any fungal attack.

A tea made of Korean mint flowers and a leaf or two, is warming and relaxing and aids the circulation. It has been found to help with digestive tension, nervousness, anorexia and fear. The tea is particularly helpful for extreme shock where the person is literally shaking from head to toe. A few sips of the tea sweetened with honey, will quickly restore calm and speed up the circulation to remove toxins from the body. In the case of flu and other viral infections, take Korean mint tea with 2 000 mg of vitamin C at the first sign of aching muscles, sore throat and fever; this is often so effective that the infection dwindles to nothing.

Korean mint antifungal lotion

1 cup fresh Korean mint leaves and flowers
1 cup tea tree flowers and sprigs
10 cloves
2 cups water

Boil the fresh leaves and flowers with the cloves for 10 minutes. Leave the lotion to cool, then strain and dab frequently over the infected area or use as a wash for athlete's foot.

Korean mint cream for skin or nail fungus

1 cup fresh Korean mint leaves and flowers
1 cup good aqueous cream
2 teaspoons tea tree essential oil
1 teaspoon lavender essential oil

Simmer the Korean mint and aqueous cream in a double boiler for 20 minutes, stirring frequently. Strain, and discard the mint. Add the tea tree and lavender oils, and mix thoroughly. Spoon the cream into a sterilised jar. Massage gently into the fungal infection two or three times a day.

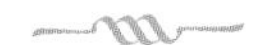

CULINARY USES

Korean mint party punch

SERVES 12

I make a delicious party punch with Korean mint over the Christmas season when it grows so prolifically.

Juice of 4 lemons
1 cup honey
2 litres boiling water
2 cups Korean mint leaves and flowers
2 litres mango juice or mango
and orange juice mixed

Mix the lemon juice with the honey and set it aside for an hour or two. Pour the boiling water over the Korean mint leaves and flowers and allow the mixture to cool, then strain and add the lemon and honey mixture and the fruit juice. Mix well and chill. Immediately before serving, add crushed ice and sprinkle with a few Korean mint flowers and tiny leaves.

COOK'S NOTE

I use Korean mint flowers to decorate many drinks and dishes, from pasta and desserts, to cakes and even roasts, as it cleanses the palate so beautifully.

Korean mint and mushroom stir-fry

SERVES 4

The typically liquorice-like taste of the Korean mint makes it a marvellous addition to celery and mushrooms. This vegetarian dish is so quick and easy to prepare that I keep a packet of mushrooms in my fridge and celery and Korean mint growing close to the kitchen door.

2 finely chopped onions
3–5 thinly sliced leeks
3 tablespoons olive oil
1 cup Korean mint flowers, lightly broken up
1 packet thinly sliced mushrooms
1 head of celery, about 6 stalks, chopped
Juice of 1 lemon
Sea salt and cayenne pepper to taste
1 cup water
Dash of Worcestershire sauce
1 cup grated mozzarella cheese

Brown the onions and leeks in the olive oil with the Korean mint flowers. Add the mushrooms and brown them lightly, then add the celery, lemon juice, salt and cayenne pepper. Stir-fry gently. Add the water and let it sizzle quickly, while stir-frying all the time (this makes a superb sauce). Lastly, add the dash of Worcestershire sauce and the mozzarella cheese. Serve hot with brown bread and butter, mashed potatoes or brown rice, and a green salad.

Mutton pot roast with Korean mint

SERVES 6–8

This roast makes an interesting change for Sunday lunch. It needs to be cooked slowly and succulently in one of those heavy cast iron pots with a good lid.

6–10 mutton chops, as lean as possible
Olive oil
4 large onions, thinly sliced
3 large red or green sweet peppers, thinly sliced
Sea salt and black pepper to taste
Juice of 2 lemons
6 large potatoes, peeled and cut into quarters
6 large carrots, peeled and cut into strips
1 cup Korean mint flowers, stripped off their stalks
A few Korean mint leaves
¾ cup sultanas
2 cups chopped celery
1 litre water
½ cup chopped parsley
4 cups fresh garden peas

Brown the meat on both sides in a little olive oil. Add the onions and brown. Gradually add all the other ingredients except the parsley and peas. Adjust the seasoning, cover, and turn down the heat to simmer. Add water as needed, and taste every now and then. I often add another dash of lemon juice or more salt and pepper. Simmer gently, stirring occasionally until the meat is tender and the vegetables cooked. Boil the peas separately with a sprig of mint. Serve the meat in its big cast iron pot with the peas and parsley sprinkled over it, together with brown rice.

Lavender

Lavandula × *intermedia* 'Margaret Roberts'

Native mainly to the Mediterranean area and cultivated throughout the world, lavender was used by the early Romans in their bath houses, as a strewing herb, and as a beauty aid. There are many varieties of lavender, all exquisitely scented, but not all edible. The best variety to use in any number of dishes, cosmetics and beauty products is the Margaret Roberts lavender. This variety cross-pollinated in the Herbal Centre gardens and was named by the nursery industry. Versatile and easy to grow, it adapts to cold winters and can tolerate a fair amount of frost and intense heat. This lavender flowers throughout the year. It has the typical English lavender look of long stems and whorls of flowers up the stem, and is delicious in the kitchen, and beautiful as a long-lived cut flower.

CULTIVATION

All lavenders require full sun and deeply dug, well-composted soil in which to thrive. The Margaret Roberts lavender grows large and needs about a metre between each row and plant in order for it to produce a continuous mass of flowers – and the more you pick, the more it flowers. This variety needs to be watered twice weekly, three times a week in summer. I replace the bushes every three or four years and am eternally grateful for this exceptional plant and its continuous flowering.

MEDICINAL USES

Lavender stalks can be burned in the fireplace to disinfect, deodorise and perfume the room (include a few flowers too), and sprigs of lavender rubbed onto kitchen counters will discourage flies. Skin ailments respond beautifully to lavender's antibacterial properties and throughout history lavender has been used for its calming and soothing effect. Lavender helps to ease sore throats, rheumatic aches and pains, depression, headaches and sleeplessness.

To make lavender tea, pour a cup of boiling water over ¼ cup fresh flowers. Allow the tea to stand for five minutes, then strain and sip slowly. It is excellent for nervous anxiety as well as a wonderful deodoriser and underarm wash – all that was needed to keep fresh in medieval times!

Crush fresh lavender flowers, inhale the rich scent, and rub crushed leaves and flowers on the temples; this will immediately soothe a pounding headache and relieve dizziness and fainting. Rub fresh lavender sprigs on children's pillows to ease restlessness and add a small bunch of fresh flowers tied in muslin to the bath to help unwind after a hectic day.

Lavender massage cream is ideal for dry skin, cracked heels, rheumatic aches and pains, sore tired feet and to calm irritable children.

Lavender massage cream

1 cup fresh Margaret Roberts lavender flowers
1 cup good aqueous cream
1 tablespoon almond oil
10 drops pure lavender essential oil

Simmer the lavender flowers and aqueous cream in a double boiler for 15 minutes, stirring occasionally. Strain out the flowers and allow the cream to cool for 10 minutes. Add the almond oil and lavender essential oil, spoon into a sterilised jar and keep well sealed.

Lavender and oats scrub for dry itchy skin

3 cups lavender flowers, stripped off their stems
4 cups large flake oats
3 cups Epsom salts
2 or 3 squares of fine muslin or cheese cloth (30 × 30 cm)
Ribbon

Mix the flowers, oats and Epsom salts together. Spoon about ¾ cup of the mixture into each muslin square and tie up into a sachet using ribbon. Store the remaining scrub mixture in a tin with a tight-fitting lid for future use. To use the scrub-filled sachet, hook it over the hot-water tap to soak it thoroughly, then lather it up with soft glycerine soap and rub over the skin, particularly thoroughly over

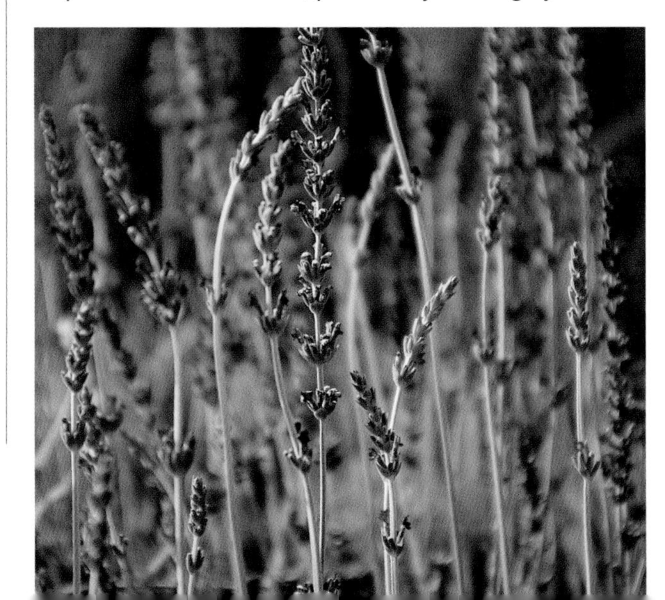

the feet and legs. Hang it up to dry and repeat the next day. After two applications, discard the scrub mixture, wash the muslin square, refill it and repeat. It is a real treat! I make this easy scrub every winter and find it soothing, softening and comforting for the skin, and I use it lavishly.

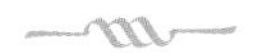

CULINARY USES

Cajun potatoes with lavender

SERVES 4

This potato dish makes a delicious accompaniment to fish and chicken dishes. I also serve it with crusty brown bread and feta cheese. It is satisfying, filling and healthy.

½ cup olive oil
2 large onions, peeled and thinly sliced
6 medium potatoes, peeled and thinly sliced
½ cup water
Juice of 2 lemons
1½ cups tomato puree
Black pepper and sea salt to taste
2 tablespoons Margaret Roberts lavender flowers
2 tablespoons chopped parsley

Heat the olive oil in a large pan and fry the onion until lightly golden. Add the potatoes and stir-fry. Add the water and all the other ingredients except the parsley. Cover and simmer for a few minutes, checking every now and then to see if the potatoes are tender. Stir gently. Serve piping hot with chicken or fish, sprinkled liberally with parsley.

Lavender biscuits

MAKES ABOUT 24

These biscuits make an excellent tuckbox filler and keep well in a sealed tin.

4 tablespoons soft butter
4 tablespoons castor sugar
1 cup cake flour
2 teaspoons baking powder
1 beaten egg
2 tablespoons fresh lavender flowers, stripped off their stalks

Cream the butter and sugar together until light. Add the flour, baking powder and beaten egg, and lastly the lavender flowers. Knead to a smooth consistency, adding a little extra flour if necessary. Pat the dough out gently

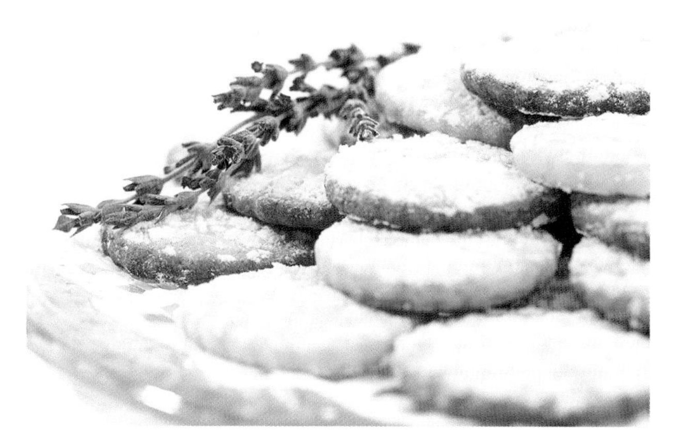

on a lightly floured board and cut into shapes. Place the biscuits on a well-greased baking sheet and bake at 180°C for about 10 minutes or until the biscuits are lightly golden and firm. Remove at once and dust with icing sugar.

Lavender cheese squares

SERVES 4

This is one of my favourite recipes for a teatime snack, a lunch dish with soup, or served as a supper dish with avocado salad.

6 slices brown bread
Butter
2 teaspoons lavender flowers, stripped off their stems and calyxes
½–¾ cup mayonnaise or chutney
1½ cup grated mozzarella cheese
A little chopped parsley
Cayenne pepper

Toast the bread, and butter the slices while still hot. Mix the lavender flowers into the mayonnaise or chutney and spread onto the toast. Sprinkle the mozzarella cheese liberally over the slices, sprinkle with parsley and dust with cayenne pepper. Place under the grill for about four minutes, or until the cheese starts to bubble. Cut into squares and serve hot.

COOK'S NOTE

Few people think of cooking with lavender, but just a little gives a wonderfully fresh taste and enhances flavours so remarkably that inventing dishes with lavender can become an engrossing hobby! The flowers can be sprinkled over a fruit salad, and the leaves can be added to stews and braised meat dishes. Lavender is also an excellent addition to marinades for game. For best flavour, use *Lavandula × intermedia* 'Margaret Roberts'.

Linseed

Linum usitatissimum • **Flax**

Linseed is an ancient plant that has been cultivated since at least 5000 BC as a source of flax or linen fibre. At that time flowers and seeds took second place to the fibre content of the stems, but the Greeks were well aware of the extraordinary medicinal content of the plant. Pliny the Elder (AD 23–97) wrote about linseed's virtues: 'What department is there to be found of active life where linseed is not employed? And, in what production of the Earth are there greater marvels to us than this plant?'

CULTIVATION

Linseed is an easy and fast-growing annual that enjoys full sun and deeply dug, well-composted soil. Sow the seeds by scattering them over an area, then rake them in and soak the ground with a gentle spray. Mulch the ground with a light layer of leaves to help keep it moist until the seedlings are sturdy, and water twice-weekly. In no time you will be able to pick the small, heavenly blue flowers. You can plant linseed all year, except in the coldest months.

MEDICINAL USES

Flax is becoming one of the wonder plants of the new century and medical research is concentrating on this easy-to-grow plant. New evidence proves that the seeds and flowers contain enzymes that hugely benefit the whole urinary system, including the kidneys. The seeds are rich in mucilage and unsaturated fats, and are a world-renowned remedy for constipation, digestive irritation and digestive sluggishness.

A poultice of crushed flowers and warmed seeds relieves painful boils, and crushed flowers moistened with milk have been used as a soothing poultice for rashes, grazes and sunburn since the Middle Ages. Flax flower lotion is still used in country districts in Europe today as a soak for tired aching feet. Gypsies found that placing crushed flax petals on a spot or pimple helped to soothe inflammation. They dried the blue flowers for winter use and used them in a tea for chilblains, chills, circulatory problems, cold feet and for treating coughs, chest ailments, sinusitis and the aches and pains of rheumatism. To make the tea, pour a cup of boiling water over ¼ cup flowers and let it stand for five minutes. Strain, sweeten with honey if liked, then sip slowly.

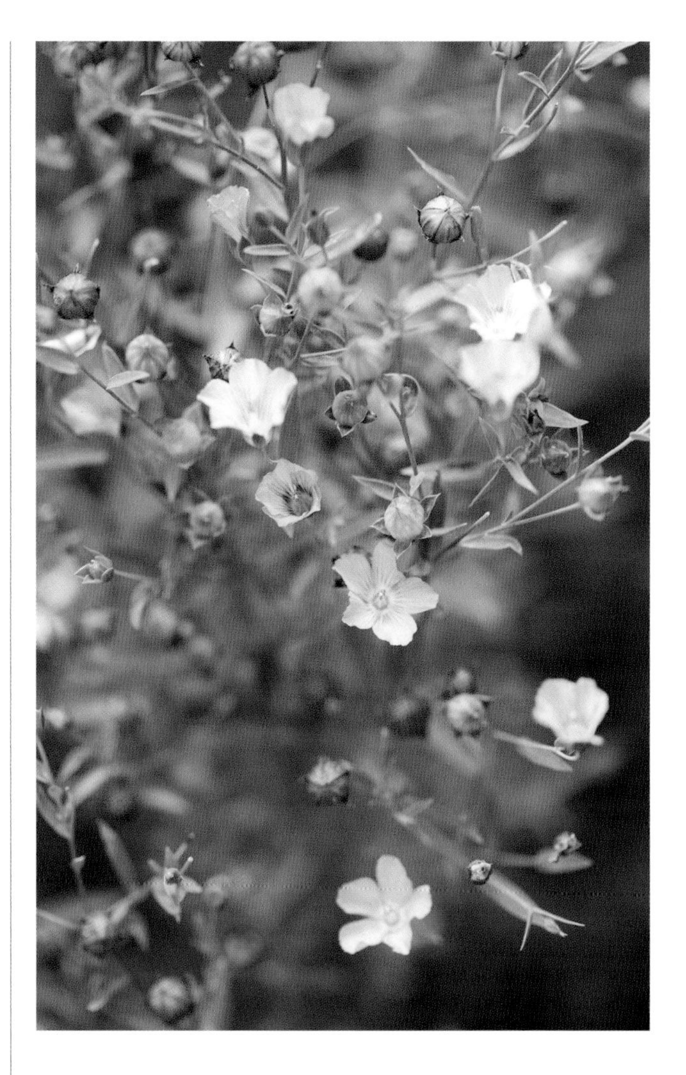

Gypsy linseed tea

Take this tea for circulatory problems, chest ailments and rheumatism.

2 tablespoons linseed
2 tablespoons fresh flax flowers
(or 1 tablespoon dried flowers)
6 cloves
Rind of half a lemon
1 litre cold water
Juice of 2 lemons
3 tablespoons honey
Pinch or two of cayenne pepper

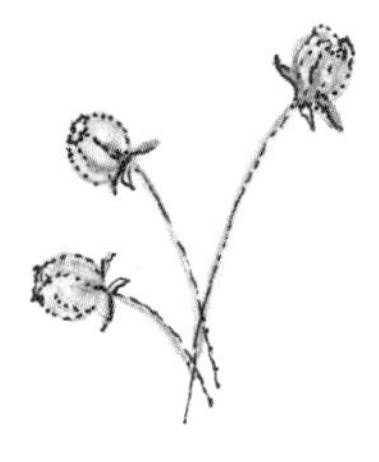

Place the linseed, flax flowers, cloves and lemon rind in the cold water, and simmer covered for 15–20 minutes. Strain and add the lemon juice, honey and cayenne pepper. Take half a cup three or four times during the day. Warm the tea up each time – but not in a microwave!

Flax flower lotion

3 cups flax flower tops, buds included
2 litres water

Gently simmer the flowering tops in the water for 10 minutes with the lid on. Set the lotion aside and cool until pleasantly warm before using as a soak for tired feet, or as a wash over itchy areas. Use also as a spritz spray for sunburned skin.

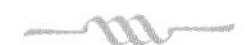

CULINARY USES

Flax flower chocolate sauce

SERVES 6–8

This sauce is spectacular over ice-cream, rice pudding or over a plain cake, and is probably my most talked-about dessert!

250 g plain milk chocolate, broken into pieces
2 tablespoons butter
4 tablespoons water
4 tablespoons thin cream

Melt the chocolate in a double boiler, stirring occasionally. Add the butter and beat gently. Add the water, mix well, and remove from the heat. Finally add the cream, beating all the time. While the sauce is still warm, pour it over the cake or pudding and immediately press in several flax flowers that have been pulled gently out of their calyxes. When they are cool and set, the flowers look like tiny blue cups and no one ever knows what they are!

Flax flower and potato soup

SERVES 4–6

Filling and sustaining, this is an exceptional soup for supper when you are overtired. It keeps well in the fridge. Try it warmed or chilled.

1 medium onion, finely chopped
A little olive oil
500 g leeks, sliced and trimmed
1 green pepper, finely chopped
500 g potatoes, peeled and roughly diced
1 litre chicken stock
Sea salt and black pepper to taste
1 teaspoon freshly grated nutmeg
1 teaspoon paprika
½ litre milk
150 ml thin cream (optional)
½ cup flax flowers, calyxes removed

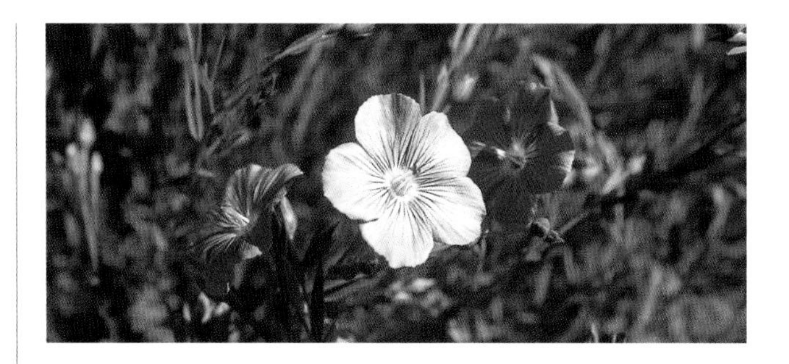

Brown the onion in the olive oil; add the leeks and green pepper, and cook for five minutes, stirring frequently. Add the potatoes and stock. Bring to the boil and simmer for 10 minutes or until the vegetables are cooked. Allow to cool a little. Pour into a liquidiser and blend. Return to the pan, add the sea salt, pepper, nutmeg, paprika and milk and heat thoroughly. Finally, stir in the cream if you are serving the soup hot, or chill the soup before adding the cream and stir in the cream just before serving. Pour into individual soup bowls and decorate with floating flax flowers and chopped parsley.

Spaghetti and tomato with linseed

SERVES 4–6

This quick supper dish is dead simple to make.

500 g spaghetti
1 large onion, peeled and chopped
1 clove garlic, finely chopped (optional)
A little olive oil
4 large tomatoes, skinned and chopped
2 tablespoons brown sugar
Sea salt and freshly ground black pepper
½ cup linseed
6 finely chopped sweet basil leaves
Freshly grated parmesan cheese
½ cup flax flowers

Bring four litres of salted water to the boil, add the spaghetti and boil rapidly until *al dente* or just tender. Meanwhile fry the onion and garlic in a little olive oil, add the tomatoes and stir-fry. Add the sugar, sea salt and pepper and the linseed, and stir well until the tomatoes have softened. Remove from the stove and keep hot. Strain the pasta and return it to the pan with one tablespoon of olive oil mixed in. Add a little sea salt and black pepper and stir until the pasta is well coated. Add the tomato sauce, mix in the chopped basil leaves and pour into a deep bowl. Sprinkle with the parmesan cheese and dot with the flax flowers. Serve immediately.

Lucerne

Medicago sativa • **Alfalfa**

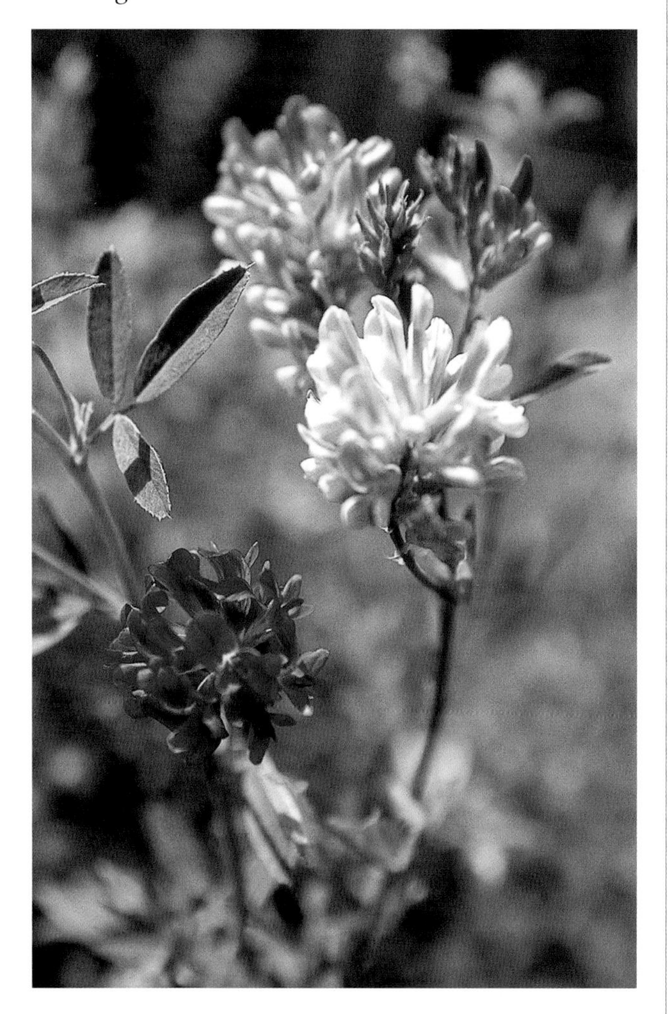

Lucerne is one of the oldest of all cultivated plants. The ancient Arabs called it the 'father of all foods', and used it as a feed for their magnificent horses which were fleet-footed, brave and supple. Today this long-lived perennial is grown all over the world as fodder for horses and cattle. It makes a pretty garden subject, too, as its mass of mauve-blue flowers attract a host of butterflies in early summer.

CULTIVATION

Lucerne is very easy to grow and requires little attention. Cut back the long flower-bearing stems 3–4 times a season to encourage tender new shoots. Lucerne needs full sun and compost-enriched soil. Because it is cut so often for baling as cattle food, it needs constant feeding, so a good dressing of compost two or three times a year is important. Water twice-weekly in summer and every 10 days in winter.

MEDICINAL USES

Nutritional experts rate lucerne as one of the most important food supplements known to humankind. It is rich in silica, manganese, calcium, iron, potassium, magnesium, sodium and vitamins A, B, C, E, K and the rare vitamin U, as well as being the only plant in the world other than comfrey that contains vitamin B_{12}.

To make lucerne tea, pour a cup of boiling water over ¼ cup fresh leaves and flowers and steep for five minutes. Strain and sip slowly. Sweeten with a touch of honey if desired. The tea is of tremendous benefit to those under extreme stress or suffering from a loss of energy, over-exhaustion, anxiety and panic attacks. A cup taken daily for a week and then on alternate days will do much to relieve modern-day tensions and ease desperation.

Fresh lucerne leaves, flowers and the tiny, threadlike alfalfa sprouts in the diet give an immediate energy boost, flushing toxins from the body and helping to absorb vitamins and minerals. One winter the Herbal Centre garden staff put this to the test. Half the staff ate a large daily salad of lucerne sprigs and flowers, dandelion leaves and flowers, buckwheat leaves and flowers, celery and parsley leaves, land cress, and a squeeze of lemon juice. They sometimes added nasturtium leaves and flowers, chopped chives, clover leaves and flowers, and pansies and borage flowers for variation. Needless to say, not one of the 'salad eaters' got a cold or flu that winter and every one of the 'non-salad eaters' did!

Lucerne is vitally important for convalescents who need easily assimilated nutrients and it should be added to their daily diet in the form of teas and soups, with the fresh leaves and flowers added to salads. Lucerne also has substantial oestrogenic activity, which is good news for treating menopause symptoms and irregular menstrual cycles.

Lucerne wash for insect bites, stings and inflammation

This soothing wash is vital for people working in gardens, where a bite or sting is an everyday occurrence.

Lucerne flowering sprigs
Soapwort flowering sprigs
Water

Boil a large pot of lucerne and soapwort flowering sprigs in enough water to cover, for 30 minutes. Cool for 20 minutes, then strain. Fill spritz spray bottles with this soothing brew, or soak cloths in it, for binding over the inflamed areas, and also use it to wash with.

Lucerne energy drink

SERVES 1

This drink is a quick pick-me-up and a boost for the immune system, and can take the place of a meal when you are very tired.

1 banana, peeled
½ cup lucerne leaves and flowers
1 apple, peeled and cored
1 tablespoon sunflower seeds
½ cup stoned dates, cut into pieces
½ cup sultanas, soaked
1 cup fresh fruit juice, e.g. mango, orange or litchi

Whirl all the ingredients in a liquidiser, then sip slowly straight away, adding a little water if it is too thick.

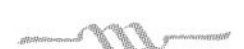

CULINARY USES

Iced avocado and lucerne soup

SERVES 4

A delicious lunchtime dish, this soup is a quick energiser and easy to make. Prepare it no more than an hour before serving as the avocados discolour quickly.

2 ripe avocados
Sea salt and black pepper to taste
2 sticks celery, finely chopped, leaves included
Juice of 1 lemon
2 cups plain Bulgarian yoghurt
½ cup lucerne flowers and a few leaves, finely chopped
1½ cups good chicken stock
½ teaspoon cayenne pepper
1 tablespoon parsley, finely chopped

Peel and cut up the avocados, add the lemon juice, sea salt and pepper, and mash finely. Add the rest of the ingredients except the parsley, whipping smoothly until they are well blended. Chill in the refrigerator, resting the bowl on a bed of ice. Serve the soup chilled in individual bowls, sprinkled with parsley and decorated with lucerne flowers. This soup is particularly good served with salty biscuits.

Lucerne flower and vegetable tempura

SERVES 4

These Japanese-inspired fritters make an unusual snack and are quick and easy to make.

Batter
1 teaspoon salt
½ teaspoon cayenne pepper
1 cup flour
1 extra-large egg
½ –⅓ cup warm water

Vegetables and flowers
2 carrots, peeled and cut into strips
1 large onion, sliced
  and rings separated
1 cup mangetout peas, topped
  and tailed
2 cups lucerne flowers, stems
  still attached
2 cups sliced button mushrooms

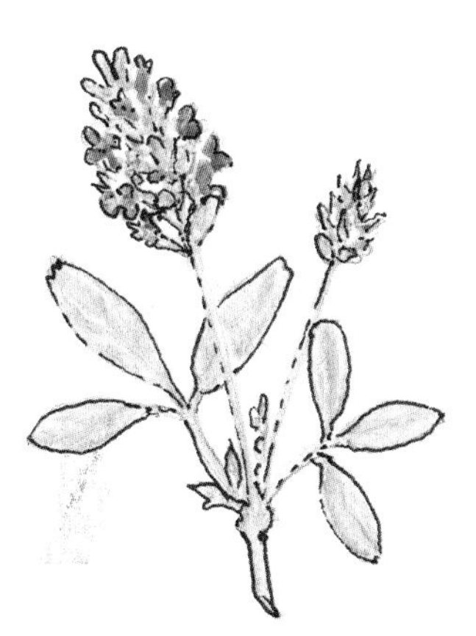

Sweet ginger sauce
2 tablespoons clear honey
1 tablespoon hot water
¼ cup finely grated fresh ginger
3 tablespoons soy sauce
2 tablespoons red wine

To make the batter, mix the salt and cayenne pepper into the flour, break the egg into it and mix again. Add the warm water and mix to a light batter, adding a little extra water if necessary. Have a large flat pan ready with hot sunflower oil.

Dip each vegetable and flower individually into the batter and then place in the pan. Do four or five pieces at a time. Fry until crisp and golden, remove with a slotted spoon, and drain on kitchen towel.

To make the hot ginger sauce, dissolve the honey in the hot water. Place all the ingredients in a screw-top jar and shake well. Pour the sauce into a bowl and serve as a dip with the hot tempura.

COOK'S NOTE

Pick lucerne leaves and add to salads just before serving so that they do not wilt (wilting will build up flatulence!). Grow alfalfa sprouts too, as lucerne seed is one of the quickest and most delicious of the sprouting seeds to cultivate.

Marigold

Tagetes patula ● *T. erecta*

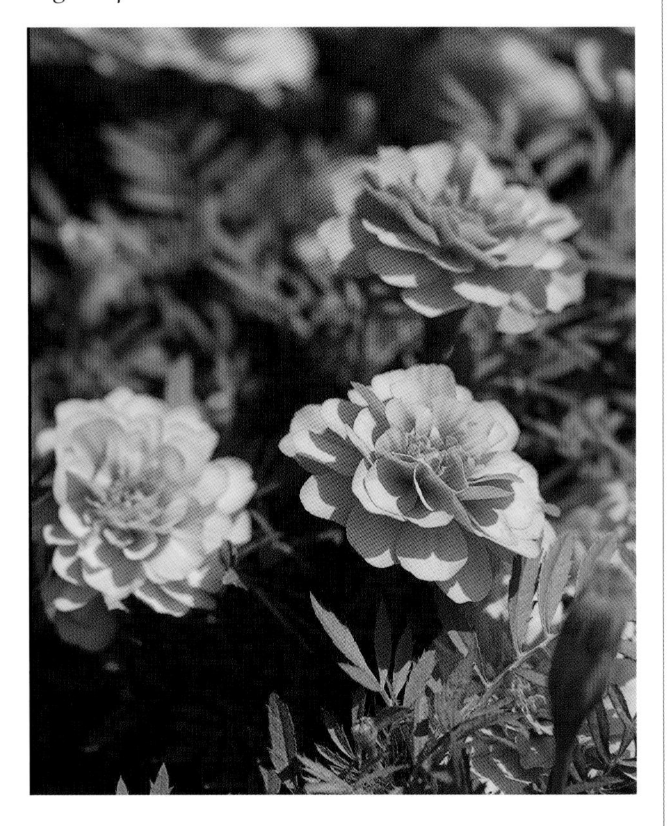

CULTIVATION

Propagate from seed, as marigold is a summer annual. Sow in spring where it is to grow, in deeply dug well-composted beds in full sun. Also sow seeds in trays for pricking out and planting, spaced 30–50 cm apart depending on size. Water three times per week. Harvest flowers continuously as the more you pick the more they produce. Marigolds are an asset next to anything – they literally fight off insect attack, offer shade and often support. Even delicate plants thrive near them. They are exceptionally useful in treating nematodes, white fly, red spider, mildew and even the resistant mealie bugs.

I have grown my best tomatoes with tall marigolds, and spread the seed thickly between rows of raspberries and fruit trees, keeping the soil moist and well composted for weeks on end. Cut marigold plants make a superb 'straw' for strawberries and no crickets, slugs, snails or beetles will venture near them, and by growing small marigold plants between strawberries you will have a bumper crop of perfect fruit. Try plantings between rows of beetroot, green peppers, bush beans and cherry tomatoes.

The 'Mary-gold' was named in honour of the Virgin Mary as from a distance it was mistaken for *Calendula officinalis* (p. 42), and thus the brightly coloured 'Mary-gold' became 'marigold'. In Europe the name refers to calendula, while in Africa it refers to the strong-smelling spectacular African marigold, *Tagetes erecta*, and also the French marigold, *T. patula*! Such confusion – and all because of the beautiful bright orange colour!

The French marigold, *T. patula*, is native to Mexico, not France. It was brought into Spain as a strong insect repellent to save grain in the early 16th century when trade in plants became the craze. From there it entered the trade routes as an insect repellent. The African marigold, *T. erecta*, also derives from Mexico, and was misnamed like its close cousin.

By the end of the 16th century India was one of the favoured traders of the African marigold. Indian people threaded the orange flowers into garlands used during celebrations and religious ceremonies. Today modern cultivars grace most summer gardens in South Africa; they are also planted between summer vegetables and under fruit trees and vines as effective insect repellents.

MEDICINAL USES

Used for centuries as a safe medicine, the brilliant petals of the marigold make an excellent tea that is a safe diuretic, flushing toxins from the kidneys and bladder and easing water retention and swollen feet. To make the tea, pour a cup of boiling water over ¼ cup fresh petals and a piece of leaf. Let the tea stand for five minutes, stir once or twice, and strain. Add a squeeze of lemon juice and a touch of honey if desired. The Mexicans and Spaniards add half a teaspoon of aniseed and two cloves, lightly crushed, as a daily tea for indigestion, colic, flatulence and heartburn.

In the 17th and 18th centuries, hot marigold tea with aniseed was served as an after-dinner drink at inns, and dried marigold petals were sprinkled over rich indigestible dishes. Later the Spaniards served hot marigold teas made with a dash of brandy or whisky as a nightcap to aid sleep.

Marigold baths were used to relieve rheumatism and the aches of old age, and compresses of warmed petals wrung out in hot cloths were used over arthritic and rheumatic joints. Whole plants were laid on mattresses covered with a blanket to relieve aching backs.

The Mexicans still use hot compresses of marigold petals on horses with sore legs or backs, and drenches were once made to rid livestock of ticks, fleas and lice.

Marigold bath for rheumatism

14 large marigold flowers and a few leaves
5 litres of water

Boil the marigold in the water for 20 minutes. Add the brew to a bath of warm water to ease rheumatism and the aches and stiffness of old age.

CULINARY USES

Marigold mixed spice

¾ cup dried marigold petals
½ cup crushed coriander seed
½ cup fennel seed
½ cup dried oreganum
¾ cup dried thyme
½ cup celery seed
1 cup coarse sea salt
½ cup black peppercorns

Mix the ingredients together thoroughly and spoon into a pepper grinder. Grind slowly and taste as you go. This spice is a taste sensation, delicious on fish with a squeeze of lemon juice and some grated lemon zest. It is also perfect with chicken, hardboiled eggs and mayonnaise, and with cheese and newly baked brown bread it becomes the Mexicans' favourite lunch!

> COOK'S NOTE
> **Dried marigold petals can be used in soups, stews, sauces and with mixed spices. To dry them, spread the petals, split from their calyxes, on sheets of brown paper in the shade. Turn them daily. Once dry, store them in glass jars with well-fitting lids.**

Marigold and mango stir-fry

SERVES 4–6

This is a quick Mexican supper dish that everyone loves; it can be varied using whatever vegetables you have in the kitchen. Add a little chilli if you are a chilli-lover.

3 tablespoons olive oil
2 onions, finely chopped
¾ cup marigold petals
2 large sweet potatoes, coarsely grated
1 yellow pepper, finely chopped
2 or 3 young and tender green mealies, cut off the cob
1 brinjal, cut into cubes, skin included
2 large mangoes, peeled and sliced
Juice of 1 lemon
1 tablespoon chopped fresh oreganum
1 teaspoon sea salt
1 teaspoon paprika

Heat the olive oil in a heavy-bottomed pot and fry the onions until golden brown. Add the marigold petals and stir-fry quickly. Now add all the other ingredients, one at a time. Stir-fry gently as each ingredient goes in. Check that the mixture is not too dry and have a small jug of water nearby. Turn the heat down, cover the pot, check there is enough water and cook until everything is soft and tender. The mango cooks down to a sauce and the secret is to never let it dry out. Serve hot and fragrant with rice or millet.

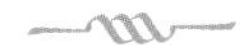

OTHER USES

Marigold flea-repelling lotion for dogs

Boiling water
1 large bucketful roughly chopped marigold flowers with stems and leaves
Chopped khakibos leaves, stems and flowers (if available)

Pour enough boiling water over the marigolds and khakibos to completely submerge the plants, and leave covered to draw overnight. The next morning strain, wring a cloth out in this strong brew and wipe over the dogs to get rid of fleas. Place marigold sprigs in the dogs' beds, with khakibos under the pillow – the fleas will flee and the itching and scratching should come to an end!

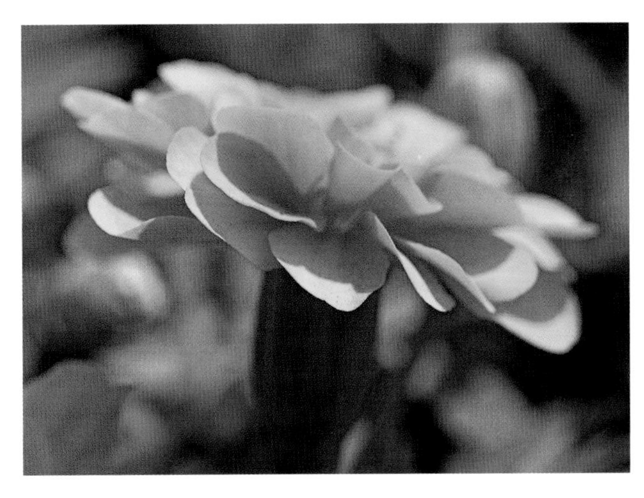

Milk thistle

Silybum marianum

CULTIVATION

Remove the seeds carefully from the dry ripe seed heads, and sow in individual seed trays filled with fine compost. Germination is quick and reliable and the tiny seedlings can be pricked out and transplanted gently into individual bags filled with rich moist compost as soon as they are big enough to handle. Keep the bags in light shade and check daily to keep them moist.

Prepare beds in full sun using deeply dug richly composted soil. Plant the seedlings 1 m apart as the flowering heads will reach 1.5 m in height and the plants need space. Run a hose into the bed in a gentle trickle so that the water reaches the roots. Twice-weekly is often enough, but check in hot weather.

Milk thistle is a robust annual, sometimes a biennial. Seedlings appear in spring, so be on the lookout for them as they can be transplanted only when they are very small and young. Once you have grown milk thistle you will always have it!

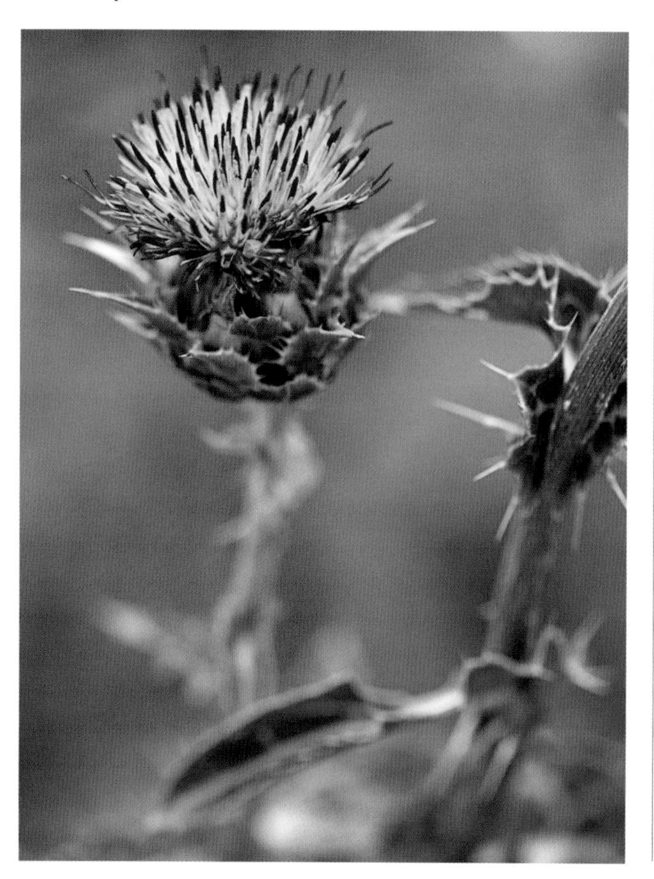

Milk thistle has been used for literally thousands of years. Although its ancient uses were recorded in the early herbals and pharmacopoeias, it was only in the 1970s that German researchers discovered the exceptional flavolignans, collectively known as silymarin, that protect the liver so effectively by rejecting toxins and blocking their entry through cell membranes. When the liver is under stress, be it through excessive intake of alcohol, coal-tar drugs such as painkillers (codein, aspirin), chemotherapy, or antibiotics, milk thistle comes to the rescue.

Milk thistle was recorded as a vegetable in its native Europe and Asia, and was cultivated in fields around the Mediterranean. The flowers were picked young and de-thorned, and became a valuable addition to soups and stews. Monks used the pink thistle tufts on the tops of the flowers to make a medicinal tea taken to restore internal health, to ease nausea and biliousness and to lift depression associated with liver damage. In 1597 *The Herball of General Historic of Plants* recorded milk thistle as the treatment for 'melancholy diseases'.

Today hepatitis is a common ailment and milk thistle has become a valuable treatment under medical supervision. Cirrhosis of the liver is also common now, often due to alcohol and drug abuse, and the fields of milk thistle grown in many countries are gaining in size as the pharmaceutical industry expands. Over-the-counter milk thistle formulations in capsule and tablet form are readily available in pharmacies today.

MEDICINAL USES

Milk thistle scavenges free radicals and boosts protein synthesis in the liver to repair damaged cells, especially after drinking. It is literally the best cure for a hangover and a 500 mg capsule bought from the chemist taken three times during the day after over-indulgence will help to repair and detoxify the overloaded liver. However, excessive drinking is dangerous and the liver can become so damaged that nothing can save it.

Milk thistle counters the absorption of toxic substances such as paraffin, and even inhaled poisons like insect sprays; however the correct dose must be administered immediately by a doctor. It will speed up recovery following chemotherapy and help to limit the liver damage and side-effects of chemotherapy once the cycle is complete and the patient is undergoing rest and recovery.

A cup of milk thistle tea once or twice daily will help to restore the liver to health. To make the tea, pour a cup of boiling water over ¼ cup fresh sliced flowers, with the spines removed. Allow the tea to stand for five minutes, stir well, strain, and sip slowly. Milk thistle seeds can be removed from the dried flower heads and stored in sealed glass jars. A teaspoonful or two of the seeds added to cleansing teas with fennel flowers, aniseed and coriander seed, or even simply with a squeeze of fresh lemon juice and a little honey will help to keep the arteries clear of cholesterol and the liver free of fatty build up from rich food.

Milk thistle is used in homeopathic medications to treat the liver, gall bladder, gall stones and depression, and is considered one of the most important remedies of the 21st century!

Milk thistle flower drink

This drink is used for easing depression, cleansing the liver, and after chemotherapy.

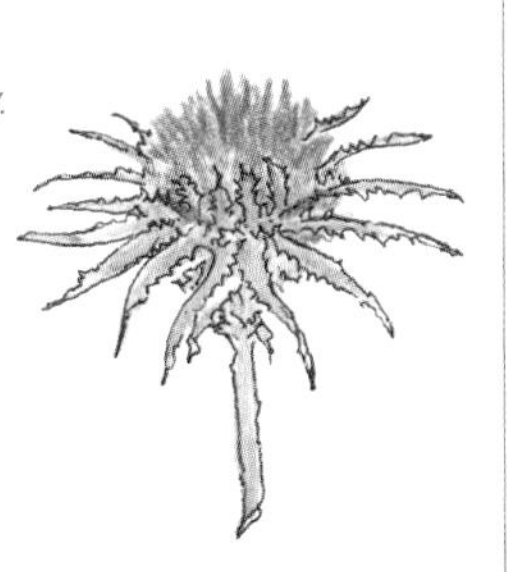

4–6 milk thistle flowers, roughly cut
1 litre unsweetened grape or apple juice
1 teaspoon aniseeds
1 teaspoon linseeds, lightly crushed
10 lucerne flowers and buds
Ice and iced water

Simmer milk thistle flowers and fruit juice with the lid on for 20 minutes. Add the aniseeds, linseeds, and lucerne flowers and buds. Leave it covered and allow it to cool. Strain, discard the flowers and seeds, add a little iced water and serve with crushed ice. Sip slowly. Make it fresh daily; it is literally an investment in health. Add carrot juice with pineapple for a change.

CULINARY USES

Milk thistle vegetable soup

SERVES 4–6

I found this age-old recipe in an old herbal and often make it in winter when the new milk thistle plants appear. It is delicious and a tonic for the liver.

½ cup olive oil
4 onions, finely chopped
3 cups fresh celery, leaves included, finely chopped
1 small-medium-sized cabbage, thinly sliced
3–4 cups milk thistle leaves and young flowers, prickles cut off, and finely chopped
3–4 cups spinach leaves

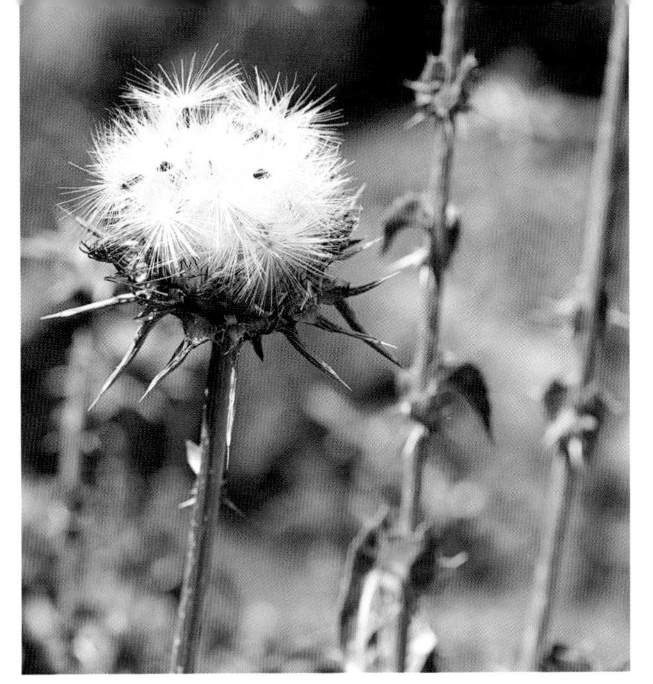

½ cup fresh flowering thyme sprigs, finely chopped
¾ cup pearl barley
2 litres good chicken stock
Sea salt and red cayenne pepper to taste
Juice of 2 lemons

Heat the olive oil in a heavy-bottomed pot. Brown the onions; add the chopped celery and stir-fry. Next add the shredded cabbage and stir-fry, followed by all the remaining ingredients except the salt, red pepper and lemon juice. Simmer the soup for 40 minutes or until the barley is tender. Add a little water if it is too thick and finally add the lemon juice, salt and red pepper to taste. Serve it in big bowls with freshly baked brown bread. I try to make this soup often as it is so important to keep the liver clear of toxins; on the days that I make it I also drink milk thistle tea with slices of lemon (see medicinal section).

COOK'S NOTE

When the flower heads are young and tender, snip off the thorns and boil the flowers as you would globe artichokes. Serve them with butter, salt and black pepper and lemon juice.

Add fresh chopped milk thistle leaves to tomato sauces, tomato bredies and mutton stews that include carrots, tomatoes and sweet potatoes. Thinly sliced leaves, with their spiny edges cut away, can be steamed into a delicious 'spinach' served with a rich cheesy white sauce as a popular 'peasant food'. Be creative as the leaves and flowers are rich in vitamins and minerals the body needs.

Mint

Mentha species

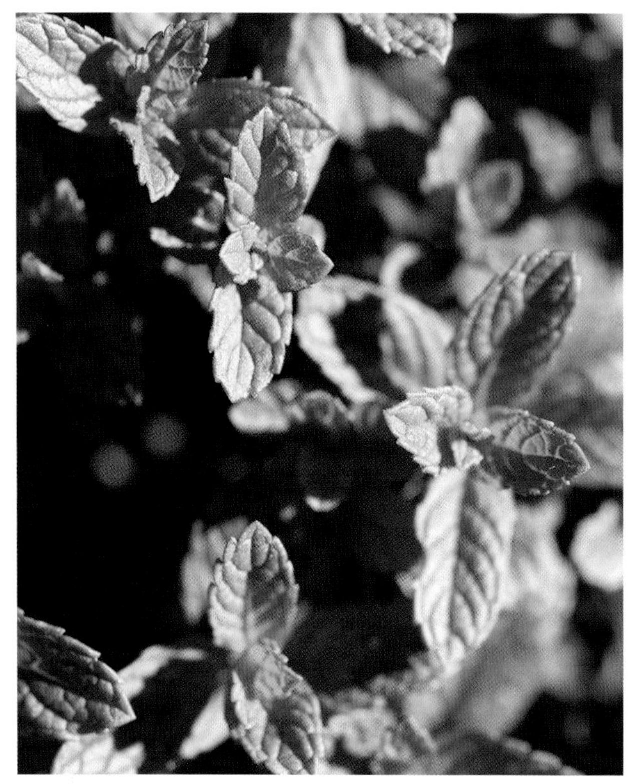

Garden mint

The *Mentha* genus comprises an incredibly rich diversity of species that originated in Europe and now occur worldwide. I have chosen just a few of my favourites to write about here, all with edible flowers, and all differing slightly in taste. Apple mint, *Mentha suaveolens*, is perfect for mint sauce and is more tasty, I find, than most other mints; black peppermint, *M. piperita* 'Nigra', has a strong peppermint flavour and is excellent for stimulating the brain; eau de cologne mint, *M. piperita* var. *citrata*, as its name suggests, smells and tastes of eau de cologne and is best with fruit salads and desserts; spearmint or garden mint, *M. spicata*, is most delicious with ice-cream; and chocolate mint, *M. spicata* var. *piperita*, has delectable chocolate overtones.

CULTIVATION

All mints need moist, rich soil and do best in partial shade in damp areas, but will also flourish in full sun as long as their roots are in water or very moist soil. Propagation is by means of roots pulled off the mother plant and planted immediately into wet soil. The mints constantly seek new ground, so it is a good idea to edge the bed with plastic or plant the mint in tubs to prevent them from spreading uncontrollably. Provide a rich dressing of compost twice a year to prevent the mint bed from becoming depleted.

MEDICINAL USES

All the edible mints are anti-inflammatory, antiseptic, antibacterial, antispasmodic, antiflatulent and effective stimulants. A mint tea, made by standing a thumb-length sprig in a cup of boiling water for five minutes, eases digestion and provides relief from abdominal discomfort and stomach upsets. During exam time a cup of peppermint tea works wonders to help concentration and ease nervous energy. During menopause, peppermint flower tea will relieve hot flushes and help ease digestive problems, take away a bloated feeling and help heartburn and a rapidly beating heart. Peppermint tea will also relieve cold and flu symptoms. Chew a sprig of any mint and the flower to sweeten the breath, and use the mint tea as a gargle and mouthwash to clear mouth and gum infections.

Mint lotion will soothe itchy, inflamed areas, mosquito bites and rashes, and if added to the bath it will soothe sunburn, windburn and chapped winter skin.

Mint lotion

Use this lotion for itchy, sunburned and chapped skin.

3 cups mint flowers and leaves (especially peppermint and spearmint)
3 litres water

Boil the mint flowers and leaves in the water for 10 minutes. Allow the lotion to cool, then strain and pour into a spritz bottle and spray the area or dab on with cotton wool pads soaked in the brew. Alternatively, add to the bath for a relaxing soak.

Mint footbath

3 litres mint lotion
3–4 drops peppermint essential oil

Make the mint lotion as per the recipe above. Add the peppermint essential oil and soak the feet for 10 minutes. This will soothe tired feet beautifully. It can also be used as a spritz spray to repel mosquitoes.

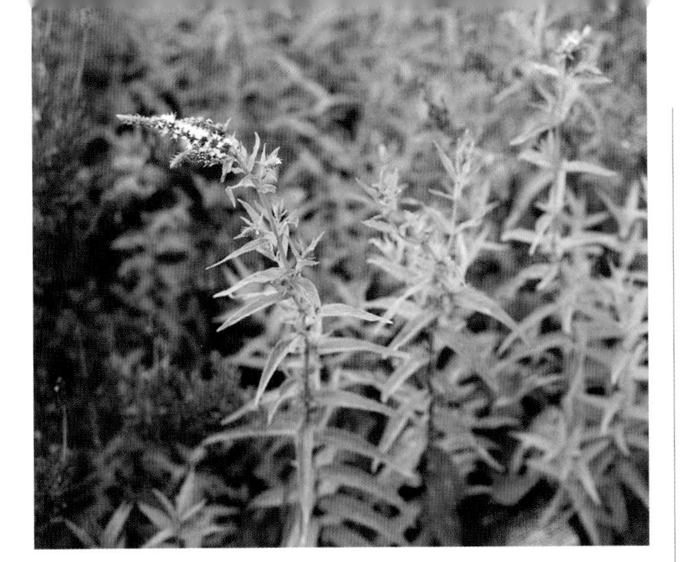

Spearmint

Mint digestive tea

This tea is great for colic, flatulence and bloating.

1 cup mint flowers and sprigs
½ tablespoon aniseed flowers and seeds
½ tablespoon caraway flowers and seeds
½ tablespoon fennel flowers and seeds
1 litre water

Simmer the ingredients together for 20 minutes. Cool for 10 minutes, then strain. Sweeten with a touch of honey and sip slowly. Keep excess in the fridge and warm a cup as and when needed.

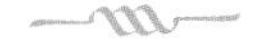

CULINARY USES

Chocolate mint mousse

SERVES 4

Use the leaves and flowers of chocolate mint (M. spicata *var.* piperita) *in this recipe.*

250 g plain dark chocolate, broken into little pieces
1 tablespoon finely chopped chocolate mint leaves and flowers
4 eggs, separated
1 cup cream, lightly beaten
1 tablespoon good filter coffee
½ cup thick cream, whipped for decoration
Chocolate mint flowers for decoration

Break up the chocolate and melt it with the mint leaves and flowers in a double boiler. Beat the egg whites into soft peaks. Beat the egg yolks and stir carefully into the melted chocolate. Add the cream and stir well. Add the dissolved coffee. Finally, fold in the egg whites. Spoon into pretty dishes, decorate with the whipped cream and sprinkle with chocolate mint flowers. Serve chilled.

Watermelon and mint dessert

SERVES 6–8

This is one of my favourite summer desserts. It is so easy to prepare and makes a refreshing end to a dinner party on a hot summer's night.

1 medium-sized watermelon
½ –1 cup white or castor sugar
¾ cup chopped spearmint leaves and flowers

Cut the watermelon in half, with a zigzag edge. Scoop out the flesh in neat balls using a melon baller and remove the pips where possible. Keep chilled until ready to serve.

Meanwhile mix the sugar with the chopped spearmint leaves and flowers (pull the flowers off their stems and break them into tiny pieces). When you are ready to serve, layer the watermelon balls with the mint and sugar mixture in one half of the watermelon shell. Pile the watermelon balls high and end with a layer of sugar and mint. Decorate with sprays of mint leaves and flowers.

Mint and mushroom supper dish

SERVES 4

This satisfying vegetarian dish is easy to prepare.

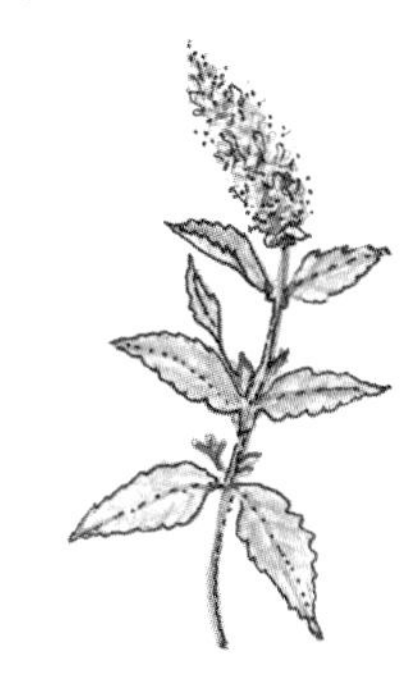

4 cups button mushrooms
4 medium onions, peeled and sliced
4 large tomatoes, peeled and sliced
Sea salt and black pepper to taste
½ cup finely broken-up mint flowers and chopped leaves
1 cup good vegetable stock
2 cups fresh wholewheat breadcrumbs
1 cup grated mozzarella cheese
Mint flowers for decoration

Arrange the mushrooms in an ovenproof baking dish, cutting the larger ones in half if they are too big. Top with onion rings and tomatoes, sprinkle with salt and pepper and the mint flowers and leaves. Add the stock. Mix the breadcrumbs and mozzarella cheese together and sprinkle over the dish. Bake at 180°C for about 20 minutes or until the onions and mushrooms are tender and the topping lightly browned. Decorate with mint flowers and serve piping hot with brown rice.

Moringa

Moringa oleifera • **Drumstick tree**

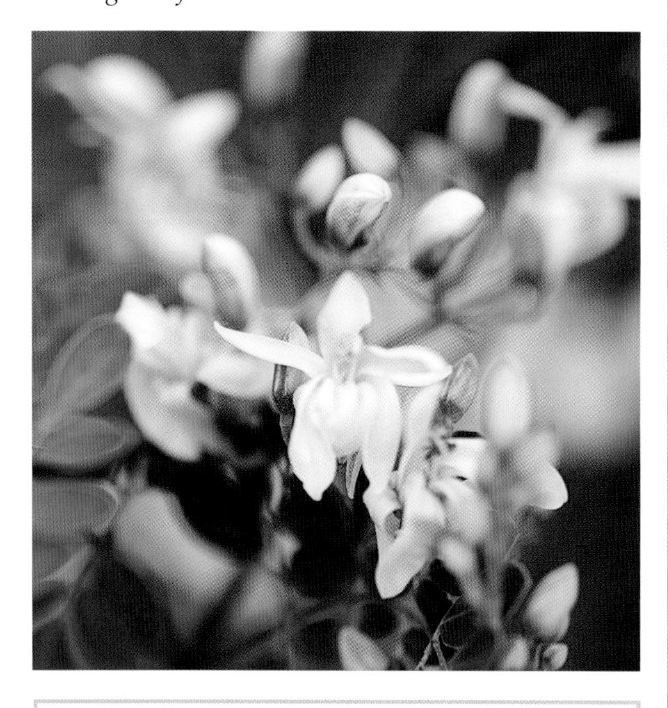

This small, dainty, shrub-like tree with its creamy white, sweetly scented flowers and light green, fern-like foliage is attractive enough to be a focal point in a tropical or subtropical garden. It is native to India, where it has long been cherished and respected not only for its dainty appearance, but also for its importance as a nourishing staple food. In many Indian households moringa is on the daily menu in one form or another: the leaves are cooked with tomato and onions as spinach; the pods are used in traditional sauces and chutneys, soups and stews; and the flowers are used in stir-fries and puddings. All parts of the tree are rich in protein, vitamins and minerals, including calcium, phosphorus, vitamin C, iron and folic acid, as well as beta-carotene, which is essential for healthy vision.

CULTIVATION

The moringa needs full sun and does well even in a neglected corner, pushing up its pretty fragile branches against all odds. I planted a specimen in a deep, well-composted hole and it grew 4 m in height in one year!

Propagation of the moringa is by seed. Once the pod ripens, it splits to reveal about 10 winged seeds. Rub the seeds on a stone to weaken the casings and plant the seeds in individual bags in moist sand. Germination takes about two months. The moringa has a long tap root and the seedlings do not like to be disturbed once established, so when planting them out into their final positions in full sun, be very careful how you slit the bag and lower the plants into the hole. Make a big 'dam' around the sapling and flood it with water once or twice a week until it is well established. Thereafter a weekly watering will ensure an abundant crop of leaves and flowers. The moringa can grow 3 m in a year.

MEDICINAL USES

Medicinal uses of the leaves and flowers have been well recorded in India's pharmacopoeias. They stabilise blood pressure, purify the blood, and build strong bones and teeth due to their high calcium content. The juice of the leaves followed by coconut water is an acknowledged remedy for dysentery and diarrhoea, and the leaves added to carrot juice makes an effective diuretic.

The roots are used as a heart medicine and to bring down fever; oil from the seeds is used for gout and rheumatism; the gum from the trunk helps with dental caries and gum ailments; a poultice of leaves soothes glandular swellings and headaches; leaves and flowers help prevent infections of all kinds, especially throat, chest and skin infections; and the juice of the leaves will clear blackheads and pimples. What a plant!

To clear river water of organic pollution, add 1 cup dried powdered moringa seeds to one bucket of river water.

Moringa flower tea

This excellent brew is useful for treating chest and mouth infections and can be used as a wash for skin.

1 cup moringa flowers and buds
1 moringa leaf, well pressed down
4½ cups water

Simmer all the ingredients for 20 minutes with the lid on, stirring frequently, crushing the flowers. Strain. Drink a cup with a little honey and a good squeeze of lemon juice for a sore throat, gum infection, mouth ulcer, bleeding gums, a cough and phlegm on the chest. Warm up a cup of this excellent brew at a time and drink the litre during the day. For rashes, itchy inflamed insect bites, infected scratches, grazes and cuts, use the tea as a wash, lotion or spritz spray. The tea can also be used in a poultice. Soak a pad of cotton wool in the brew and bind it in place with a crêpe bandage. Refresh the poultice three times a day, using a freshly soaked pad.

CULINARY USES

Moringa health salad

SERVES 4

This basic salad can be varied with vegetables in season. The mung beans and alfalfa sprouts are an excellent addition.

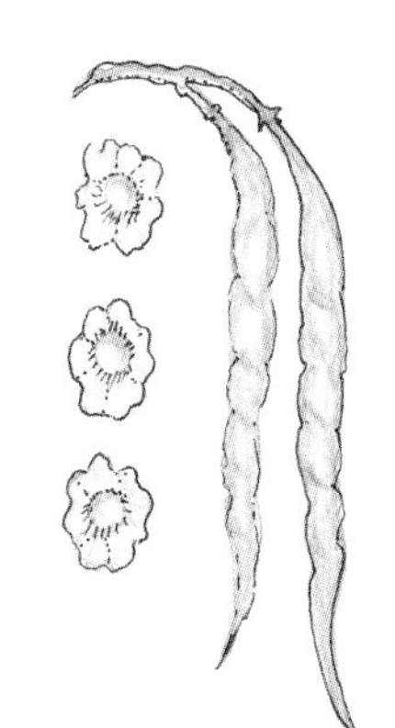

2 cups moringa leaves and flowers, stripped off their stems
1 cup chopped celery
1 cup chopped green pepper
1 cup chopped peeled cucumber
2 cups watercress leaves
1 cup cooked fresh asparagus spears
2 cups diced pineapple
1 cup diced mangetout or sugar snap peas
2 cups butter lettuce or kale leaves
Mung beans (optional)
Alfalfa sprouts (optional)

Mix all the ingredients together lightly. Serve with lemon juice and sprinkle with finely chopped parsley. Decorate with moringa flowers.

Chickpea and moringa flower supper dish

SERVES 4

This traditional moringa recipe was given to me by an Indian homeopathic doctor who believes that we should be enjoying this magical tree in some form at least twice a week.

2 cups chickpeas
2 bay leaves
1 large onion, finely chopped
Olive oil
2 tomatoes, skinned and chopped
2 cups moringa flowers and leaves
2 teaspoons fresh origanum
1–2 tablespoons freshly grated ginger
2 tablespoons soy sauce
2 tablespoons runny honey
2 tablespoons lemon juice
2 tablespoons good fruit chutney

Soak the chickpeas overnight. In the morning place them in fresh water with the bay leaves and boil until tender. Discard the bay leaves and drain. Meanwhile, fry the onion in a little olive oil. Add the tomatoes and stir-fry quickly. Add the moringa flowers and leaves, origanum and freshly grated ginger. Mix the soy sauce, runny honey, lemon juice and chutney together, and stir this into the simmering tomato mixture. Finally, add the chickpeas and stir well so that they are coated with the fragrant mixture. Serve hot with crusty brown bread and decorate with fresh moringa flowers.

Moringa flower fruit dessert

SERVES 4

This recipe is especially loved by children, and is a nourishing standby for those who have no appetite. Add or substitute the fruit with fruit in season, such as peaches, nectarines, mangoes, litchis or grapes.

1½ cups sago
2 cups milk
¾ cup honey
1 stick cinnamon
2 apples, peeled and grated
2 pears, peeled and grated
2 bananas, thinly sliced
1 cup moringa flowers, removed from their stalks

Simmer the sago in a double boiler with the milk, honey and cinnamon for about an hour, or until tender. Add more milk if necessary. Meanwhile, prepare the fruit and keep it covered so that it does not discolour. As soon as the sago is tender and transparent, remove the cinnamon stick and fold in the fruit and moringa flowers. Serve hot with plain yoghurt or a little cream, decorated with moringa flowers.

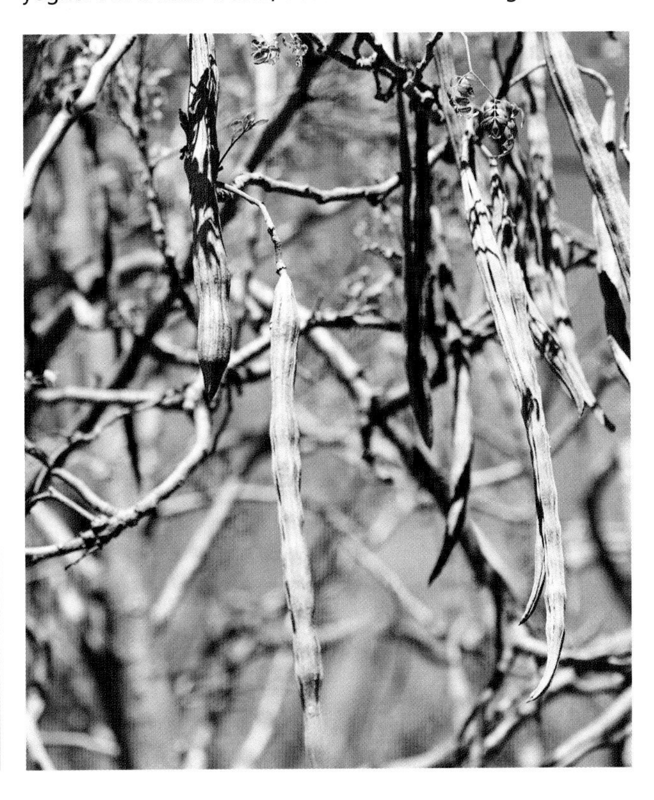

Mullein

Verbascum thapsus ● **Verbascum** ● **Aaron's rod** ● **Our Lady's taper**

Native to Europe, this beautiful tall biennial once enjoyed pride of place in many gardens but in modern times it has sadly been all but forgotten. In its first year it forms a large rosette of huge, soft, downy, grey-green leaves; in medieval times people suffering from cold feet were advised to line their slippers with these furry leaves on winter nights! In the second year a tall spire of brilliant yellow flowers is produced, and a mass of tight buds. The spire can reach well over 1 m in height and makes mullein an eye-catching border plant. The flowers appear all summer long until finally the spike dries off, scattering a multitude of seeds. In days gone by the tall flowering spike was dried, dipped in tallow and burned as a taper, usually in funeral processions, but also on feast days and in religious ceremonies.

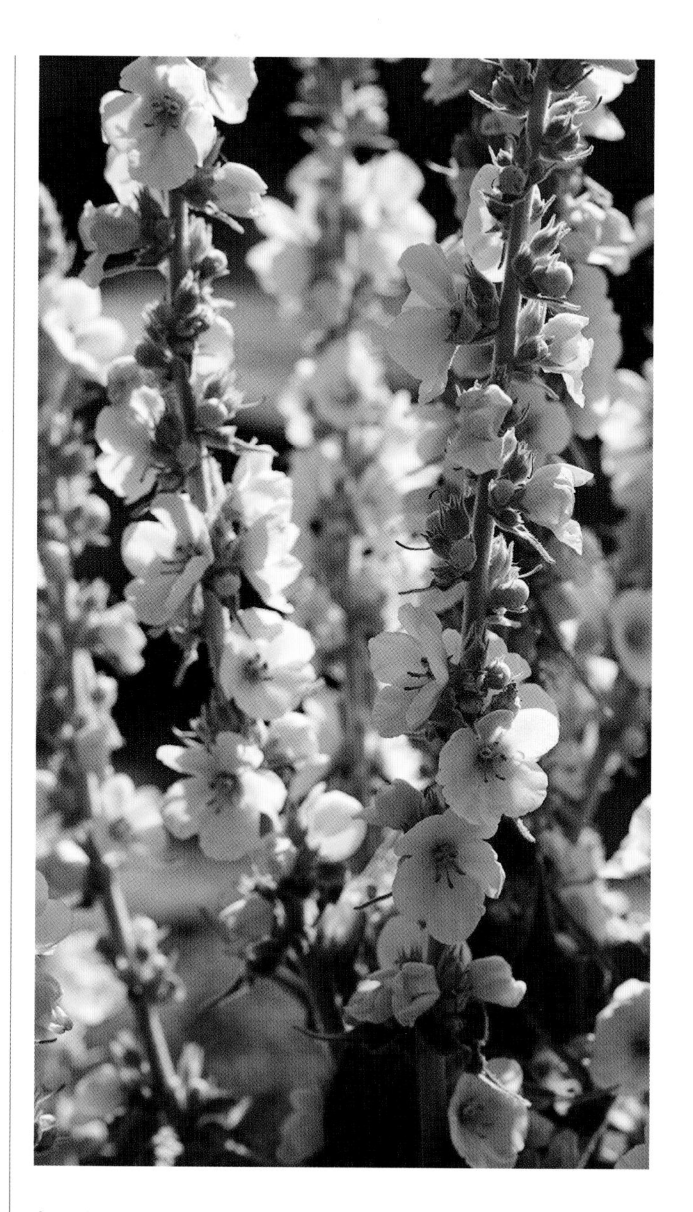

CULTIVATION

Mullein requires full sun and is unfussy as to soil type. Although it prefers well-drained, compost-rich soil, it will grow easily in the most inhospitable places and needs no attention whatsoever other than a good weekly watering. Transplant the seedlings when they are still small but just big enough to handle as they have a long tap root that does not like to be disturbed. Both flowers and leaves can be dried for winter use, although I find that the plant survives the frost and strong cold winds well.

MEDICINAL USES

Since the first century AD, mullein has been used as an expectorant to treat coughs and pleurisy. A syrup made from honey and mullein was used to treat chest conditions, coughs, bronchitis, pneumonia and chronic catarrh, and it was added to fruit dishes for children suffering from colds. A poultice of warmed leaves was used to ease muscular aches and rheumatic pains, and an ointment made with leaves and lard was found to be excellent for haemorrhoids and varicose veins.

Modern science has proved that this easy-to-grow plant is indeed amazingly beneficial for a wide variety of illnesses, including respiratory ailments, hay fever, sinusitis, feverish chills (it promotes sweating), eczema and earache. Mullein can be taken as a tea for all these ailments, once or twice a day. To make the tea, pour a cup of boiling water over ¼ cup fresh leaves and a couple of flowers. Allow the tea to infuse for five minutes, and then strain. It is also useful as an antiseptic wash for wounds and infected grazes and scratches.

Mullein cough syrup

1 cup mullein flowers and a few small leaves taken off the flowering spike
3 cups water
Rind of half a lemon
3 tablespoons lemon juice
3 tablespoons honey

Simmer the flowers and leaves in the water with the lemon rind for 15 minutes with the lid on. Strain, and discard the leaves, rind and flowers. Add the lemon juice and honey. Mix well. Drink ½–¾ cup at intervals through the day (about five times a day), and make fresh batches of the syrup frequently.

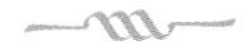

CULINARY USES

Strawberry and mullein mousse

SERVES 4–6

This delectable dessert is perfect for a summer lunch.

3 cups hulled, sliced strawberries
½–¾ cup castor sugar
2 eggs
¾ cup castor sugar
1 tablespoon gelatine
½ cup warm water
1 cup fresh cream, whipped
1 cup mullein flowers, pulled from their calyxes

Sprinkle the strawberries with ½–¾ cup castor sugar and leave them to stand for two hours. Beat the eggs with ¾ cup castor sugar until creamy. Dissolve the gelatine in the warm water and stir into the egg and sugar mixture. Fold in the whipped cream. Gently add the strawberries, and lastly the mullein flowers. Pour into a glass dish and set in the fridge, or pour into individual glass dishes. Serve decorated with a few fresh strawberries and mullein flowers.

Stuffed marrow with mullein flowers

SERVES 4–6

1 large green marrow
6 potatoes, peeled and halved
3 onions, peeled and halved

Stuffing

2 onions, chopped
450 g topside mince
1 cup breadcrumbs
2 tomatoes, peeled and chopped
2 carrots, finely grated
1 tablespoon fresh thyme
1 cup mullein flowers
½ cup raisins
Sea salt and black pepper to taste

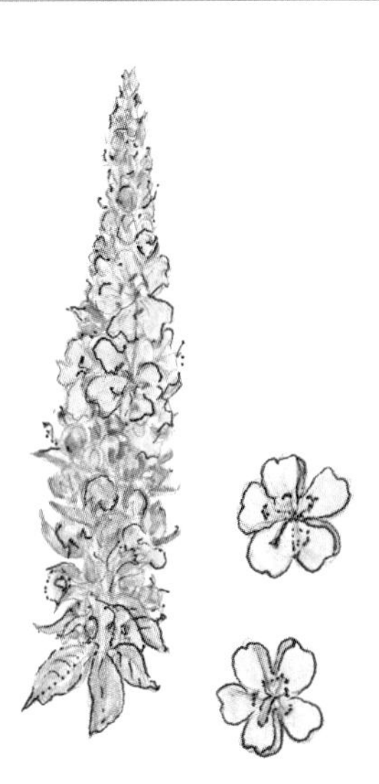

1 green pepper, finely chopped
½ cup parsley
A little sunflower oil

Peel the marrow with a potato peeler if the skin is tough. Cut off the ends and remove the seeds. Peel and halve the potatoes and onions.

To make the stuffing, sauté the onions, add the mince, and brown lightly. Add the breadcrumbs and the rest of the ingredients. Add a little water and simmer until done. Spoon the mixture into the marrow and use toothpicks to hold the ends in place. Place on a baking tray. Tuck the potatoes and onions around it. Dribble with a little oil and bake at 200°C for about 30 minutes or until the vegetables are cooked. Serve with brown rice and peas and decorate with fresh mullein flowers.

Mullein and carrot lunch dish

SERVES 4

I make this recipe every summer and it always draws compliments.

8–10 carrots, peeled and thinly sliced lengthways
1 large onion, finely chopped
A little olive oil
2 cups thinly sliced mushrooms
1 cup milk
2 cups cooked butter beans
½ cup brown sugar
½ cup honey
Sea salt and black pepper to taste
1 cup mullein flowers
½ cup parsley

Croutons

4 slices wholewheat bread
½ cup butter or sunflower oil

Cook the carrots in salted water until tender, then drain. Meanwhile, fry the onion in a little olive oil, add the mushrooms and milk, and simmer gently. Add the butter beans, sugar and honey and stir in the drained carrots. Add the salt and pepper and stir gently so as not to break up the carrots. Finally, add the mullein flowers and spoon into a serving dish.

To make the croutons, cut the wholewheat bread into small squares and fry them in a little butter or sunflower oil in a flat pan, turning them frequently. Drain them on absorbent paper. Add the hot croutons to the carrot dish and sprinkle with parsley. Serve with a green salad.

Mustard

Brassica alba ● *B. nigra*

Black and white mustard crops have been grown since medieval times and mustard is still cultivated around the world for use medicinally and as a condiment. From its native Middle East and Mediterranean areas, its popularity spread through India, China and Burma across to America. Mustard is rich in minerals, including high levels of phosphorus as well as calcium, iron, potassium, and vitamins A, B and C. Today mustard is being researched for its ability to boost the immune system.

CULTIVATION

Mustard is such an easy crop to grow that it seems a pity so few gardeners consider it. A fast-growing annual, it needs full sun and fertile soil, rich in humus. As a child I grew mustard and cress on wet cotton wool and it was a wonderfully rewarding experience, one that modern children seem to hardly know. Keep sowing new rows of mustard so that you can reap the seeds and use the new flowers and leaves at the same time. The plant can literally be eaten when only 1 cm high, and as a garden subject its bright yellow flowers will bring you pleasure and good health, and butterflies too!

MEDICINAL USES

Mustard seeds, leaves and flowers are a marvellous circulatory stimulant and a noteworthy alkaline food. Mustard greens (the flowers and young tender seeds included) compare very favourably with other leafy green vegetables, with the added advantage that they do not have a high oxalic acid content, which robs the body of nutrients. Mustard's alkaline nature aids digestion, and it is both a good antispasmodic herb and a diuretic. It has been used for centuries to treat bronchitis and pleurisy; it is believed to have antiseptic properties; and it helps to relieve arthritis, rheumatism and urinary tract ailments. The old-fashioned mustard foot bath recommended in our grandmothers' day at the first sign of a feverish cold or flu is really effective.

Fresh mustard leaves and flowers in a daily salad make an excellent tonic, but for treating constipation, bronchitis and pneumonia there is no better medicine than a mustard soup. The flowers and leaves can also be used to make a superb immune-building drink.

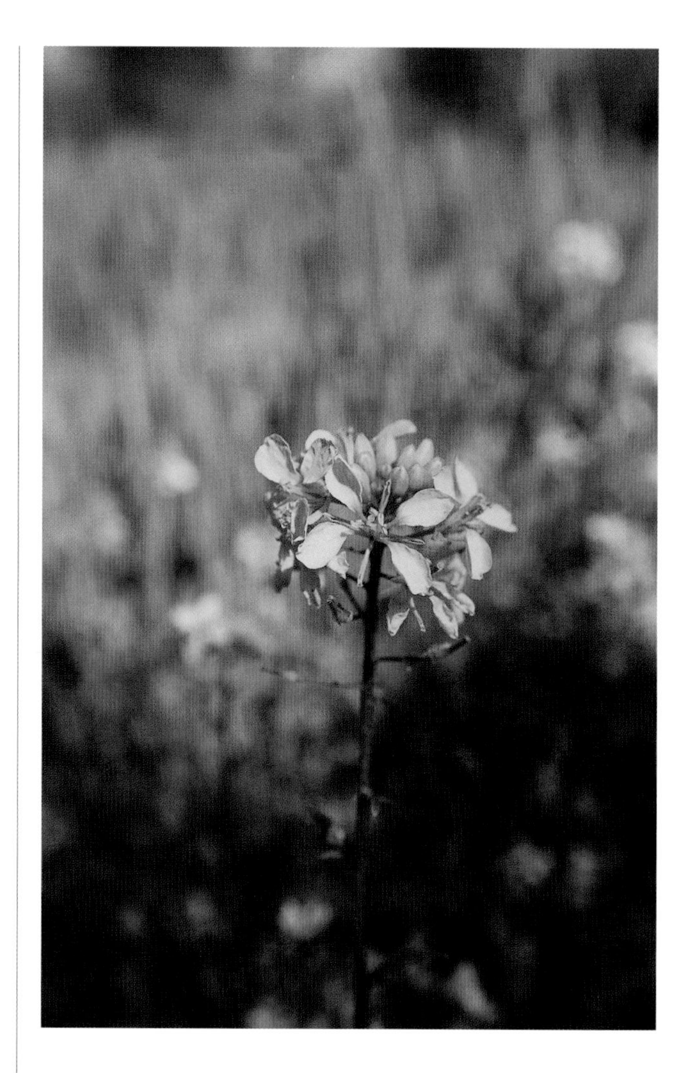

Mustard foot bath

4 tablespoons mustard seeds and flowers
2 litres hot water

Crush the seeds and flowers and mix into the hot water. Soak the feet for 10 minutes. In addition to aching feet, this bath helps with fatigue, coughs and colds.

Mustard tonic soup

Take this soup when suffering from urinary tract infections, bronchitis or pneumonia.

2 cups mustard flowers and leaves
1 cup chopped celery
½ cup parsley
1 cup beetroot leaves
1 litre water

Simmer the mustard, celery, parsley and beetroot leaves in the water for 10 minutes. Liquidise and season with lemon juice only. Take about a cupful, hot, twice a day. It is a comforting tonic and helps to get rid of phlegm.

Immune-building mustard drink

1 cup mustard flowers and leaves
½ cup parsley
1 carrot
1 apple
1 cup grape juice

Blend the ingredients together in a liquidiser until smooth, and drink twice a day.

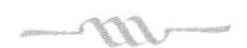

CULINARY USES

Homemade mustard

MAKES 1–2 BOTTLES

Use this mustard as a spread on sandwiches, or serve it as a delicious condiment with cold meat or warm chicken, fish and meat. It makes a superb gift too.

2 tablespoons whole mustard seeds
4 tablespoons honey
1 cup white grape vinegar
2 tablespoons dry mustard powder
(or crush your own seeds in a food processor)
2 tablespoons olive oil
2 tablespoons fresh mustard flowers
2 tablespoons chopped fresh tarragon

Soak the whole mustard seed with the honey and vinegar overnight. The next morning add the remaining ingredients and mix well. Spoon into a glass jar with a well-fitting lid and keep refrigerated.

Mustard flower pickle

MAKES ABOUT 4 BOTTLES

Keep this delicious pickle for at least three weeks before eating. Serve it with cold meats, salads, sandwiches and pasta. The vegetables can be varied according to what is in season.

4 cups cucumber, peeled and thickly sliced
2 cups cauliflower florets
4 cups small pickling onions
4 cups green peppers, cut into strips
1 cup red peppers, cut into strips
2 cups mustard flowers
2 tablespoons mustard seeds
2 cups brown sugar
4 cups brown grape vinegar
1 tablespoon sea salt

Wash the vegetables thoroughly in salted water and pack them attractively into glass jars with the mustard flowers. Boil the mustard seed with the sugar, vinegar and salt for 15 minutes with the lid on. Pour the hot mixture over the vegetables until the bottle is full. Seal immediately and store in a dark cupboard.

Mustard flower vegetable curry

SERVES 6

This is a warming, substantial dish that can be easily varied according to what is in season.

2 cups sliced onions
½ cup olive oil
2 cups peeled, diced potato
1½ cups peeled, sliced carrots
2 cups chopped tomatoes
2 cups cauliflower florets
2 cups sliced green beans
1 litre good vegetable stock
½ cup grated fresh ginger
2 teaspoons ground coriander seeds
1 teaspoon cayenne pepper
1 teaspoon turmeric
½ cup pecan nuts
½ cup seedless raisins
1 cup mustard flowers
½ cup desiccated coconut
½ cup honey
Sea salt to taste

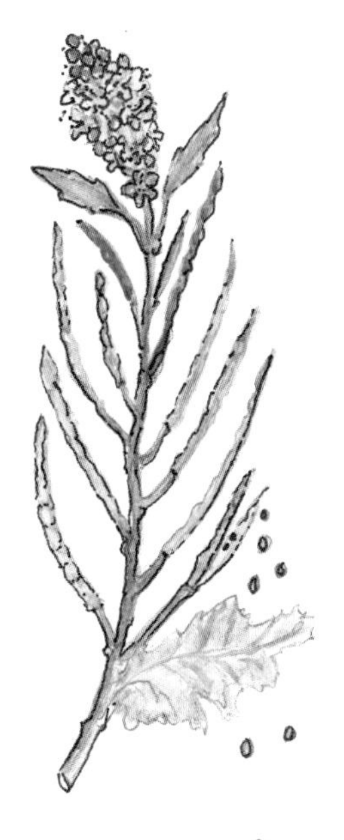

Brown the onions in the oil in a large pot. Add all the vegetables and stir-fry briefly. Add the stock and simmer. Mix the spices with a little water. Add the spice mixture, nuts, raisins, mustard flowers, coconut, honey and salt. Simmer with the lid on until the vegetables are tender. Serve decorated with fresh mustard flowers and brown rice.

Myrtle

Myrtus communis

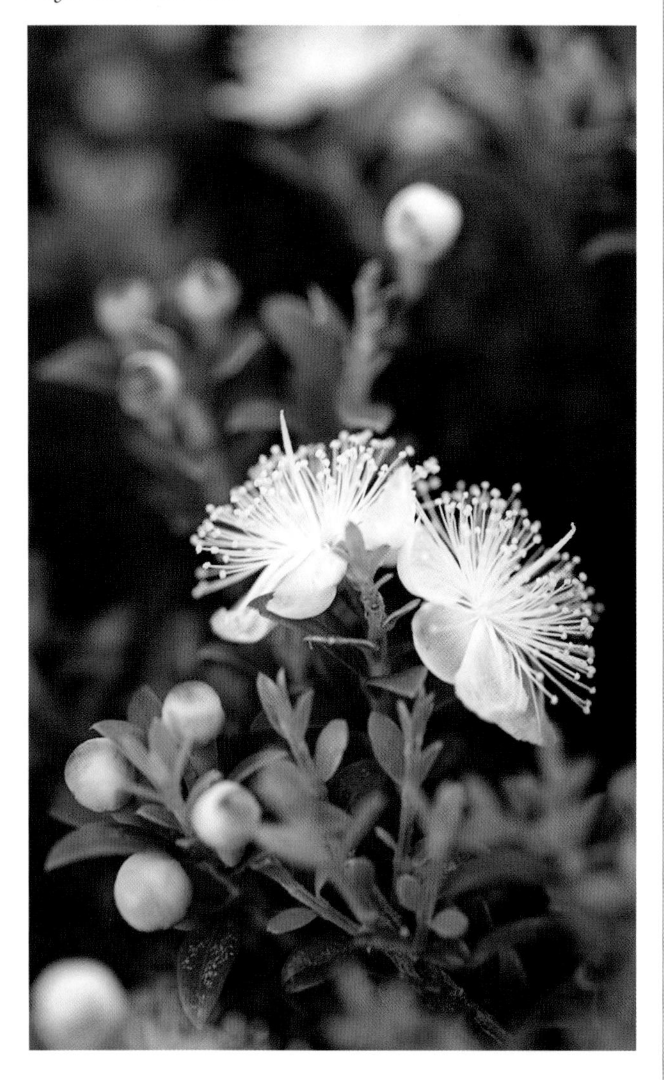

In ancient times myrtle was dedicated to Venus, the Roman goddess of love, and it was carried in bridal bouquets to symbolise love and constancy. Myrtle is native to the warmer, temperate climates of southern Europe, and has been used for over 2 000 years as a flavouring, a perfume, a cosmetic and a medicine. The more one grows myrtle the more impressed one becomes, as the entire plant is usable. In Chile, myrtle seeds and dried flower buds are used to make a type of coffee, and the flowers are used in pickles. The aromatic leaves and stems are important ingredients in potpourris, as well as being a good insecticide.

CULTIVATION

Myrtle is easily cultivated, but slow-growing. It grows 1–3 m in height, and with its evergreen, glossy leaves, it can be placed in an eye-catching position in the garden as it never has an off period. It makes a superb, tough hedge and takes clipping and pruning beautifully. It needs full sun, well-composted soil and a deep weekly watering to do really well. Propagation is by means of cuttings, which root easily.

MEDICINAL USES

Myrtle buds and flowers have been found to contain quite high quantities of vitamin C, malic and citric acid and an array of minerals. Both leaves and flowers are astringent and antiseptic. The leaves have a marvellous skin-cleansing action and can be made into a lotion that soothes skin rashes, oiliness and problem skins. The same lotion makes an excellent wash for infected bites as it is both antiseptic and astringent. Recent research has revealed that myrtle contains a substance that has a substantial antibiotic action, which explains why it is so quick to clear up infection and why it is effective in treating acne. Taken as a tea, it helps to relieve urinary tract disorders. To make the tea, pour a cup of boiling water over ¼ cup of flowers. Let it stand for five minutes, then strain and sip slowly, with a touch of honey if desired.

A poultice of flowering sprigs soaked in hot water and bound over a sprain or bruise as hot as is comfortable, will immediately disperse the haematoma and lessen the tension and swelling over the sprain. For many years I made a beautiful myrtle vinegar that I found to be helpful for sprains and bruises in my physiotherapy practice.

Myrtle antiseptic lotion

Use this lotion for rashes, problem skin and infected bites.

2 cups myrtle flowering sprigs
2 litres water

Boil the flowering sprigs in the water for 10 minutes. Cool and strain. Use on cotton wool pads as a toner for oily spotty skin, as a spray to keep the skin moist, or as a wash on infected bites.

Myrtle vinegar for sprains and bruises

Myrtle flowering sprigs
White grape vinegar

Fill a bottle with myrtle flowering sprigs and top it up with white grape vinegar. Stand the bottle in the sun for 10 days. During that time strain out the old sprigs and replace with new ones twice so that the minerals and vitamins in the myrtle leach into the vinegar. Finally, rebottle and press one myrtle sprig into the bottle for identification. Add the vinegar to the bath or use on a warmed cloth over bruises and sprains to ease the pain.

Myrtle flower massage cream

Use this wonderful cream for bruises, sprains, aching legs and feet. I make it for cyclists – it is excellent for cramps and strained ligaments.

2 cups flowering myrtle sprigs
1 cup good aqueous cream
1 tablespoon almond oil
1 tablespoon flax seed oil
2 teaspoons vitamin E oil

Simmer the sprigs and aqueous cream together in a double boiler for 20 minutes. Strain into a glass bowl and add the oils. Mix well and spoon into a sterilised glass jar with a well-fitting lid. Massage in very lightly and gently. Cover the area with a small towel soaked in myrtle brew. To make the brew, fill a pot with myrtle sprigs and flowering sprigs, add enough water to cover, and simmer for 20 minutes. Strain. Soak the towel in the brew as hot as can be tolerated and cover with another thick towel to retain the heat.

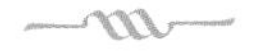

CULINARY USES

Myrtle pepper

MAKES 2 BOTTLES

This deliciously spicy pepper is very easy to prepare and makes a super gift for the keen cook.

1 cup dried myrtle flowers
1 cup dried myrtle flower buds
½ cup coriander seeds
½ cup peppercorns
½ cup dried paprika pieces
  or ¼ cup powdered paprika
½ cup powdered nutmeg
½ cup dried thyme

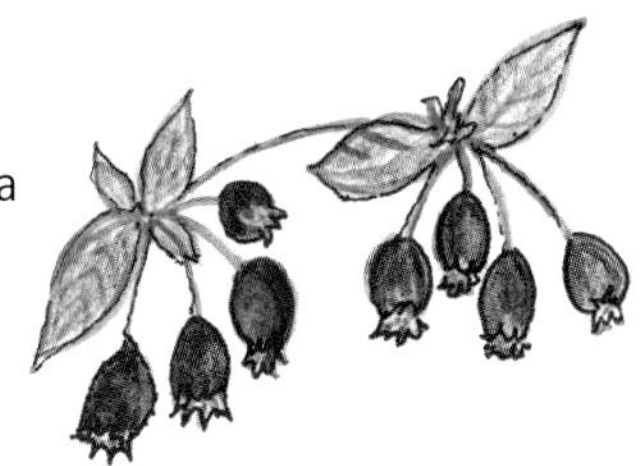

Mix the ingredients together and store in a screw-top jar. Shake the pepper thoroughly, and spoon small quantities into a grinder. Leave a little space at the top of the grinder so that the mixture can be shaken every now and then. Grind onto savoury dishes such as pasta, egg, cheese and potato dishes.

Myrtle and cheese spread

SERVES 6

Use this tasty spread as a sandwich filling or on toast as a supper dish, or serve on crackers as a snack.

2 cups finely grated cheddar cheese
1 cup smooth cottage cheese
2 teaspoons mustard powder
1 cup mayonnaise
½ cup myrtle flowers, calyxes removed
1 teaspoon freshly ground black pepper
1 tablespoon finely chopped capers
  or nasturtium seeds
1 teaspoon celery seed
1 tablespoon finely chopped tarragon
Juice of 1 lemon

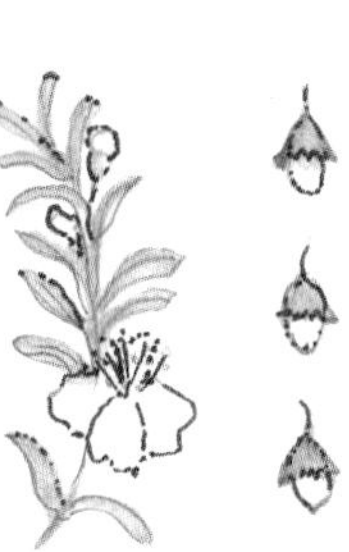

Mix the ingredients together well, making sure that everything is blended thoroughly. Spread on toast, top with tomato slices and place under the grill until it bubbles.

Apple and myrtle stir-fry dessert

SERVES 4

This quick dessert is so appreciated that I often make double the quantity. It is ready in five minutes, so the secret is to have all the ingredients ready before you start.

1 tablespoon butter
5 apples, peeled and coarsely grated
½–¾ cup sugar
Juice of 1 lemon
½ cup sunflower seeds
½ cup crystallised ginger, cut into small, thin pieces
½ cup chopped pecan nuts
½ cup myrtle flowers, calyxes removed
½ cup apple juice

Heat the butter in a pan or wok, and add the apple. Stir-fry quickly, then add the sugar and mix well. Next add the lemon juice and all the other ingredients and stir well. Should it become too dry, add a dash more apple juice. Serve piping hot with whipped cream.

Nasturtium

Tropaeolum majus

The nasturtium originated in South America, particularly Bolivia and Peru, and is now a familiar summer annual all over the world. It was introduced to Spain in the 16th century and was recorded by a well-known herbalist, Gerard, in London in the 1590s. With its pleasant peppery taste it has become a favourite herb and today nasturtium seeds are marketed worldwide and beautiful cultivars abound, from the more compact bush nasturtiums to double-flowered ones, in a breathtaking array of colours. The bright orange sprawling nasturtium that we all grew up with is happily still around, but the colours of the latest cultivated varieties now include brilliant yellow, cream, wine red and every combination and shade in between.

This season I was delighted to count 21 different colours and combinations along my pergola walk, all of which were self-sown from a single packet of seeds sown two summers previously!

CULTIVATION

Growing nasturtiums is child's play – indeed they are a rewarding crop for children to grow! Merely loosen a bit of soil in full sun and press the big seeds into it, keep the soil moist, and within a few days the succulent little seedlings will appear. They thrive in literally any soil, although if the soil is too rich you will have masses of leaves at the expense of flowers. In a protected area nasturtiums are biennial, but as they seed themselves with such ease, I pull out the old plants and let the new young ones take over.

MEDICINAL USES

All parts of the nasturtium plant may be used. As a child I was taught to eat a nasturtium leaf at the first sign of a sore throat, another leaf an hour later, and a third leaf an hour after that. Only years later did I learn that nasturtiums are high in vitamin C and that they contain a natural antibiotic. They are still used today in South America as a treatment for bladder and kidney ailments, for coughs, colds and flu, and for sore throats and bronchitis. These flowers contain a variety of vitamins and minerals and have been used through the centuries to treat scurvy and blood disorders.

COSMETIC USES

In ancient South America, the nasturtium was used as a hair-growth stimulant. Medical science has now proved that the juice from the flowers and buds stimulates the tiny capillaries of the scalp!

Nasturtium, nettle and rosemary hair tonic

This useful tonic can be used to promote hair growth and treat itching scalp and dandruff.

1 cup nasturtium flowers and stems
1 cup nettle tops
1 cup rosemary sprigs
2 litres water

Boil the herbs in the water for 20 minutes. Cool and strain. Massage the brew into just-shampooed hair, working it well into the scalp. Rinse off with water mixed with a dash of apple cider vinegar. Make it fresh each time. The hair tonic can also be combed into the hair.

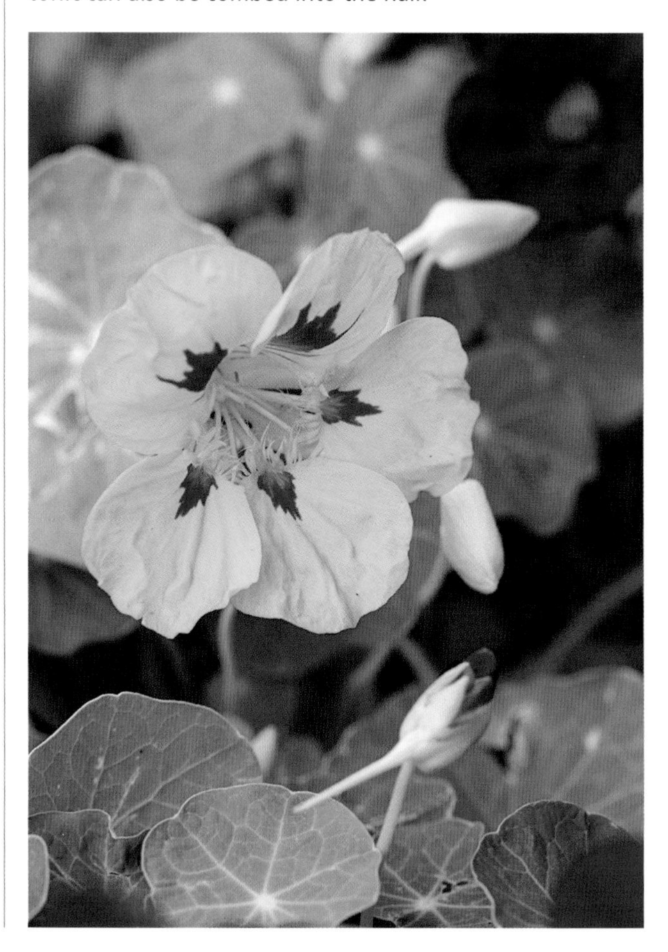

A tea of stevia flowers and buds will soothe sore throats, bleeding gums and mouth ulcers, tighten the gums and clear fever blisters. To make the tea, pour one cup of boiling water over ¼ cup of flowers, let it stand for five minutes and then strain and sip slowly. Stevia cream soothes cracked sore lips and dry skin around the lips and nose. It also helps to heal fever blisters, and it will stop any cracking and bleeding while the blisters heal.

Stevia flower gargle

This gargle is useful for treating mouth ulcers. It is very effective when made fresh and used three times daily.

1 cup boiling water
½ cup stevia flowers, buds and leaves
¼ teaspoon powdered clove

Pour the boiling water over the flowers, buds and leaves. Leave to cool for 10 minutes. Press the leaves and flowers well into the water. Strain. Add the powdered clove and stir in well. Swirl the liquid in the mouth.

Stevia flower cream for fever blisters and cracked lips

1 cup good aqueous cream
1 cup chopped stevia buds, flowers and few stems
2 teaspoons vitamin E oil
2 teaspoons grapeseed oil

Simmer the aqueous cream and stevia in a double boiler for 30 minutes, stirring frequently. Cool, strain through a fine sieve, and stir in the vitamin E oil and grapeseed oil. Spoon into a sterilised jar with a well-fitting lid and use liberally and frequently on the area. I tried this cream on a blister on my foot and found it excellent too.

CULINARY USES

Stevia flower lemonade

This is a perfect sugar-free summer drink!

Juice of 10 lemons
2 cups stevia flowering sprigs
1 litre water

Pour the lemon juice into a large jug, and set aside. Boil the stevia in the water for 20 minutes. Let it cool (covered). Add two cups of the strained stevia tea to the lemon juice. If more sweetness is needed, add a cupful at a time. When the syrup is pleasantly sweet, pour it into a glass bottle and store it in the fridge. To serve, pour ¼ glass of the lemon syrup, top up with crushed ice and water, and taste. Add more syrup if needed until you get it perfect!

> COOK'S NOTE
> **Fresh stevia leaves and flowers are delicious in drinks, desserts, cheese cakes and syrups, either finely chopped fresh, or dried, or made into a syrup by simmering one cup of fresh flowers and buds in half a litre of cold water for 20 minutes. Let the syrup stand and cool, keeping it covered. Store it in a well-corked glass bottle in the fridge. Use as a sweetener in drinks and desserts – taste as you go, a little goes a long way!**

Stevia flower rice pudding

SERVES 4–6

For a rich and creamy comfort food, this easy dessert has to be it!

4 cups milk
2 cups Basmati rice
½ cup finely chopped stevia flowers and buds
¾ cup sultanas, soaked in hot water for 20 minutes
1 cup thin cream

Gently simmer the milk, rice and stevia on low heat in a heavy-bottomed pot, stirring frequently with a wooden spoon. Once it starts to thicken, add the sultanas and stir thoroughly. Now add the cream a little at a time, or serve the cream at the table, poured over the pudding. Serve with strawberries, raspberries or sliced peaches for a celebration lunch or dinner. The secret lies in the long slow cooking that thickens the milk and softens the rice.

> COOK'S NOTE:
> **In order to replace sugar in your favourite recipes, start by halving the sugar and replacing it with finely chopped stevia flowers, buds and some leaves. For example, when cooking apricots, replace one cup of sugar with half a cup of stevia, simmer together and taste. Keep notes, and adjust!**

Strawberry flowers

Fragaria vesca ● *Fragaria* species

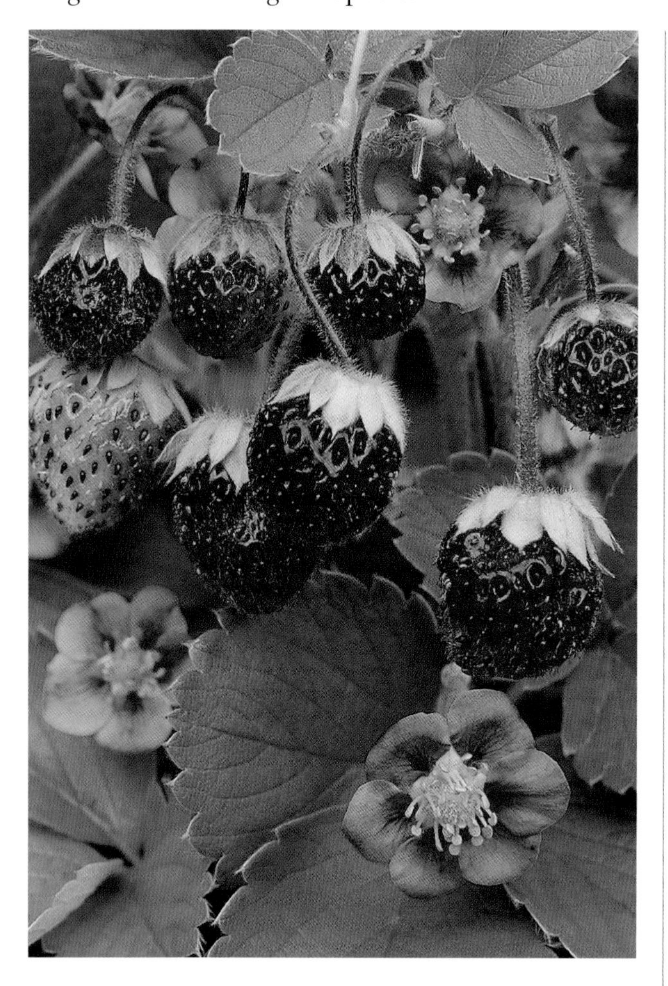

The strawberry is unlike any other fruit in that the seeds are on the outside, and the fleshy fruit is actually the receptacle or pod. It is indigenous to Europe and America, and cultivation began in the early 14th century, using *fraises du bois*, literally 'strawberries of the forest', as the mother stock. The largest fruiting plants were kept from these original crops, selected on the basis of flavour and sweetness. There are now literally hundreds of cultivated varieties of strawberry, particular to each country and therefore suitable for all climates. Many modern strawberries are based on *Fragaria chiloensis* and *F. virginiana*, which are indigenous to America. The exquisite 'Pink Panda' is a hybrid with bright pink flowers.

CULTIVATION

Growing strawberries is easy. All varieties require rich, well-composted soil, full sun, a deep twice-weekly watering, and a straw mulch once the fruits start to form. Pine needles and pine bark make a superb mulch, and the strong scent of the pine needles is a natural insect repellent. Set plants 40 cm apart and replace the mother plant every alternate year with new young runners.

MEDICINAL USES

A tea made from strawberry leaves and flowers is considered to be beneficial to the liver, kidneys and bladder, and in America it is often prescribed for cystitis, and for mouth ulcers and gingivitis. In the past, strawberry tea was used to treat typhoid, and today this same standard brew is used in the treatment of diarrhoea, gastric ailments and jaundice. To make the standard brew, boil one cup of boiling water over ¼ cup fresh strawberry leaves and a few flowers. Leave the tea to stand for five minutes, then strain and sip slowly.

The fruit of the strawberry is exceptionally rich in vitamins A, C and K, as well as folic acid, beta-carotene and potassium, and to a certain extent so are the leaves, flowers and root. The strawberry has been used medicinally since ancient times, particularly for treating diabetes, cancer and uricaemia, and modern science has found that all parts of the strawberry plant have antiviral and antibacterial properties. Fresh fruits rubbed on the teeth are said to whiten them and clear any gum infections.

Strawberry tonic wine

MAKES 1 BOTTLE

This one of the most loved tonic wines from the 17th century. It is believed to ease all stomach ailments, fevers and coughs, to comfort the liver and to make the heart merry!

1 cup strawberry fruits
1 bottle good red wine
2 cinnamon sticks
3 tablespoons honey
½ cup strawberry flowers
½ cup strawberry leaves

CULINARY USES

Nasturtium salad vinegar

MAKES 1 BOTTLE

This is a delicious, easily made salad dressing with an almost addictive bite. It can also be used in stir-fries, and the pickled flowers are delicious too. Some cooks make the vinegar in a wide-mouthed jar packed with nasturtium flowers so that the flowers can be fished out easily to flavour soups, sauces, stews and gravies. Nasturtium vinegar in a decorative bottle with a personalised label makes a wonderful gift.

Several nasturtium flowers and buds
Nasturtium leaves
10 nasturtium seeds
2 tablespoons sesame seeds
1 tablespoon mustard seeds
2 tablespoons runny honey
Brown grape vinegar

Pack the nasturtium flowers and buds and a leaf or two into an attractive 750 ml bottle. Add the nasturtium seeds, sesame seeds and mustard seeds. Dribble in the honey and finally top with good-quality brown grape vinegar. Shake gently, store out of the sun, and leave to mature for about one month before using. Give the bottle a gentle shake daily in order to disperse the ingredients. It will keep for several years in a cool place.

Nasturtium cheese dip

SERVES 6

This is a lovely spread or dip served with crudités, savoury biscuits, toast or crisps, and it gives cold meat and chicken a gourmet touch.

1 cup finely grated Gouda cheese
1 cup cream cheese
½ cup white wine
½ cup finely chopped celery
1 tablespoon Worcestershire sauce
½ cup finely chopped green pepper
¾ cup finely chopped nasturtium flowers and leaves
Juice of 1 lemon

Mix all the ingredients together and pile into a bowl. Stand the bowl on a large glass plate and surround with the toast, crisps or crackers and decorate with nasturtium flowers.

COOK'S NOTE

Ripe nasturtium seeds packed into small bottles of vinegar make a superb substitute for capers, and they give a delicious bite when sliced finely into stir-fries. Note that capers are not nasturtium seeds but are the flower buds of an unrelated shrub, *Capparis spinosa*, which grows in the Mediterranean region.

Grilled aubergine salad with eggs and nasturtium flowers

SERVES 6

This deliciously sustaining Greek-style lunch or supper dish makes an easy meal when you have guests, served simply with baked or boiled potatoes or crusty bread.

2 medium-sized aubergines, stalks removed and sliced thinly lengthways
½ cup olive oil
2 green peppers, thinly sliced lengthways
6 hard-boiled eggs, shelled
Sea salt and black pepper
8 anchovy fillets, chopped
Lemon juice
1 large avocado, peeled and diced
1 cup nasturtium flowers
8 spring onions, split in half lengthways
Olive oil
Balsamic vinegar
½ cup finely chopped parsley

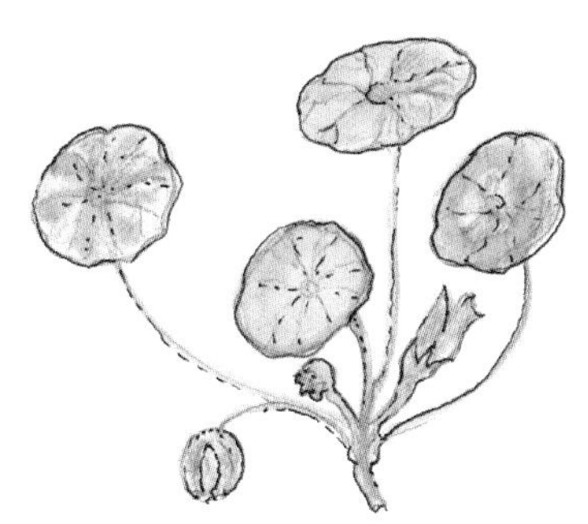

Brush the aubergines with a little olive oil and place them under the grill for about 10 minutes (check!). Add the green peppers and dry-grill them, turning them until they are charred all over. Slice the hard-boiled eggs in half and sprinkle them with crushed sea salt, black pepper and the chopped anchovy fillets. Place the peppers in a plastic bag to sweat, and when they are cool, remove the skins. Squeeze a little lemon juice over the avocado to prevent it from turning brown. Arrange all the ingredients on a large platter and tuck in the nasturtium flowers and spring onions. Drizzle with a little olive oil and balsamic vinegar. Sprinkle with chopped parsley.

For an alternative dressing, combine two tablespoons of olive oil, the juice of one lemon, two tablespoons of honey and one tablespoon of chopped pickled nasturtium seeds in a screw-top jar. Shake well and pour over the salad just before serving.

Orange blossom

Citrus species

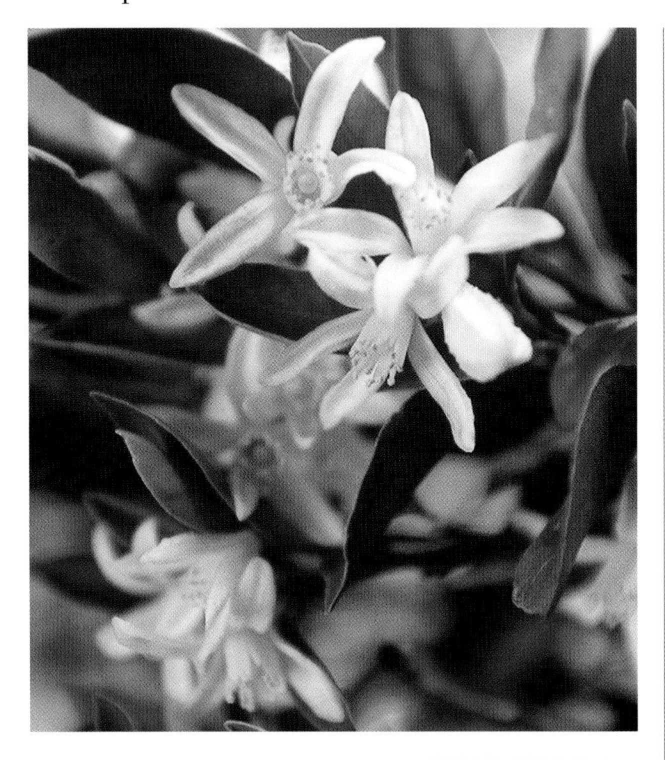

Citrus trees have been in cultivation since the first centuries of civilisation. Originally from China and southeast Asia, the earliest species moved westwards via the trade routes to India, then Arabia and finally to the Mediterranean. Roman records from Palestine in the first century mention citrus, and from then on citrus trees were cultivated in Italy and the rest of the Roman world. In 1002, citrus trees were established in Seville in Spain, and the famous Seville orange, valued for its bitter taste in marmalade, is still cultivated today. Lemons were cultivated in Egypt by the 10th century and from then on citrus trees were established in warmer regions around the world.

CULTIVATION

Any number of cultivated varieties of citrus are now available to gardeners worldwide, from tiny kumquats, calamondins and chinottos, which do exceptionally well in tubs and make enchanting patio plants, to tangerines, limes, rough-skinned lemons, ruby grapefruit and blood oranges. They are evergreen, easy to care for and incredibly rewarding to grow. A deep watering twice-weekly is imperative, and it is important to apply a good dressing of compost every four months and to check for pests and leaf curl.

MEDICINAL USES

All citrus fruits are high in vitamin C, and particularly lemons are excellent for treating excess acidity in the body. Citrus fruit ease constipation, clear catarrh and blocked noses, and their high vitamin C and beta-carotene content makes them vitally important for our daily health. Calcium, phosphorus and magnesium are present in the fruit, and to some extent in the flowers.

Orange blossom has been found to be sedative, antispasmodic, and an excellent remedy for depression, anxiety, nervous debility, grief, fear and insomnia. A tea made from fresh orange blossom will aid sleep and act as a natural tranquilliser. To make orange blossom tea, pour a cup of boiling water over one tablespoon of fresh flowers, or half a tablespoon of dried flowers. Let the tea stand for 3–5 minutes, then strain, sweeten with a touch of honey if desired, and sip it slowly for any of the above ailments and for poor circulation, as a natural blood cleanser, for premenstrual tension, fatigue, palpitations and stress.

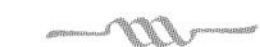

COSMETIC USES

Orange blossom is astringent and contains a skin-softening oil that is effective in refining coarse, oily skin. It can be made into a tonic lotion to clear oily skin and to brighten tired skin, and it can be dabbed onto spots, rough areas and open sores.

Orange blossom tonic lotion for oily skin

1 cup orange blossoms
4 orange leaves
1½ litres water
2 tablespoons apple cider vinegar

Simmer the orange blossoms and leaves in the water for 15 minutes, in a pot with a well-fitting lid. Set the lotion aside to cool, then strain. Add the apple cider vinegar and pour into a sterilised bottle and cork well. Shake for one minute. Use as a skin tonic to clear oily skin and dab it frequently onto spots, rough areas and open sores.

CULINARY USES

Iced tea with orange blossom sugar

SERVES 4–6

Served in tall frosted glasses on a summer afternoon.

1 litre boiling water
1 teabag
1 tablespoon orange flowers
1 litre iced water
Juice of 1 lemon
Orange blossom sugar to taste (see recipe)
1 lemon or orange, thinly sliced

Pour the boiling water over the teabag and leave the brew to stand for three minutes. Remove the teabag and allow the tea to cool. Float the orange blossom in the iced water. Add the iced water and lemon juice to the tea and sweeten to taste with orange blossom sugar. Pour into a glass jug, and float the lemon or orange slices on top plus several fresh orange blossoms. Serve chilled with a little crushed ice. Individual flowers can be frozen into ice cubes and served with the iced tea.

Orange blossom sugar

In days gone by this wonderful old-fashioned sugar with its lingering, haunting scent and taste would have been kept in a silver sugar casket and used with iced tea, jasmine tea, or in eggnogs, custards or cream.

1 kg white sugar
1 cup orange or lemon blossom
1 whole nutmeg, cracked with a mallet or using a pestle and mortar
1 stick cinnamon
1 tablespoon roughly crushed allspice berries (pimento)

Mix all the ingredients together and store in a large, sealed screw-top glass jar. Shake daily.

Orange blossom fairy butter

Fairy butter dates back to 1736, when it was highly fashionable to use it to ice buns and cakes. This modern version of the recipe can be used as a cake filling or icing on top of a plain sponge cake. I have used it to ice a wedding cake (orange blossom is a traditional wedding flower) and found it to be superb.

2 eggs
2 cups icing sugar
Juice of 1 lemon
1 teaspoon vanilla essence
Dash of brandy or your favourite liqueur
½–¾ cup orange blossom, calyxes removed, petals finely chopped
Fresh orange blossom, for decoration

Whisk the eggs well with the icing sugar until creamy. Add the lemon juice. Beat well. Add the vanilla essence, and a dash of brandy or liqueur, and beat thoroughly. Lastly, fold the orange blossoms in lightly. Spread the icing onto the cake and decorate with fresh orange blossom.

Orange blossom sago pudding

SERVES 4

This is one of those absolutely delicious old-fashioned puddings that is perfect for a springtime Sunday lunch.

1 cup sago
2 cups hot water
3½ cups milk
¾ cup sugar
1 cinnamon stick
½ cup orange blossom, removed from their calyxes
250 ml cream, whipped
Ground cinnamon

Soak the sago in the hot water for an hour, then strain. In a double boiler, heat the milk, sago, sugar and cinnamon stick, and simmer on a low heat for about 2½ hours, or until the sago is swollen, transparent and tender. When you are ready to serve, remove the cinnamon stick and stir the orange blossoms in lightly. Spoon into individual dishes, smother with whipped cream and dust with ground cinnamon. Decorate with orange blossoms.

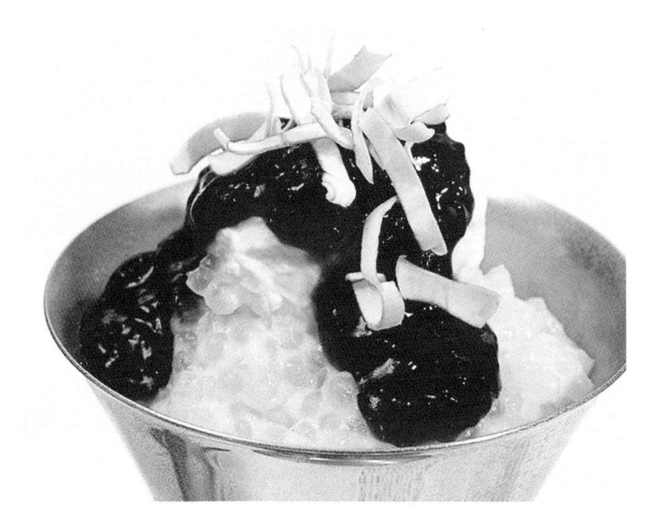

Pansy & viola

Viola lutea • *V. tricolor*

'Pansies with their happy faces, grow with joy in sunny places.' No garden is complete without an edging or planting of pansies and violas. The exquisite garden pansy (*Viola × wittrockiana*) hybrids available today probably derived from *Viola tricolor*, *V. lutea* and possibly *V. altaica*. The beautiful markings of these three original pansies were so admired by gardeners and botanists during the 19th century that pansy societies were founded to hybridise and improve the species. The array of species available today is breathtaking in its variety of colours and markings, and there is a huge selection of seed available. The tiny heartsease, *V. tricolor*, the forerunner to the viola and pansy hybrids we know today, originated in Europe and Asia, but has now spread all over the world. Violas, or 'little pansies', as they are often known, are an enchanting small-flowering variety and were originally hybridised by James Grive in 1863 from show pansies crossed with *V. cornuta*, which come from the Pyrenees, and *V. lutea*.

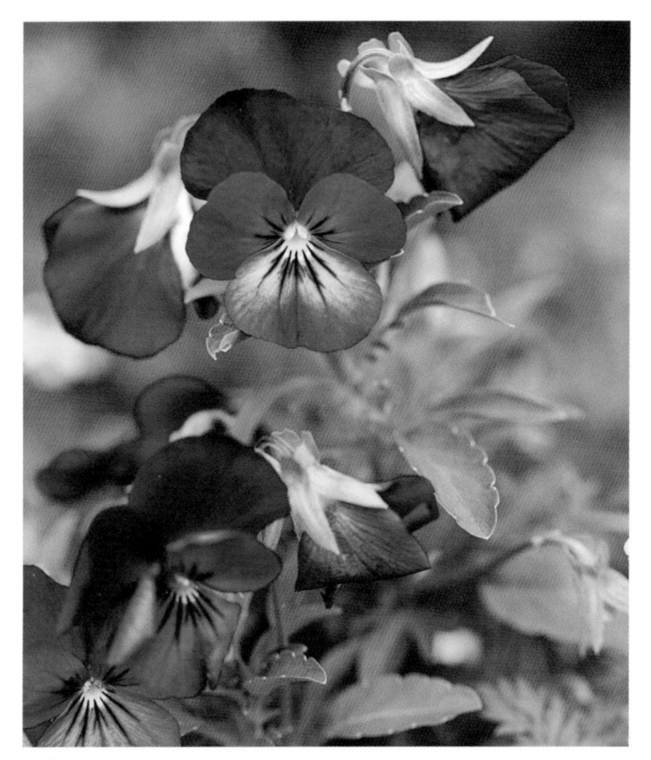

Viola

CULTIVATION

Pansies require little attention other than well-dug, compost-rich soil, a twice-weekly watering and frequent dead-heading to ensure a longer flowering period. Plant in early winter as the pansy is a cold-weather annual.

MEDICINAL USES

The tiny heartsease has been used in herbalism for matters of the heart, hence its name; it is also used to treat high blood pressure, indigestion, and skin ailments such as eczema, rashes and inflammation. It can also be used to treat coughs and colds, stiff, sore joints, gout and rheumatoid arthritis. To ease rheumatism and aches and pains, add a strong infusion to the bath.

A tea made from flowering *V. tricolor* sprigs and one or two garden pansies can be used as a treatment for high blood pressure. Add ¼ cup flowers to a cup of boiling water; leave the tea to stand for five minutes, then strain. Take one or two cups daily until the blood pressure normalises, thereafter have one cup on alternate days or twice-weekly.

CAUTION: Do not take pansies and violas medicinally for prolonged periods, as this can cause nausea and vomiting. Always allow an 8–10-day break after using these flowers for two weeks.

Viola bath infusion for arthritis

4 cups *V. tricolor* flowering sprigs and pansies
2 litres water

Boil the flowering sprigs and pansies in the water for 10 minutes. Cool for five minutes, strain and add to the bath. This infusion will help to ease aches and pains. Do this two or three times a week; it is infinitely soothing. Also take a cup of tea made from *V. tricolor*.

Viola skin cream for eczema, rashes and inflammation

1 cup *V. tricolor* flowering sprigs
1 cup aqueous cream
2 teaspoons vitamin E oil

Pound the flowering sprigs to a paste, mash in the aqueous cream until it is fully incorporated, then warm in a double boiler for 15 minutes, stirring frequently. Strain through a fine sieve and mix in the vitamin E oil. Spoon into a sterilised screw-top bottle. Keep in the fridge and apply frequently.

CULINARY USES

Strawberry and pansy granita

SERVES 6–8

This dessert must be made the day before so that it can freeze well.

2 kg ripe strawberries, hulled
300 g castor sugar
Juice of 1 lemon
250 ml thick cream
125 ml sweet sherry
Fresh pansy flowers

Liquidise the strawberries with the sugar and lemon juice. Place in a measuring jug and top up with water to 1.5 litres. Taste and add more sugar if necessary. Pour into a shallow tray and freeze. Take the tray out every 30–40 minutes and break up the ice crystals with a fork. Do this four or five times or until you have a tray of strawberry ice crystals.

The following day, whisk the cream before serving the dessert. Pile the strawberry crystals into individual bowls, push a pansy or two down the side, dribble with sherry, top with whipped cream and decorate with pansies. Serve immediately.

Almond pansy macaroons

MAKES ABOUT 18

These are simple to make and delicious served with ice-cream, custard, as a tea biscuit or with after-dinner coffee.

4 tablespoons castor sugar
4 tablespoons ground almonds
2 egg whites, stiffly beaten
1–2 drops vanilla essence
Fresh pansy flowers

Line a baking sheet with greaseproof paper and paint it with a little sunflower oil. Mix the sugar and almonds together and fold into the egg whites with the vanilla essence. Drop small spoonfuls onto the greased paper, well apart. Bake for 10–12 minutes at 180°C until faintly golden brown. Cool for a few minutes, then lift off with a spatula and cool on a wire rack. Store in an airtight tin.

COOK'S NOTE

When you are ready to serve the macaroons, mix a little icing sugar with water, and paint the mixture on the backs of fresh pansy flowers. Press the pansies onto each macaroon and arrange the macaroons attractively on a glass plate, decorated with more pansy flowers.

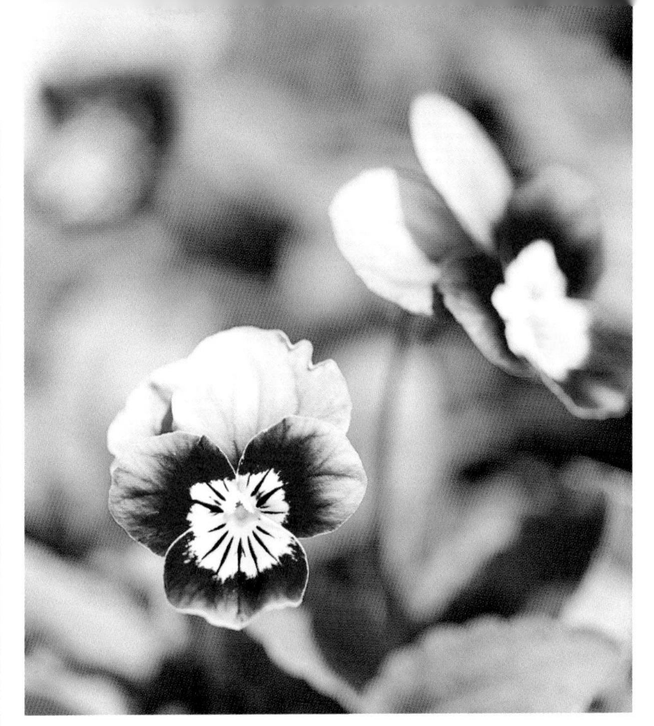

Pansy

Pansy and asparagus cheese bake

SERVES 6–8

I make this dish in spring when fresh asparagus and pansies are both at their best.

750 g fresh green asparagus spears
2 cups milk
2 eggs, well beaten
2 tablespoons flour
1 cup grated Gouda cheese
Sea salt and black pepper to taste
1 medium onion, finely chopped
1 cup brown breadcrumbs
1 tablespoon mealie-meal
2 tablespoons finely grated Parmesan cheese
1 tablespoon butter
10 heartsease flowers or other violas

Cut the asparagus spears into 2-cm lengths and cook them in boiling salted water. When just tender, drain and arrange in a glass baking dish. Whisk the milk into the eggs, followed by the flour, sweet-milk cheese, and the salt and pepper. Finally, whisk in the chopped onion. Mix the brown breadcrumbs, mealie-meal and Parmesan cheese together. Pour the egg mixture over the asparagus and top with the breadcrumb and parmesan mixture. Dot with butter and bake at 180°C for about 20 minutes or until the egg mixture is set and the cheese topping starts to brown. Decorate with violas just before serving.

Pea

Pisum sativum • **Garden pea**

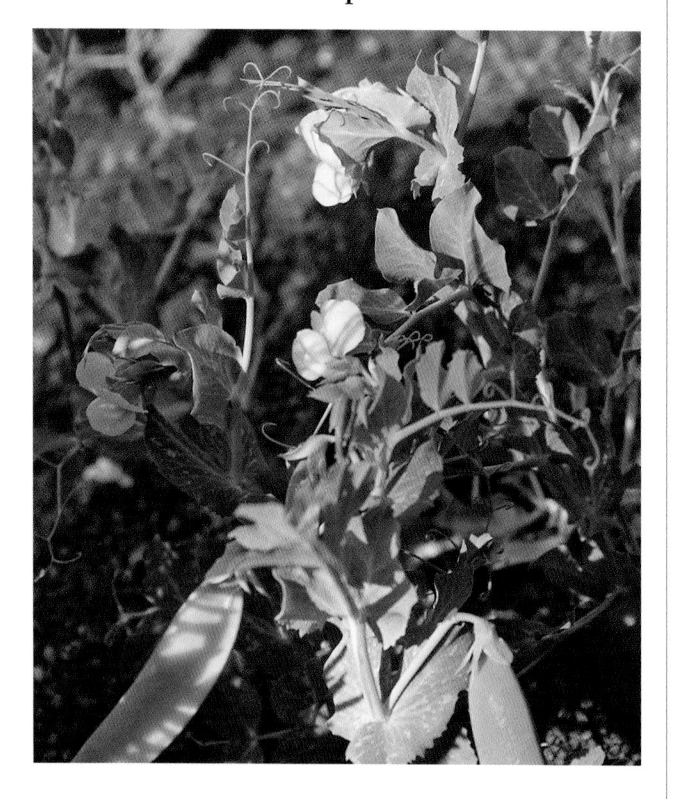

The pea is a robust and rewarding crop, perhaps as old as wheat and barley, and has been eaten as a green vegetable for over 7000 years! It originated in the Mediterranean basin as both a food and a medicine.

Ancient pharmacopoeias show that peas were recorded in Swiss Bronze Age burial sites around 5000 BC, and the ancient Greeks and Romans used peas in great quantities in soups and gruels and as trade. Herbal records indicate that peas were used as a winter medicine for respiratory ailments, and that trade in pea greens for medicinal purposes surpassed trade in pea greens as a food!

In the Middle Ages monks grew peas in their cloister gardens and made hot pea soups for coughs and colds and to treat the many ailments that benefitted from them. In 1602 dried peas were taken to America on the Mayflower and soon became a lucrative trade. A little later, a French gardener developed the first tender-podded climbing pea, and this became a favourite gourmet food in the court of Louis XIV. Today peas are grown commercially in the cool temperate regions of the world, not as greens or edible flowers, but as ripe pods, and about 20 million tons are grown and distributed per annum.

Personally I have focused on growing the old antique or heritage varieties of pea. I use the whole plant, including the succulent flowers, which are mostly white but also palest pink. These old-fashioned garden peas are, I believe, the healthiest peas of all! However get to know all cultivated varieties – sugar snaps, *petit pois* and *mangetout* included – as peas are a health food everyone can relish!

CULTIVATION

Sow the seeds 30–50 cm apart in deeply dug richly composted soil in full sun and in a wide furrow so that a hosepipe can be inserted at one end. Sow in March or early April and set a trellis, fence or lattice for them to climb onto as they are essentially climbers. Watch over the young pea shoots as birds, cutworms, monkeys and squirrels love them! I cover them with leaves to camouflage them and crisscross sticks over the area. Give them a long slow twice-weekly watering; as the days shorten, once-weekly is usually sufficient. For the winter plantings I have successfully grown peas next to carrots, turnips, radishes and lettuce.

To sprout peas, soak a cupful in a bowl of warm water and leave overnight. The next morning spread the peas in a shallow dish lined with wet cotton wool. Keep the peas moist by spritz-spraying them frequently, and allow them to grow in good light. I place the tray in sunlight for a short while every now and then to keep them mildew free. When the sprouts are 3–4 cm high pull them up and eat them fresh and succulent with salads and stir-fries.

MEDICINAL USES

Green peas and their flowers are rich in protein, phosphorus, zinc, manganese, potassium, magnesium, vitamins B, C and K, folic acid and amino acids. The whole pea plant should be eaten at least three times a week during the winter months to act as an invigorating tonic, to fight infections and boost the immune system.

Peas, flowers and leafy sprigs have long been a respected folk remedy for detoxifying the liver, and clearing digestive ailments, bloating and cramps. To make a soothing hot tea, pour a cup of boiling water over half a cup of pea flowers and one teaspoon of caraway seeds. Leave the tea to stand for five minutes. Stir it well and sip slowly, chewing the seeds and eating the flowers for full benefit. This acts as a tonic for the whole system, and taken after a heavy rich meal, it will quickly relieve indigestion. Pea flowers and mint also make an excellent digestive tea – pour a cup of boiling water over half a cup of mint sprigs mixed with pea flowers. Let the tea stand for five minutes, strain and sip slowly.

In Asia young tender pea shoots, known as *tou mio*, are stir-fried with other vegetables, adding an enormous number of vitamins, minerals and amino acids to the diet.

Pea flower tonic soup for the digestive system

SERVES 4

For irritable bowel syndrome, indigestion, bloating cramps, this easy-to-make mild soup will become a panacea.

4 cups flowering tips of the pea vine, flowers, leaves, tendrils
2 cups chopped fennel leaves, stems, flowers
2 cups chopped celery
2 teaspoons aniseeds
2 teaspoons caraway seeds
2 litres chicken stock
Juice of 1 lemon
½ cup chopped parsley
Sea salt to taste

Boil up everything together in a heavy-bottomed pan. Cook for about 40 minutes, then liquidise. Serve hot.

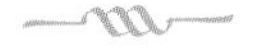

CULINARY USES

Pea flower soup

SERVES 4-6

This soup takes some beating on a cold winter's day!

½ cup olive oil
6 leeks, carefully cleaned and thinly sliced
2–3 large potatoes, peeled and coarsely grated
8–10 cups finely chopped pea tendrils, leafy sprigs and flowers
1 teaspoon crushed cumin seed
Sea salt and black pepper to taste
2 litres strong chicken stock
Juice of 1 lemon

Heat the oil in a heavy-bottomed pot. Fry the leeks with the grated potatoes for a few minutes, stirring frequently. Add the pea shoots and flowers and the cumin seed, sea salt and pepper, and lastly the chicken stock. Simmer the soup until tender. Add the lemon juice and taste; a little more salt or lemon juice may be needed. For a smooth soup, use a stick blender and whirl to a smooth consistency. Serve piping hot decorated with fresh pea flowers, a grinding of black pepper and homemade brown bread.

Pea flower relish

2 × 500 g JARS

This relish is delicious served with chops, sausages or baked potatoes, or even with cheese on bread rolls, and it keeps well in the fridge.

4 cups pea flowers and a few tendrils
2 onions, sliced into rings
12 radishes, topped and tailed and quartered (add more if there is space)

Sauce
1 cup dark grape vinegar
¾ cup honey
¼ cup hot water
2 teaspoons mustard powder
2 teaspoons coriander seeds, lightly crushed

Pack the jars with layers of pea flowers, onion rings and radishes. Simmer the sauce ingredients together for 10 minutes, and pour the hot sauce over the bottled ingredients. Seal and label the jars – do not open them before the relish has matured for two weeks!

COOK'S NOTE

The more you pick pea flowers the more they grow, plus they are one of the best winter salad ingredients. I find that butter lettuce, pea flowers and tendrils, thinly sliced radishes, and a big squeeze of fresh lemon juice makes a most satisfying winter salad. Served with hardboiled eggs, homemade mayonnaise, and homemade brown bread, this is a meal fit for a king!

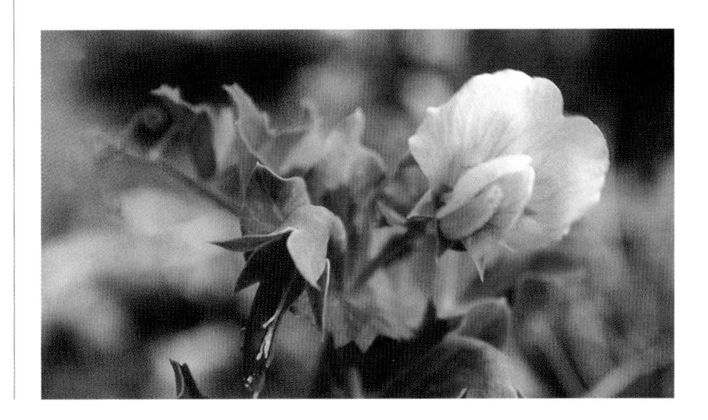

Peach blossom

Prunus persica

Three hundred years before Christ, the Greek philosopher Theophrastus wrote about the peach, naming it perske after Persia, which he thought to be its country of origin, and Dioscorides mentioned the peach in the first century. It is in fact native to China, where a huge number of cultivated varieties exist today. It took many centuries for the peach to reach Europe, and in 1629 the first peach trees were sent to America where they flourished, and from there they spread rapidly around the world.

CULTIVATION

It is important to choose a variety of peach that will do well in your area as there are a vast number of cultivated varieties available today. I tend to choose the earliest of fruiting peaches as this eliminates the need to spray. Tansy planted under the trees will help to prevent insect attack. Peach trees need rich, well-composted soil in full sun and can be pruned into attractive small trees that are perfect even in a small garden. Peaches fruit on young shoots, so pruning is not difficult. Merely shaping the tree in its first few years will ensure a practical, attractive shape in years to come.

I am saddened by the decline in popularity of peach, plum, fig and apricot trees compared with a mere 50 years ago, when every garden had at least one or two kinds of fruit tree. Their brief early spring flowering is a delight to the eye, and the first sign that spring is on the way.

MEDICINAL USES

Organically grown peaches are a superb health food. Rich in vitamins A and C and beta-carotene, the fruit (and to a lesser extent the blossom) is alkaline in the body and helps to eliminate toxins. It is important that peaches are eaten fresh, as the sugar and sulphur content in tinned and dried fruit are best avoided, and they should be unsprayed and organically grown. Easily digestible, they are particularly important for the elderly and they combine beautifully with other fruits. In 17th century Italy peach blossom was made into a poultice for bruises, rashes, eczema, grazes and stings.

Tea made from the leaves or blossoms is a marvellous detoxifier for the kidneys, and the significant calcium, phosphorus and iron content has a tonic action on the blood. Even today in rural areas around the world peach blossom tea (and peach leaf tea when the leaves appear in early summer), is made to ease kidney ailments and urinary tract infections and to clear the body of toxins, especially after a debilitating illness. To make the tea, pour a cup of boiling water over ¼ cup fresh or dried blossom. Allow the tea to stand for five minutes, then strain. Sweeten with honey if liked or add a slice of lemon, and in the case of an aching kidney area, add a few thin slices of fresh ginger.

CAUTION: Do not use the ornamental flowering peach – only the blossom of the fruit-bearing peach is used medicinally.

Peach blossom vinegar for wasp stings

I have made this remedy every spring for many years, especially when my children were little. If it is applied immediately after the sting, there will be very little swelling. The secret is to keep applying the vinegar-soaked cloth to the stung area.

1 bottle clear grape vinegar
1 cup peach blossoms, calyx and petals

Press the peach blossoms, calyx and petals into the vinegar. Cork it securely and give it a daily shake. After two weeks it will be potent. I leave the blossoms in the vinegar and with time they become almost translucent. When stung by a wasp, quickly soak a paper towel or a wad of cotton wool in the vinegar and apply it to the area. Frequently resoak the poultice in the peach blossom vinegar. Also suck two Nat Mur tissue salt tablets every 10 minutes for an hour.

CULINARY USES

Springtime peach blossom sundae

SERVES 1

Treat yourself to this exquisite dessert as soon as the blossoms appear, as they are present so briefly. This springtime sundae is so visually lovely that it is almost a shame to eat it!

2 scoops vanilla ice-cream
1 banana
1 tablespoon chopped pecan nuts
Glacé cherries
Cinnamon
½ cup fresh peach blossom petals

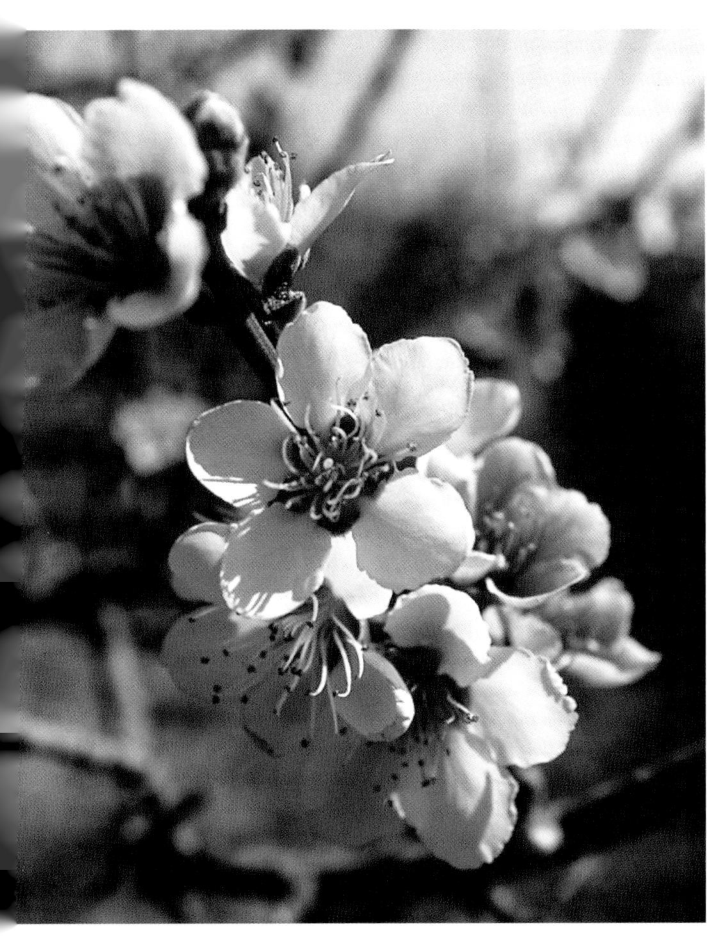

Place the ice-cream in a pretty glass bowl. Slice a banana in half lengthways and place the halves on either side of the ice-cream to form a little boat. Sprinkle with the nuts and dot with cherries. Dust with cinnamon and sprinkle liberally with the peach blossom petals. Add strawberries or mulberries and whipped cream for variation.

Peach blossom spring fruit salad

SERVES 4

During winter we tend to yearn for a refreshing fruit salad. This one is made from the first spring fruits.

4 pears, peeled and diced
2 cups strawberries, hulled and sliced and sprinkled with honey
2 cups mulberries, stalks removed and sprinkled with honey
2 apples, peeled and finely grated
2 bananas, peeled and thinly sliced
1 small pineapple, finely grated
½ cup pear juice
1 cup cream
¾ cup peach blossom petals

Mix the fruits and juice together. Whip the cream, place the fruit salad in individual glass dishes, add a good dollop of cream, and sprinkle lavishly with peach blossom petals.

Grilled mushrooms with peach blossom

SERVES 4

This is a quick-and-easy supper dish. Ring the changes with different sauces such as fresh tomato sauce, green pepper and onion sauce, or cheese sauce. The peach blossom gives a light and delicate taste to the otherwise fairly strong flavours.

8 large brown mushrooms
Butter
Juice of 1 lemon
1 large onion, peeled and finely chopped
Olive oil
2 cups peeled, diced tomatoes
2 tablespoons honey
2 teaspoons chopped fresh oreganum
1 cup chopped celery
Sea salt and pepper to taste
¾ cup peach blossom petals
Chopped parsley

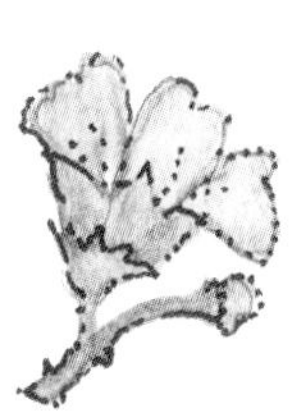

Place the mushrooms stalk side up on a flat baking dish and dot with butter. Squeeze the lemon juice over them. Place under the grill for about 10 minutes. Meanwhile, make the sauce. Brown the onion in a little olive oil, add the tomatoes and simmer until tender. Stir in the honey. Add the oreganum, celery and seasoning and stir for a minute or two. Pour the sauce over the mushrooms, and sprinkle with the peach blossom petals and a little chopped parsley. Serve with brown rice.

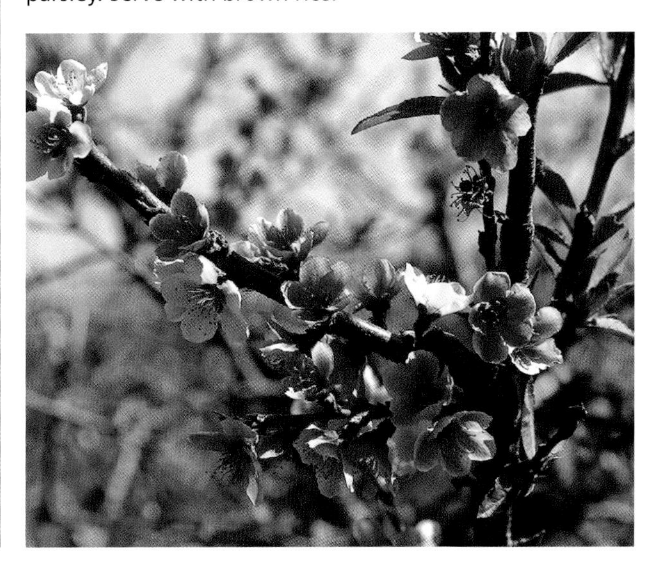

Pineapple sage

Salvia elegans ● *S. rutilans*

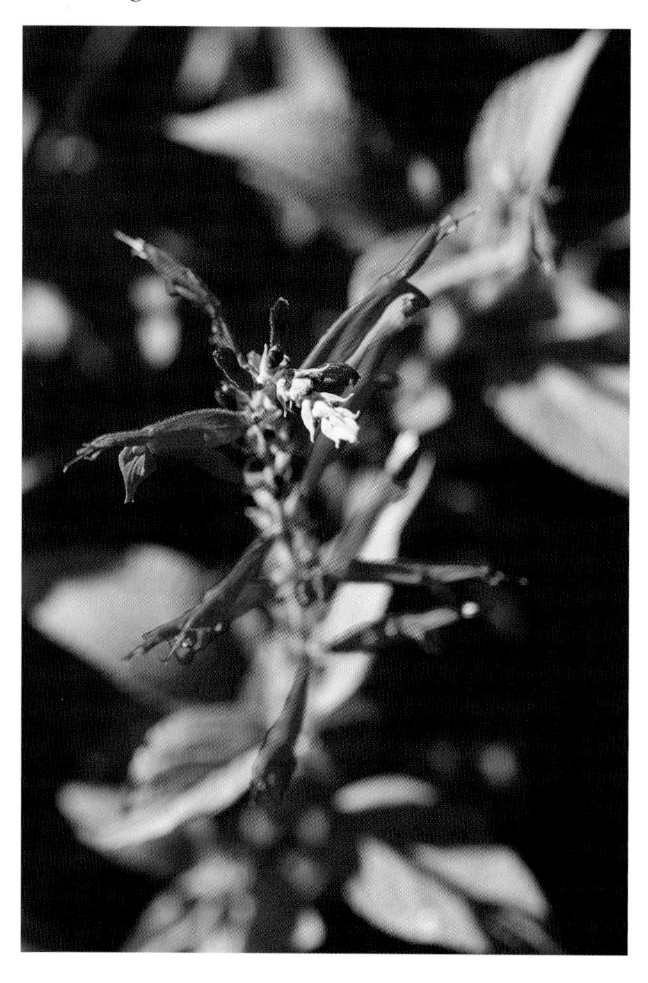

The sages are a huge family comprising hundreds of species, some of which are annual, some biennial and some perennial (pineapple sage is perennial). It is a deliciously scented and flavoured sub-shrub, originating in Mexico and other parts of South America. In ancient times pineapple sage was used in sacrificial ceremonies as a gift to the gods. The stems were rubbed onto floors and pillars to impart their exotic fragrance, and bunches of pineapple sage were burned on ceremonial fires to ward off evil spirits. Water flavoured with pineapple sage flowers was drunk at ceremonies to cleanse the body before imbibing potent drinks made from prickly pears and other fermented fruits, and it was also taken afterwards to help relieve hangovers.

CULTIVATION

Pineapple sage can reach 1 m in height in favourable conditions. It is frost-tender and sun-loving, and forms a striking feature in the garden with its abundant multi-stemmed growth. A twice-yearly dressing of compost and a deep weekly watering is all it requires. In late winter cut back all the flowering stems to ground level to encourage tender new shoots. The strong, unmistakable pineapple scent is attractive to butterflies, and just one blazing bush will draw a host of multi-coloured butterflies to the garden. To propagate pineapple sage, dig out small tufts of rooted new shoots with a sharp spade and transplant immediately into well-dug, well-composted soil 1 m apart in full sun. Do not let the new little clumps dry out, and mulch the ground around them with dry leaves to protect them against changes of temperature.

MEDICINAL USES

Pineapple sage is a member of the great Laminaceae family; like *Salvia officinalis*, it has antibiotic properties, and a tea made from the flowers and a few leaves is an effective treatment for chesty coughs, colds and blocked noses. Infuse ¼ cup of fresh flowers and leaves in a cup of boiling water and allow the tea to stand for five minutes, then strain and sweeten with honey. When lemon juice is added to the tea it makes an effective gargle; this was once popular with chanters and singers in religious ceremonies, who believed that it strengthened the voice.

A poultice of crushed flowers will quickly soothe bee stings and mosquito bites.

Pineapple sage nose cream

For a painful, red nose, raw from endless blowing during a cold or flu, this is a gently soothing cream that will quickly repair all the redness.

1 cup aqueous cream
½ cup pineapple sage flowering sprigs
½ cup thyme flowering sprigs
½ cup comfrey leaves and flowers, finely chopped
2 teaspoons vitamin E oil
1 teaspoon tea tree oil
1 teaspoon eucalyptus oil

Simmer the aqueous cream, pineapple sage sprigs, thyme sprigs and comfrey in a double boiler for 20 minutes. Take it off the heat and allow to stand for 10 minutes. Strain and then add the three oils. Spoon into a sterilised jar. Apply frequently to the nose and also a little around each nostril. This cream is antiseptic, antiviral and antibacterial. Treasure it!

COSMETIC USES

A bundle of flowering sprigs tied in a piece of muslin and tossed under the hot water tap in the bath will soften and soothe sunburned and wind-chapped skin. The crushed flowers were once used as a cosmetic by country girls who rubbed them on their cheeks to create a blush. Mashed into a little boiling water and left to stand until pleasantly warm, the flowers were also rubbed into the nails to strengthen them and colour them lightly.

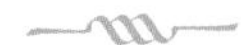

CULINARY USES

Pineapple sage and grapefruit health breakfast

SERVES 1

1 large ruby grapefruit
1 tablespoon sesame seeds
2 teaspoons grated fresh ginger root
2 tablespoons soft brown caramel sugar
½ teaspoon freshly grated nutmeg
1 tablespoon pineapple sage flowers

Carefully cut and scoop segments out of the grapefruit, place in a bowl and add the sesame seeds, ginger root, sugar and nutmeg. Mix everything together well before adding the flowers. Mix lightly. Spoon into a glass bowl and serve chilled, decorated with a few fresh flowers.

> COOK'S NOTE
> **Because of their distinctive pineapple taste, pineapple sage flowers can be added to drinks, fruit salads and desserts, and their bright red colour lends an exotic look to any dish. To make an easy dessert for a hot summer Sunday lunch, scoop balls of vanilla ice cream into a dish and cover with finely chopped fresh pineapple, sprinkled with lots of pineapple sage flowers.**

Couscous and pineapple sage

SERVES 4

Couscous is an ancient grain devised by the Berbers of North Africa from millet, and later from wheat. The national dish of Morocco, it is full of vitamins and minerals. Couscous is available in most supermarkets, and like rice, is superb served with meat, stews and spicy relishes.

2 cups couscous, the instant, commercial kind
½ cup pineapple sage flowers
1 cup finely chopped or grated fresh pineapple
½ cup finely chopped parsley
Juice of 1 lemon
½ tablespoon finely crushed coriander seeds

Cook the couscous according to the directions on the box. I usually soak the grains for five minutes in warm water and then steam them in a steamer, separating the grains with a fork. When fluffy and tender, serve on a flat warm dish, and at the last minute sprinkle with the flowers, pineapple, parsley, lemon juice and coriander seeds. Serve hot with a rich meat or chicken stew.

Pineapple sage and fresh pineapple drink

SERVES 4

This is a delicious drink for hot summer days. Ring the changes with litchi, apple or mango juice. If using mango juice, add the flesh of one peeled ripe mango to the pineapple puree.

1 large, very sweet pineapple or 2 small ones
½ cup fresh mint leaves
3 cups plain white grape juice
Honey to sweeten
Pineapple sage flowers for decoration

Peel, chop and liquidise the pineapple. Add the mint leaves and grape juice and whirl until smooth. Chill until ready to serve. Just before serving, taste for sweetness. If necessary, add a little honey and whirl again. Pour into tall glasses and sprinkle with pineapple sage flowers.

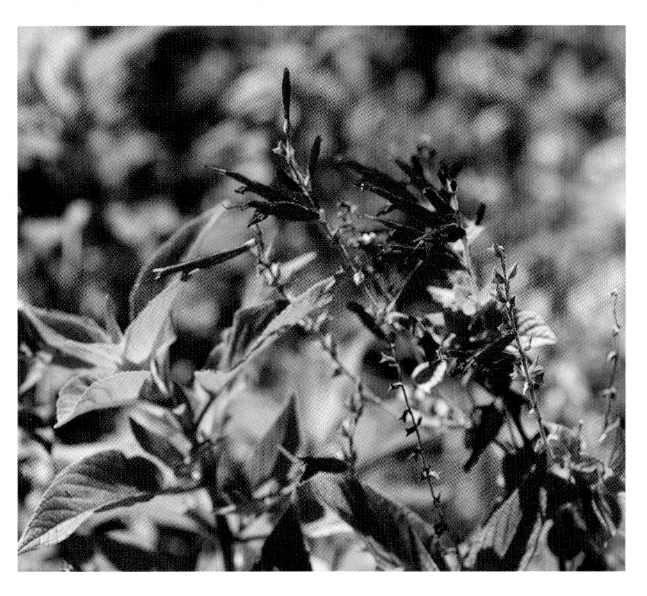

Plum blossom

Prunus domestica

The plum originated in western Asia and the Caucasus and can be dated back about 2 000 years. It was first naturalised in Greece and subsequently throughout the temperate regions of the world, and by the 15th century plums were grown widely in France and Italy. They were a staple fruit crop in Britain up until the Second World War, when their popularity waned unaccountably and plum orchards gave way to other more important food crops. From then on plums were found mostly in cottage gardens and old farmyards, and sadly many of the early cultivated varieties were lost for all time.

CULTIVATION

Plums favour a heavier, moister soil than most fruit trees, but bear well in most positions, requiring little attention other than good, rich soil in full sun, a dressing of compost twice a year, a deep weekly watering, and a winter pruning that shapes the tree. In colder areas plums do well trained or espaliered in a fan shape against a wall, and can be pruned vigorously early on, as the branches often sag under the weight of the fruit. Plant tansy underneath plum trees to keep fruit flies at bay.

Plant a plum tree near the house to enjoy its fragrance and beauty all year. Today nurseries offer self-pollinating varieties and all plums make a charming tree, with exquisite white blossoms in spring, and fruit and shade in summer. Judicious propagation has resulted in about 1 500 varieties, including prunes, and commercial plum orchards are in vogue once again.

MEDICINAL USES

All varieties of plum are rich in minerals and vitamins, but need to have ripened fully before eating to prevent acidity. They are high in phosphorus, calcium and vitamins A and C. Fresh plums have a laxative effect, and dried prunes are an even more potent natural laxative. In ancient Greek medicine, plum blossoms were used to treat bleeding gums and mouth ulcers, and to tighten loose teeth.

Mixed together with sage leaves and flowers, plum blossoms were used in plum wine or plum brandy as a mouthwash to soothe a sore throat and mouth ailments and to sweeten bad breath. As plums and sage both flower in spring, it is easy to see why they were combined in this way. Plum trees flower prolifically in spring for a brief period; during this time every year I make plum blossom vinegar, which has similar benefits in the mouth and throat.

Plum blossom vinegar

This vinegar makes a soothing gargle for treating oral infections and sore throats.

1 cup plum blossoms, fully opened, calyxes included
3 cups apple cider vinegar

Pick the blossoms when they are fully open and push them into a bottle containing the apple cider vinegar. Give the mixture a daily shake. Do this for about 10 days, then strain. Discard the old blossoms and replace with a cup of fresh flowers. Leave them in the bottle for 10 days and then strain. Use one tablespoon of the vinegar in a glass of water as a rinse, or gargle to clear mouth infections and sore throats.

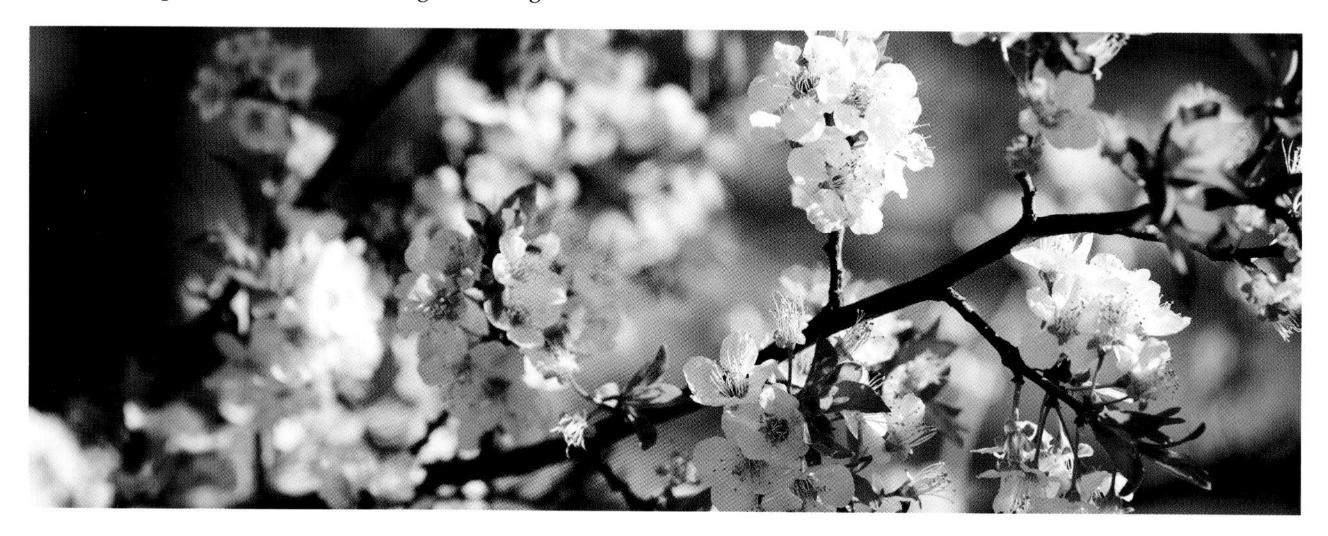

Greek plum blossom and sage mouthwash

This recipe was recorded by the ancient Greeks and is useful for treating ulcers, bleeding gums and halitosis.

1 bottle good brandy
1 cup plum blossoms
1 cup sage leaves and flowers
4 tablespoons honey

Warm two cups of the brandy with the plum blossoms, sage flowers and leaves and the honey in a double boiler for 20 minutes, stirring gently now and then. Allow it to cool for 10 minutes, then strain and add to the bottle of brandy, first pouring out some of the remaining brandy. Carefully insert the blossoms and sage, top up the bottle with brandy and cork. To use the mouthwash, dilute one tablespoon of the mixture with half a cup of hot water and swish around the mouth, a few sips at a time. Keep it in the mouth as long as possible, then swallow or spit it out.

CULINARY USES

Plum blossom and pumpkin supper dish

SERVES 4

This delicious and comforting supper was made in the old days on the farm in the early spring, when the nights were still chilly. The last of the winter-stored pumpkins would have been used to make this deliciously sustaining dish with the first spring plum blossom.

4 cups peeled, diced pumpkin
1 tablespoon butter
½ cup soft brown caramel sugar
2 teaspoons cinnamon
1 cup chopped onion
1 cup chopped celery
2 tablespoons sunflower oil
½–¾ cup plum blossom
½ cup seedless raisins or sultanas, soaked for 20 minutes in hot water
½ cup sesame seeds
½ cup sunflower seeds
1 teaspoon mustard powder
Salt and pepper to taste
1 cup grated cheddar cheese

Cook the pumpkin in salted water until tender. Drain, and mash in the butter, sugar and cinnamon. Stir-fry the onion and celery in the oil until they just start to brown. Add the plum blossom, drained raisins, sesame seeds and sunflower seeds. Season with mustard powder, salt and pepper. Finally, add the pumpkin and stir-fry until everything is thoroughly mixed. Spoon the mixture into a serving dish, sprinkle with the grated cheese, and place briefly under the grill until the cheese is melted. Serve piping hot.

Chinese plum blossom tea

SERVES 1

Plum blossom tea has almond overtones and was considered a great delicacy in 16th century China. The buds were picked in spring and dried and stored in caddies for the winter months. However, fresh blossoms are far nicer. Remember that the Chinese tea ceremony is unhurried and peaceful, which is how this delicious tea will be of most benefit.

1 cup boiling water
1 tablespoon fresh plum blossom
1 small sprig spearmint (or any other mint)

Pour the boiling water over the plum blossom and sprigs of mint. Allow the tea to draw for five minutes. Strain, sweeten with honey and sip slowly. This is an excellent after-dinner drink too, and can be added cold to jellies and jams.

Plum blossom and celery cheese platter

SERVES 4

This is delicious as a light lunch, or served in the traditional way at the end of a meal. You can combine any of your favourite cheeses, moistened if necessary with a little cream or milk to obtain a smooth consistency.

½ cup mashed feta cheese
½ cup cream cheese
½ cup soft goat's milk cheese
6 long celery sticks, washed and cut into 10 cm lengths
Sea salt and paprika to taste
½ cup plum blossoms

Mix the cheeses together in a food processor to form a smooth paste. Mound the cheese neatly in the hollow of each celery stick, and sprinkle with sea salt, paprika and plum blossoms. Serve on a bed of lettuce together with savoury biscuits.

Plumbago

Plumbago auriculata • **Cape leadwort** • **Cape forget-me-not**

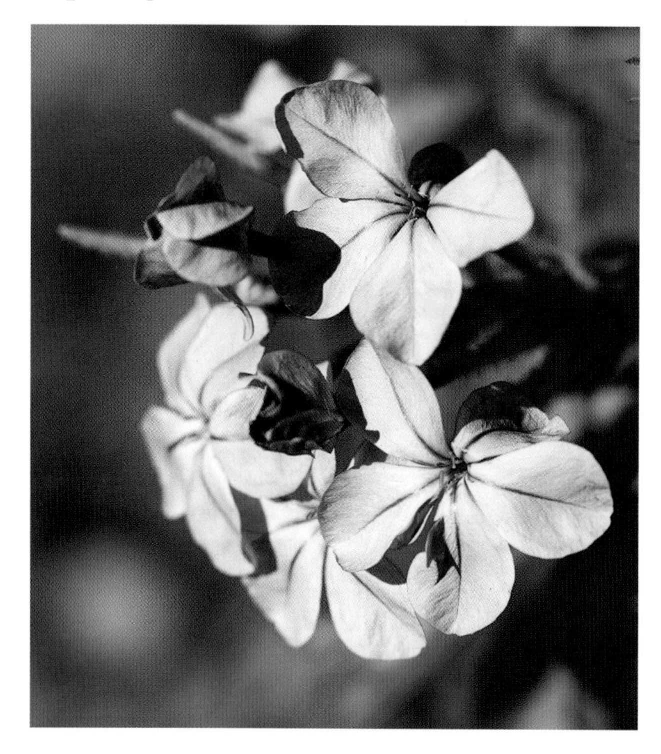

This pretty, blue-flowered, scrambling shrub is indigenous to South Africa and has become a treasured hothouse plant all over the world, beloved because of its long flowering period and the sky-blue clusters of flowers it produces so lavishly. In its wild state it grows in great swathes on banks and hillsides, clothed in magnificent blue in summer. However, it is enormously obliging and can be trained up trellises, espaliered on a wall or fence, or clipped into a pretty hedge, requiring little more than the occasional pruning and clipping back of spent flowers. A strong individual stem can be staked and side bits constantly pruned to form a beautiful blue topiary ball. It takes three years to reach perfection with regular attention, but the result is well worth the wait.

CULTIVATION

Propagation is by means of rooted pieces dug off from the mother plant. New plants should be planted in a sunny position and will tolerate even poor, dry soil, making plumbago a valuable garden plant for dry regions where water is in scarce supply. A newer cultivated variety of plumbago called 'Royal Cape' is available at many nurseries, and is being marketed as far afield as England, America and Australia. This variety is particularly suitable for large tubs and can be trained into a small topiary ball; it is especially attractive on account of its astonishingly brilliant blue flowers.

MEDICINAL USES

Plumbago flowers can be used to make a wonderfully soothing cream for sunburn, burns, spots and rashes. To heal a bruise, place fresh crushed flowers over the affected area, cover the flowers with the soothing cream and bind in place with a cloth. Relax for 10 minutes. You will be amazed at the efficacy of this old-fashioned folk treatment! A crushed flower or two placed over a slow-to-heal scratch will quickly soothe and heal it. Hold in place with a small plaster.

Healing plumbago skin cream

Use this cream to treat burns, spots, rashes and bruises.

1 cup crushed plumbago flowers
1 cup aqueous cream
4 teaspoons vitamin E oil

Mix the crushed flowers in the aqueous cream, then simmer in a double boiler with the lid on for 25 minutes, stirring well. Strain the cream through a fine sieve while it is still hot. As it cools, mix in the vitamin E oil. Pour into sterilised jars and keep in the fridge.

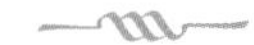

COSMETIC USES

Plumbago flowers make a soothing lotion that beats the heat, refreshes and revitalises hot greasy skin, refines large pores, and cleanses away perspiration and grime, and soothes rashes and pimples, clearing away the infection and redness.

Plumbago lotion

For sunburn, blemishes, rashes, pimples and red spots, plumbago lotion is quickly soothing and healing. Use the flowers with oats and warm water to wash greasy problem skin.

2 cups plumbago flowering heads
2 litres water
4 tablespoons rosewater

Boil the flowering heads in the water for 10 minutes. Cool, then strain and add the rosewater. Moisten pads of cotton wool with the fragrant lotion and wipe the face, or pour into a spritz bottle and spray the face, neck and arms to clear away grime and perspiration and to cool down. The lotion can also be applied to scratches, rashes and greasy skin, after the face has been washed well. It also acts as a refreshing 'air conditioner', especially if used on a long summer journey.

Crush half a cupful of plumbago flowers and use the pulp on acne spots and rashes as a gentle cleanser and scrub. Crush a further handful of flowers and continue to cleanse the face gently. The pulped flowers will help heal a rash as well. Apply two or three times a day.

CULINARY USES

Plumbago fruit jelly

SERVES 6

This lovely recipe comes from a farm in the hot, mountainous region of the Eastern Cape. It is a real winner on a summer's day.

2 tablespoons sugar
4 cups peeled, sliced peaches or nectarines
4 cups peeled, sliced prickly pears
2 tablespoons gelatine, dissolved in 1 cup warm water
2 cups peach or orange juice or water
1 cup plumbago flowers, pulled out of their sticky calyxes

Sprinkle the sugar over the peaches and arrange all the fruit in a glass bowl. Mix the dissolved gelatine and the fruit juice together. Tuck the plumbago flowers in between the fruit and gently pour the gelatine and juice mixture over the fruit. Chill. When set, serve with thick farm cream and decorate with plumbago flowers.

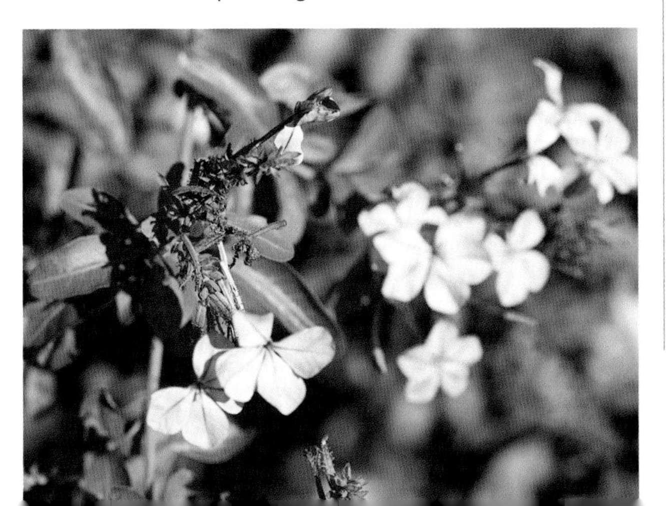

Plumbago and beetroot salad

SERVES 6–8

This is a traditional salad with a difference. It keeps beautifully bottled or in the fridge for up to two months and goes particularly well with a braai or barbecue.

10–12 well-scrubbed, medium-sized beetroots, unpeeled
1 tablespoon coriander seeds
1 teaspoon whole cloves
2 bay leaves
½ tablespoon allspice berries
1 crushed nutmeg
1 cup brown grape vinegar
1 cup brown sugar
½ cup water
½ cup plumbago flowers, pulled out of their sticky calyxes

Boil the beetroots until they are tender. Meanwhile, tie all the spices in a square of muslin and boil with the vinegar, sugar and water with the lid on for 10 minutes. Slide the skins off the beetroot and grate them coarsely. Spoon the grated beetroot into jars or a bowl, and sprinkle with the plumbago flowers. Remove the spices and pour the hot vinegar mixture over the salad. Serve it either hot or cold as a salad or relish. Decorate with more fresh plumbago flowers.

Lamb and potato pot roast with plumbago

SERVES 4–6

½ cup sunflower oil
8 lamb loin chops, trimmed of excess fat
2 large onions, peeled and sliced
6 potatoes, peeled and quartered
1 cup plumbago flowers, pulled out of their sticky calyxes
Sea salt and black pepper to taste
Juice of 1 lemon

Heat the oil in a heavy cast iron pot, and brown the chops. Add the onions and potatoes and stir-fry. When they are browned, add the plumbago flowers and just enough water to make a gravy. Season with salt and pepper and add the lemon juice. Stir frequently to prevent sticking and add a little more water when necessary. Turn down the heat, cover and simmer until the potatoes are tender. Serve piping hot with brown rice and vegetables, decorated with plumbago flowers.

Poppy

Papaver rhoeas ● **Field poppy** ● **Flanders poppy**

The bright red field poppy, *Papaver rhoeas*, has grown prolifically across Europe, Asia and the Mediterranean region for thousands of years, where it has been used as both food and medicine, and as a symbol. In the Victorian language of flowers the poppy signifies consolation. In Britain at the end of the First World War the field or Flanders poppy became the flower of remembrance for those killed at Flanders, the red petals symbolising the red of their blood. The Shirley poppy (*P. rhoeas* 'Shirley') is descended from the field poppy and is available in a wide range of colours that are breathtaking in spring. The opium poppy is quite different from the field poppy and comes in many forms, from plants with fringed petals to double- and single-flowered ones with a startling array of petal shapes and colours. Growth of the opium poppy is strictly controlled due to its potent narcotic effects. It is the source of the powerful painkillers codeine and morphine, and morphine's derivative, heroin.

Collect field poppy seed heads for dried flower arrangements and use the petals lavishly to decorate salads and fruit salads.

CULTIVATION

Sprinkle the tiny poppy seeds over moist, well-dug, well-composted soil in full sun in early autumn. Cover lightly with a scattering of small leaves to retain the moisture and keep lightly watered daily until they establish and become robust. Thereafter water twice-weekly.

MEDICINAL USES

Field poppy seeds sprinkled out of their ripe capsules were once believed to give energy and foresight and were treasured and stored for use throughout the year. Wet petals placed over a pimple or insect bite and left there to dry will soothe and take away the hot inflammation, and poppy petals steeped in vinegar make a soothing addition to the bath and will ease itches and rashes.

Poppy petal tea loosens excess mucous during coughs and colds and has remained a loved country recipe for centuries. To make the tea, steep petals from three poppies in a cup of boiling water for five minutes. Strain, and add a touch of honey or a squeeze of lemon juice.

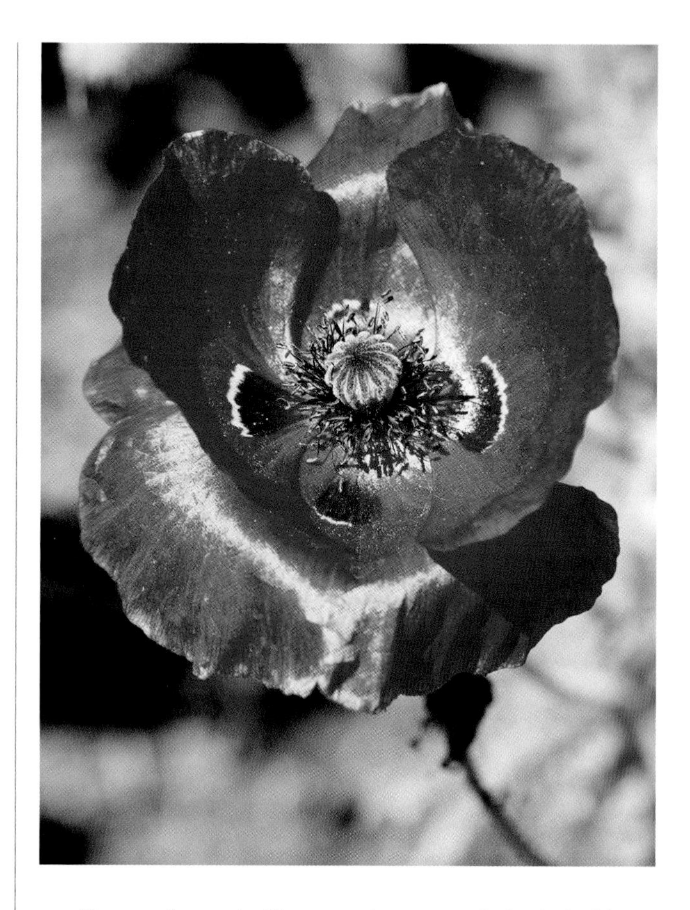

'Syrup of poppies' is an ancient remedy for irritable, paroxysmal and persistent coughs, as well as for insomnia and anxiety. I make it with elderflowers and chamomile for extra benefit.

CAUTION: The red field poppy is safe, but do not eat or use the opium poppy medicinally. All parts of it are dangerous except for the fully ripe seeds.

Poppy cough syrup

3 cups poppy petals
2 cups elderflowers, stalks discarded
2 cups chamomile flowers
2 cups raw honey
2 cups water

Simmer the ingredients in a double boiler on low heat for 20 minutes, stirring frequently to keep the flowers submerged. Let the syrup stand for 10 minutes (keep it covered). Strain the syrup through a fine strainer, pour into well-corked bottles and store in the fridge. Take a dessertspoonful in a little hot water and sip slowly – children love it! It is safe, soothing and wonderfully effective.

Poppy petal bath vinegar

This vinegar will soothe rashes and itches.

Poppy petals
1 bottle white grape vinegar

Push as many poppy petals as possible into the bottle of vinegar. The petals will colour the vinegar pink and then deep red as the vinegar blanches them. Keep the bottle in a warm place out of direct sunlight for 10 days. Give the vinegar a daily shake, then strain, discard the old petals, rebottle, add 4 or 5 fresh petals for identification, and cork well. Use half a cup in the bath, or soak a pad of cotton wool in the vinegar and dab over itchy areas.

CULINARY USES

Poppy petal muffins

MAKES 12 LARGE MUFFINS

Quick and simply delicious, these muffins are a treat for Sunday breakfast or a teatime snack.

½ cup sugar
5 tablespoons butter
Zest of 1 lemon
2 tablespoons water
2 cups cake flour
3 teaspoons baking powder
2 eggs
¾ cup milk
¾ cup plain yoghurt
2 tablespoons poppy seeds
½ cup chopped fresh poppy petals

Pre-heat the oven to 180°C. Simmer the sugar, butter, lemon zest and water in a small saucepan for two minutes, stirring until the sugar dissolves. Mix the flour and baking powder together. In a separate bowl, whisk the eggs, milk and yoghurt until creamy. Add the lemon zest and sugar mixture and whisk thoroughly. Add the flour mixture, poppy seeds and poppy petals. Stir well. Spoon into well-greased muffin pans, but do not fill them quite to the top as the muffins will rise. Bake for 15 minutes or until a skewer inserted into the middle of a muffin comes out clean. Remove from the pan and split the muffins open while still slightly warm, spread with butter and strawberry jam and top with a little whipped cream and a poppy petal. Serve immediately.

Poppy brandy

MAKES 750 ML

This potent brandy is based on a medieval recipe and can be served as a liqueur, on ice-cream, or on a sponge cake with cream. It makes a special gift. It is also delicious made with rum instead of brandy.

½ cup seedless raisins
1 tablespoon fennel seeds
1 tablespoon coriander seeds
1 tablespoon aniseed
2 tablespoons thinly sliced ginger
1 cup dark treacle sugar
1 bottle good brandy
1 cup lightly packed poppy petals and a few stamens

Pack the raisins into an empty bottle, followed by the spices and sugar. Add about two cups of brandy and shake well. Leave the mixture to stand for two hours, shaking every now and then until the sugar has completely dissolved. Add the poppy petals and stamens and the rest of the brandy. Shake well. Store the bottle in a dark cupboard for a month, giving it a shake every now and then. Resist tasting it before it is ready! Strain and pour into an attractive bottle. Discard the spices and petals.

Red salad with poppy vinaigrette

SERVES 6

A spectacular red salad, this recipe is unusual and very festive.

4 large tomatoes, sliced
2 sweet red peppers, diced
2 cups sliced strawberries
2 cups thinly sliced radishes
1 cup poppy petals

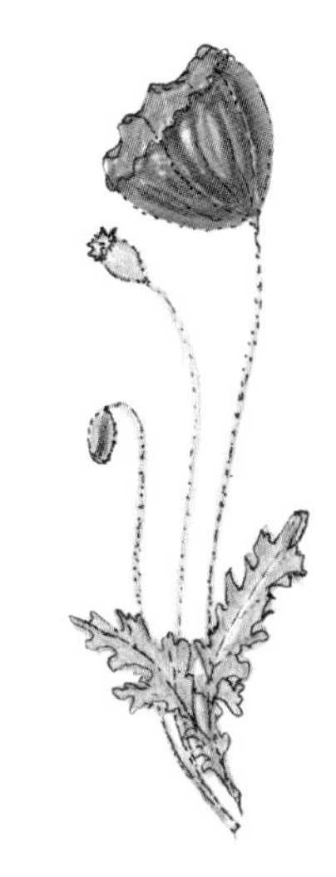

Poppy seed vinaigrette
3 tablespoons chopped fresh chives
¾ cup olive oil
½ cup brown grape vinegar
2 teaspoons mustard powder
½ cup brown sugar
2 tablespoons poppy seeds
Sea salt and black pepper to taste
2 tablespoons orange juice

Arrange the salad ingredients in a flat glass dish. To make the vinaigrette, place all the dressing ingredients in a screw-top bottle, seal well and shake. Pour the vinaigrette over the salad just before serving.

Prickly pear

Opuntia ficus-indica • **Cactus pear**

The rather prehistoric-looking prickly pear, or 'cactus pear' as it is also known, is native to Mexico and parts of North and South America, and has become naturalised in most hot dry countries around the world. It even flourishes in the great beds of volcanic lava near Sicily and in the coastal areas of the Mediterranean. The exotic, egg-shaped flowers emerge along the rims of the leaves in midsummer, their frill of bright petals topping a large, juicy, swollen calyx filled with pulp. All parts of this extraordinary plant are edible, but all are covered in tiny thorns, so careful handling is essential.

CULTIVATION

The prickly pear is easily propagated: merely chop off a leaf and push the stem end into loose, moist soil. If it is kept watered, it will sprout strong roots and continue to multiply by bearing more and more thick fleshy leaves. It thrives in heat and drought and withstands extreme conditions, seemingly unaffected by wind, hail and storms. Watch out for the brilliant red cochineal bug that was introduced to control the spread of the cactus. Brush the tiny white flecks off with a coarse-bristled brush at the first sign. Other than this pest, nothing will cause this remarkable plant to falter in its steady growth.

MEDICINAL USES

Crushed prickly pear petals can be used on insect bites to reduce the swelling and itch. Medical tests have found the petals and calyx to be rich in flavonoids, mucilage, fruit acids and sugars, as well as high quantities of vitamin C. The whole flower is astringent, and in Mexico the peeled, sliced fruit is used to reduce the pain and redness of scratches, grazes and infected wounds. The astringency stops the bleeding and tightens the surrounding tissue. The inner skin peeled from the ripening fruit (thorns removed carefully), makes a comforting dressing for wounds, burns, rashes and bites.

Because the whole flower has this remarkable astringent action, it is used in several countries to soothe and heal the gastrointestinal tract, and in cases of diarrhoea, colitis, irritable bowel syndrome, gastric ulcers, colic, heartburn and flatulence. In many rural areas the whole ripe fruit, which is the entire flower, is preserved in a syrup of honey and vinegar for the winter months (remove the thorns beforehand). In America the fruit is eaten fresh throughout the season (usually four months long) to treat an enlarged prostate gland, an effective folk remedy that has often astonished doctors. The elongated 'stem leaves' from which the other leaves grow can be used to make a splint for broken bones. Scrape off the thorns and split the stem leaf in half. Nestle the limb in it and bind in place.

A couple of leaves that have been gashed or scraped to release their oily juices can be tossed into a stagnant pool to get rid of mosquito larvae.

The flower petals soon drop off, leaving the swollen calyx or 'fruit'. This is the medicinal part, and I learned from the neighbouring farmers to make poultices using the ripe warmed fruit for bleeding or suppurating wounds.

Prickly pear wound poultice

This prickly pear poultice has been used to ease and soothe many an infected graze.

Prickly pears
Prickly pear flower petals
Boiling water

Peel the prickly pears carefully and mash the ripe pulp with a few flower petals in a flat dish.

Pour over enough boiling water to cover it and mash again. Take a spoonful or two of the pulp and gently massage it onto the graze, wearing latex gloves. Do this until all the warmed pulp is used up and is packed up over the wound. Cover with a warm wet cloth and bind in place. Leave it on for as long as it is comfortable and repeat for another day or two. The astringent properties of the swollen calyx of this thorny flower are amazing, and I have used this easy poultice to treat many injured farm animals.

Prickly pear syrup for gastric ulcers, diarrhoea and prostate ailments

10 ripe prickly pears
500 g honey
750 ml apple cider vinegar

Carefully peel the prickly pears, discarding the thorny skin. Slice them and pack into sterilised glass jars. Warm the honey and vinegar briefly, until the honey melts into the vinegar. Immediately pour this potent mixture over the sliced fruit, covering it completely. Seal immediately, label and store in a cool dark place. When needed, remove some of the fruit and leave it to drain. Eat one tablespoon daily to treat the prostate and gastric ulcers.

In some areas, the whole fruit (without the thorns) is bottled with the vinegar and honey. When needed, the thick outer skin is discarded and the fruit rinsed off before being eaten. This is done so that the sensitive digestive system can process the peeled fruit without the effects of the vinegar and honey.

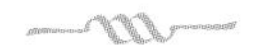

CULINARY USES

Prickly pear summer dessert

SERVES 6

This deliciously succulent fruit makes a party dessert that gets everyone talking!

20 multi-coloured prickly pears (golden yellow, light green and ruby red)
Whipped cream
Icing sugar

Peel the prickly pears and chill them for at least an hour. Slice them into 1-cm-thick rounds and arrange the slices on a glass dish. Dot with little blobs of whipped cream and dust with icing sugar. Serve chilled, and listen to the compliments!

Prickly pear salad

SERVES 4–6

1 butter lettuce
1 cup good mayonnaise
8 prickly pears, peeled and sliced into 1-cm-thick rounds
1 small pineapple, peeled and thinly sliced
2 cups green melon, scooped into balls
1 cup chopped celery
½ cup chopped basil
½ cup chopped parsley
Sea salt, paprika and black pepper to taste

Place the butter lettuce leaves neatly in a flat glass dish, starting at the edge. Spread a little mayonnaise on each leaf with a spoon. Arrange the prickly pear and pineapple slices over the lettuce. Add the melon balls and the celery pieces and spread evenly. Finally, sprinkle the chopped basil, parsley, sea salt, paprika and black pepper over the salad. Serve chilled.

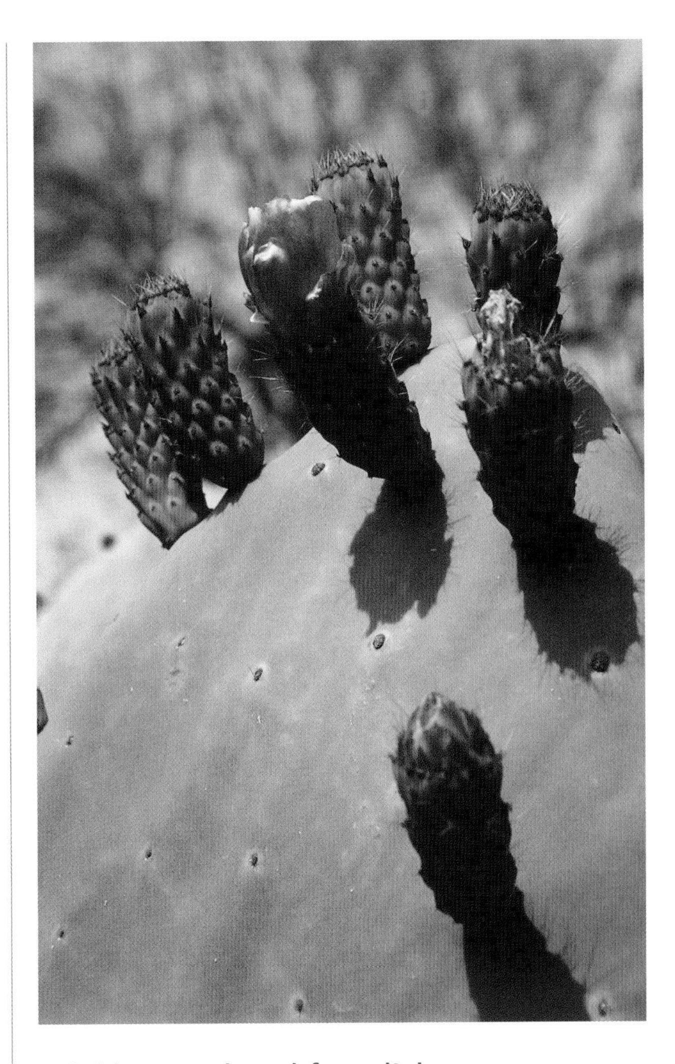

Prickly pear breakfast dish

SERVES 1

Loved by children, this cool, refreshing breakfast dish is energising and enjoyable. To ring the changes, slice half a banana with the prickly pear, or add a whole banana if you are hungry!

2 or 3 prickly pears, peeled and sliced
1 cup plain yoghurt
2 tablespoons sultanas, soaked in hot water for 1 hour beforehand
1 tablespoon chopped pecan nuts
⅔ cup cornflakes
Honey to sweeten

Place the prickly pear slices in a porridge bowl. Add the yoghurt and sprinkle with the sultanas, pecan nuts and cornflakes to add crunch. Dribble with honey and stir carefully. Enjoy this breakfast outside in the garden!

Pumpkin, squash & marrow flowers

Cucurbita species

All species of pumpkin, marrow and squash are vigorous, easy-to-grow, rambling vines. An enormous number of cross-bred and closely related species have been grown for millennia in Africa, the Americas and parts of Asia. They appeared in Europe only in the 16th century, and it was here that the huge variety we know today developed. Marrows and courgettes have more French, English and Italian origins, while the tougher, larger pumpkins were grown more widely in the Americas and Africa. Fields of mealies interplanted with pumpkins are a familiar sight in Africa, particularly the huge, flat *boerpampoen* that so resiliently withstands the rigours of the African climate and has always been a standby in times of food scarcity.

All *Cucurbita* species flower prolifically, and all the flowers are edible. The tender tips of the vines can also be eaten. They are delicious steamed or stir-fried, and along with the flowers, were considered survival foods and were believed to impart strength and fleetness of foot.

CULTIVATION

All species of *Cucurbita* are annual. Seed should be sown after the last frosts have passed, and all need full sun and well-composted soil. Space them 50 cm apart and water often until the plants are well established. Thereafter they need very little attention apart from a twice-weekly watering. They can be left to trail, or they can be trained over fences and arches. For me no summer is complete without a few vines somewhere in the vegetable garden or even in the back border.

MEDICINAL USES

Hulled pumpkin seeds liquefied with a little milk were traditionally used to treat worm infestations in both humans and animals and this remedy is still used today by rural communities around the world.

The pumpkin, and to a large extent the flowers, are rich in vitamins A, B and C, phosphorus and calcium, and also contain carbohydrate and protein. Pumpkin is an alkaline food rich in beta-carotene, and the highly nutritious inner kernels of the pips are good for the bladder and kidneys and for prostate problems.

External application of hot pumpkin over a boil or abscess was an ancient method of bringing a boil to a head, although one should take care that it is not too hot. I have used pumpkin many times on the farm over suppurating wounds, for animals as well, and I am always amazed at its healing qualities. Rural people spread mashed pumpkin over grazes and scrapes, held in place

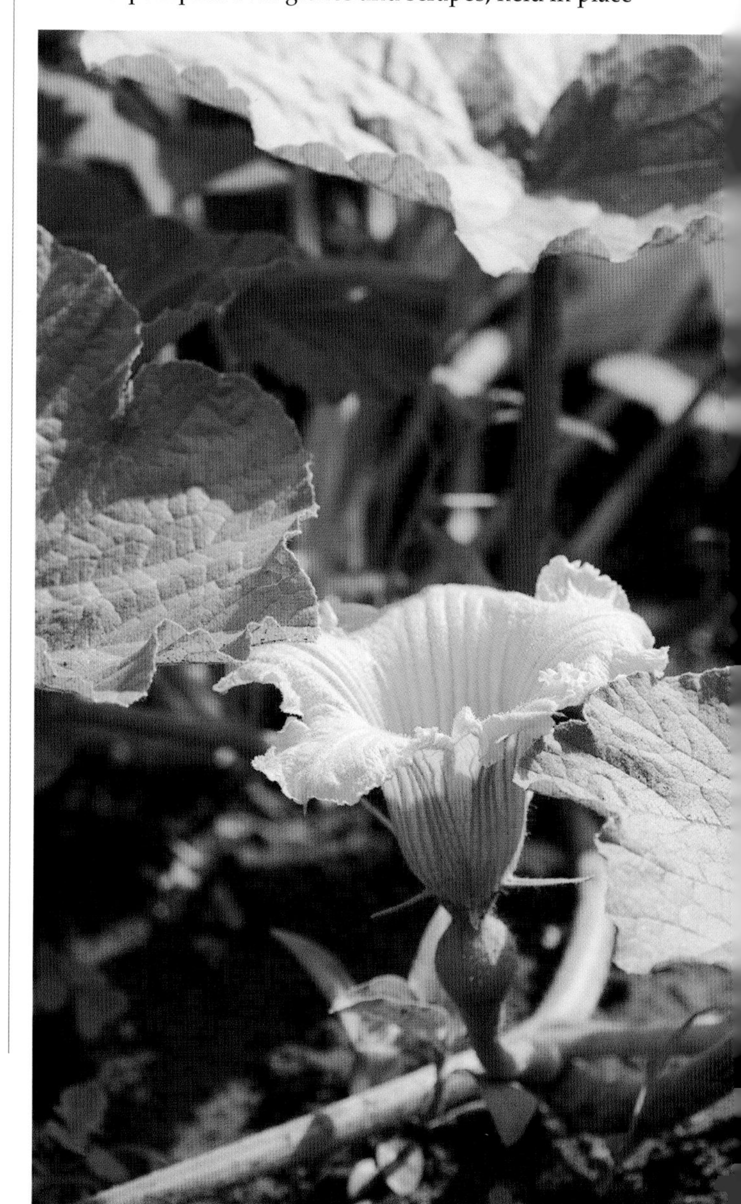

with a pumpkin flower that has been split open, and bind this in place with a crêpe bandage. The leaves are not used as they irritate the skin with their prickly texture.

CULINARY USES

Pumpkin flower soup

SERVES 4–6

This treasured standby provides a boost of energy and ensures a storehouse of health.

A little olive oil
2 cups chopped onion
2 cups chopped celery
6 cups peeled, diced pumpkin
6–10 pumpkin flowers, roughly chopped
½ cup honey
Sea salt and cayenne pepper to taste
Juice of 1 lemon
2 cups lucerne leaves and flowers (optional)
1 litre chicken or vegetable stock or water
½ cup parsley

Place a little oil in a large, heavy-bottomed pot and sauté the onions until transparent. Add the celery and stir-fry for a minute or two. Add the pumpkin, stir-fry for two minutes and then add all the remaining ingredients except for the parsley. (If you are living on a farm, lucerne leaves and flowers may be added for extra energy if you have them available.) Add the chicken or vegetable stock or water. Stir well. Cover and simmer for about 20 minutes or until the pumpkin and celery are tender. Blend in a liquidiser if you prefer, or serve the soup as it is with a sprinkling of parsley and hot crusty bread.

Stuffed squash flower salad

SERVES 4–6

This is a most acceptable salad for a summer lunch and so quick to prepare. Use any variety of squash or pumpkin flower.

12–14 squash or pumpkin flowers

Stuffing

1 tin tuna, drained and mashed
½ cup good-quality mayonnaise
Juice of 1 lemon
¼ cup finely chopped chives
¼ cup finely chopped parsley
1 tablespoon Worcestershire sauce
½ cup smooth cream cheese
½ cup finely chopped green pepper
Sea salt and black pepper to taste

Mash the stuffing ingredients together well. Spoon the mixture carefully into the squash or pumpkin flowers. Arrange the stuffed flowers on a bed of butter lettuce on a large platter, stalks facing inwards. Place slices of avocado (drizzled with lemon juice to prevent them from turning brown) and whole radishes in-between the flowers. Serve with brown bread and butter.

Baked pumpkin with stuffed pumpkin flowers

SERVES 4–6

This hearty vegetarian dish is deliciously sustaining when one is overtired.

12 pumpkin flowers
1 cup finely mashed feta cheese
1 cup finely grated cheddar cheese
Sea salt and black pepper
1 tablespoon fresh thyme
1 tablespoon fresh tarragon
A little yoghurt
A little olive oil
2 large onions, thinly sliced into rings
2 cups sliced mushrooms
6–8 thin, peeled pumpkin slices
A little brown sugar
Butter
2 cups chicken stock

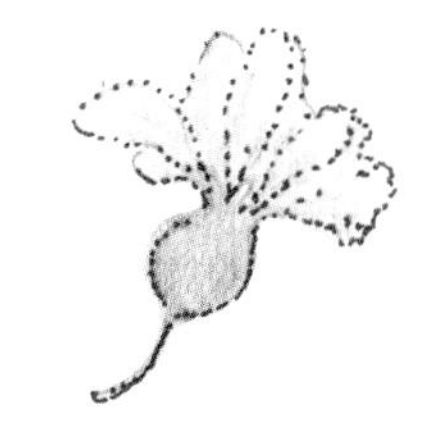

Stuff the pumpkin flowers with the feta cheese, cheddar cheese, sea salt, black pepper, thyme and tarragon, moistened with a little yoghurt. Pour the olive oil into a large baking pan. Place the stuffed pumpkin flowers in the pan. Lay the onion rings, mushrooms and pumpkin pieces on top of the pumpkin flowers. Sprinkle with a little brown sugar and dot with butter. Carefully pour the chicken stock into the pan (pour it down the side of the pan) and roast gently for about 30 minutes at 180°C until the pumpkin is tender and starting to brown. Check that it does not dry out, and add more water if necessary. Serve at the table directly from the pan. The juices will have mingled deliciously with the pumpkin flowers under all the vegetables. Serve with brown rice.

Red hibiscus

Hibiscus rosa-sinensis

Red hibiscus is one of the most loved flowers from the world's tropical and subtropical regions, and it is the most widely cultivated of the species. It has become virtually a symbol of exotic places like Malaysia, Jamaica and Hawaii.

This striking flower plays a role in many ceremonies and rituals. In Hindu ceremonies it is sacred to Ganesh, the elephant-headed deity, and even in the smallest shrines, a bright red hibiscus flower can usually be found tucked in next to the statue.

There are around 220 species of hibiscus, but only *H. rosa-sinensis* is used medicinally, in ceremonies and in rites. Also known as 'The Rose of China' and as *japakusuma* in Sanskrit, it has ancient beginnings in Ayurvedic medicine. Today it is grown commercially in India and it is being researched in that country as an emmenagogue (a herb that stimulates the menstrual flow).

Hawaiians use the flowers to make 'leis' or garlands for ceremonies, banquets and religious parades. Visitors love being decorated in this way and often take the dried flowers home as a memento.

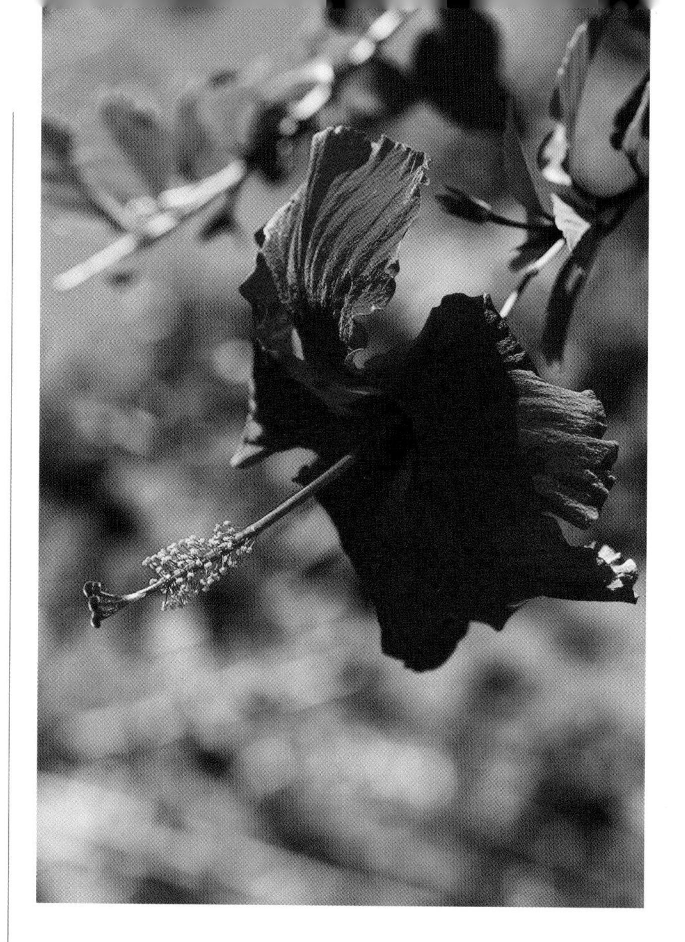

CULTIVATION

Easy and uncomplicated to grow, red hibiscus is a favourite old-fashioned plant. It has been used as a shrub, clipped and trained as a hedging plant, or left unrestrained for its constant flowers. It is also grown commercially in rows for its tough fibre-rich stems, its fresh green leaves and its startling red flowers.

Red hibiscus needs a deeply dug hole filled with compost, in full sun, and thrives with a long slow twice-weekly watering (once a week in winter). Soil must be well drained and the shrubs planted 2–3 m apart. The Hawaiians plait the branches together to make a boundary fence as the shrubs grow – they can reach 4–5 m in height if left unchecked! The plants are evergreen and demand little attention, but long branches can be pruned and they can be cut back to give shape. Use the long supple branches as support canes for other plants – they last well, stripped of their leaves. Flowers can be picked daily and used fresh.

One thing to watch out for is insect invasion. CMR beetles, scarab beetles and rose beetles all love the vibrant red of the petals. Drop the beetles into a bright yellow bucket (the beetles are attracted by the colour) half filled with water to which a tablespoon of liquid paraffin has been added. This will quickly and painlessly close the insects' breathing holes.

Today hibiscus hybrids are available in exquisite colours worldwide and nurserymen are constantly looking for new beauties, but it is only the old-fashioned red hibiscus that can be used in food and medicinally.

MEDICINAL USES

In tropical countries use of the red hibiscus stretches back to ancient times and it features in their pharmacopoeias in many well-known and loved salves, lotions and ointments. It is a valuable astringent cooling herb that soothes irritated tissues and eases minor burns, sunburn and rough red areas on the skin.

In Ayurvedic medicine the red hibiscus remains important in the treatment of menstruation and in bringing on temporary sterilisation in women, and Ayurvedic physicians use it in contraception, which is proving important, particularly in India today. Red hibiscus root is showing promising results in the treatment of venereal diseases, and further research is being done into its role in birth control, as a safe diuretic and to lower fevers.

A tea made from red hibiscus flowers has long been popular in treating cystitis, and it also acts as a digestive and stimulates kidney function to flush out toxins. To make a tonic tea for all the above ailments, pour a cup of boiling water over ¼ cup fresh hibiscus petals with two leaves and a calyx. Let the tea stand for five minutes, stirring frequently. Strain it and sip slowly. The tea can be taken cold throughout the day for cystitis. It also supplies additional vitamins.

COSMETIC USES

The fresh juice rubbed into the nails acts as a tonic and heals rough cuticles, and crushed flowers and leaves are used in lotions, creams and shampoos. Through the centuries, both the Chinese and Indians have used the fresh flowers, calyxes and stamens of the red hibiscus boiled with oil as a treatment for their beautiful shiny black hair. This famous herbal oil and hair conditioner is still sold in India under the brand name Jabakusum. It is particularly effective against dandruff, which could be the reason for its perennial popularity.

Red hibiscus flower oil for dry skin

This effective and gentle oil can be used on all skin types and has stood the test of time.

½ cup almond oil
½ cup grape seed oil
6 fresh red hibiscus flowers,
chopped roughly, stamens included and calyxes removed
1 tablespoon castor oil

Simmer the ingredients together in a double boiler for 15 minutes, stirring frequently.

Allow to cool and then strain. Pour the oil into a sterilised bottle with a well-fitting lid, and label. Use a little to treat dry skin on the neck. The oil can also be massaged into the backs of the hands, the elbows and any rough chafed places, and it will moisturise and repair damaged cuticles and cracked nails.

Not only is the red hibiscus flower used for hair growth but also for treating cystitis, cramps, fevers, coughs and herpes. In China, the juice is a valuable ingredient in mascara and shoe-blacking mixtures. The flowers are rolled up, steamed and used in the cooking of exotic dishes and for colouring foods naturally. It is no wonder there are forests of hibiscus in tropical Asia.

CULINARY USES

Red hibiscus cool drink

SERVES 4–6

6–8 fresh hibiscus flowers, with their calyxes
6 leaves
1 litre water
1 cinnamon stick
1 litre pure unsweetened apple juice

Simmer the hibiscus flowers and leaves in the water with the cinnamon stick for 20 minutes. Keep the lid on. Allow the brew to cool, then strain and chill. Add the apple juice and crushed ice, and serve. This is an excellent mild diuretic and keeps the kidneys and bladder toned.

Red hibiscus jelly

SERVES 4–6

6 hibiscus flowers, with their calyxes removed
3 cups water
4 teaspoons gelatine, mixed in a little water
1½ cups grape juice
2 cups fruit
Hibiscus petals for decoration

Boil the hibiscus flowers in the water for 10 minutes. Strain and add the gelatine mixed in a little water, plus the grape juice. Arrange any fruit of your choice – sliced peaches, de-seeded grapes, strawberries, litchis, mango squares or mixed fruit – in a glass bowl and sprinkle with a little sugar, if desired. Pour the hibiscus tea and gelatine mixture gently over the fruit, tuck in fresh hibiscus petals, and chill. Serve with whipped cream or plain yoghurt.

COOK'S NOTE

Fresh red hibiscus flowers can be cooked or steamed to colour foods a beautiful rich red, and they are a favourite in jellies, jams and syrups. Cook them with pears, apples or peaches – they will colour the fruit beautifully.

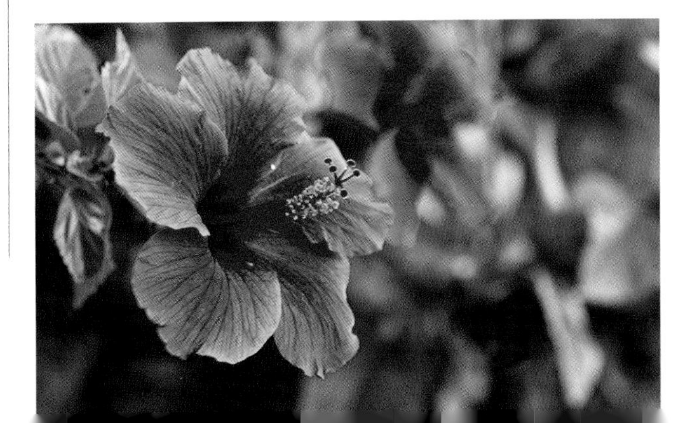

Rocket

Eruca vesicaria subsp. *sativa* • **Rock salad** • **Roquette**

Cultivated since the Middle Ages, rocket has recently undergone a huge revival in popularity. It is native to the Mediterranean area and was first prized by the Romans, who chewed the seeds and used the pungent-tasting leaves lavishly in their banquets, believing that the hot, biting taste would give them vigour and energy. Fascinatingly, rocket seeds excavated from Roman courtyard gardens have germinated after centuries of lying dormant. Rocket is still a tremendously popular herb in Italy, and it is perhaps the Italians with their culinary flair who in recent times have reintroduced it to the rest of the world.

CULTIVATION

Rocket is a fast-growing annual; once you have it in the garden it will reseed itself vigorously, often two or three times during the summer. It demands little attention, growing quickly and easily and thriving in well-composted soil in full sun, but it also does well in rocky places with poor soil and scant moisture.

MEDICINAL USES

Rocket seeds have been used through the centuries to treat bruises and sprains. A bandage was warmed (dipped in hot water and wrung out) and folded, and crushed seeds were spread inside it and held against the skin, without the seeds contacting the skin. Crushed petals were used to treat skin blemishes. The petals were pounded into a soft pulp and spread over the affected area, with the squeezed juice covering the blemish completely.

Some ancient herbals record that rocket was eaten in Elizabethan times prior to a whipping, to alleviate the pain. Given rocket's very high vitamin and mineral content, including potassium and silica, it is possible that there are some painkilling components in the leaves, although scientific research has yet to verify this.

In medieval times rocket flowers and green seeds were crushed with honey and taken a little at a time as a cough syrup. In some ancient herbal recipes, sage and parsley were included in the pungent remedy.

Medieval monks were not allowed to grow rocket in the cloister gardens as the herb was considered to be a dangerous aphrodisiac! Today it is no longer regarded as a sexual stimulant, but rocket is nevertheless considered to be an invigorating tonic herb in Europe and doctors still prescribe it for those who are overtired and anxious. To make rocket tea, pour a cup of boiling water over ¼ cup rocket flowers and ¼ cup fresh parsley. Allow the tea to stand for five minutes, then strain and sprinkle with ¼ teaspoon cayenne pepper and sip slowly.

Rocket cough remedy

This old-fashioned recipe has its roots with the monks, who made it secretly to ease the persistent coughs of the villagers. As the monks were not allowed to grow rocket, the villagers brought it to them to mix with honey and, if they were lucky, a little powdered clove. It began as a listed remedy in the monks' pharmacopoeias for coughs.

1 cup rocket flowers and leaves, chopped
½ cup honey
½ teaspoon powdered clove

Mix rocket flowers, leaves, honey and clove. Crush and pound to a paste. Take one teaspoonful at a time. Chew the mixture well and wash it down with half a glass of water.

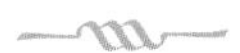

CULINARY USES

Rocket and chicken liver pâté

SERVES 4–6

Served on buttered toast, this delicious Mediterranean dish is one of the best pâtés I know and it is easy to make.

2 tablespoons butter
1 cup finely chopped onion
350 g chicken livers
Sea salt and black pepper to taste
Juice of 1 lemon
2 teaspoons fresh thyme
½–¾ cup thinly sliced, stoned olives
2 tablespoons medium-dry sherry
½ cup rocket flowers

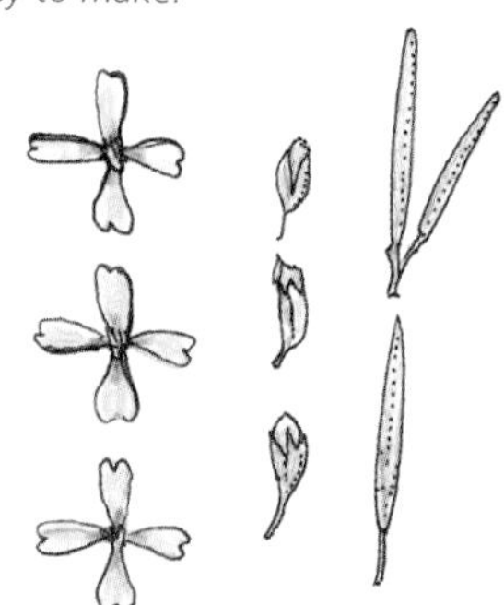

Place the butter in a large pan and fry the onions until they just start to brown. Trim the chicken livers and chop them up. Add to the onion and butter and fry gently. Add the sea salt, black pepper and lemon juice and stir well. Finally, add the thyme, olives and sherry and stir until everything is thoroughly mixed. Spoon into a glass dish and sprinkle the rocket flowers over the top. Chill and serve with toast or savoury biscuits.

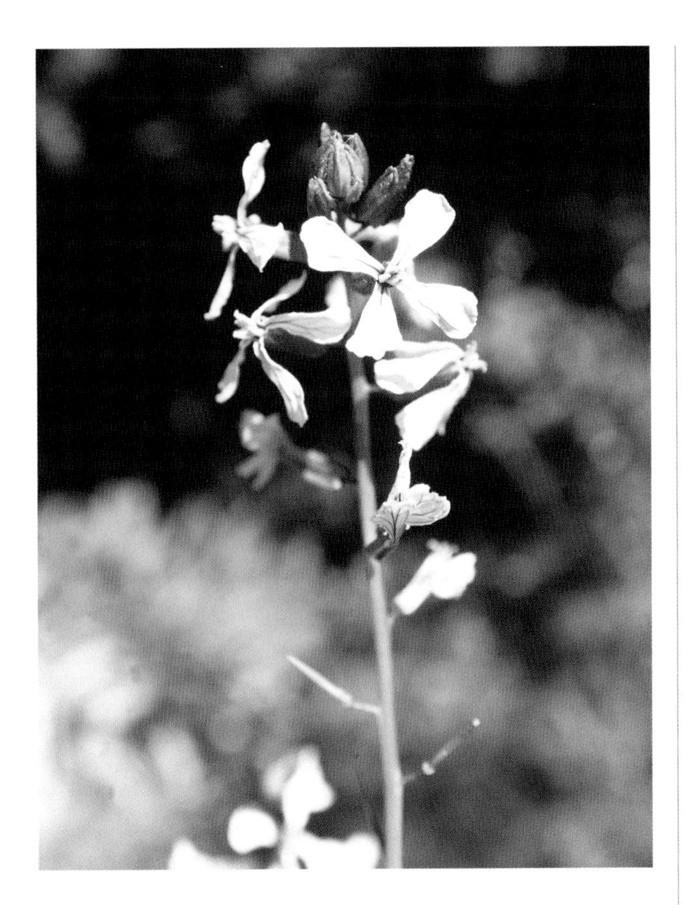

Mushroom and rocket soup

SERVES 6

Rich and tasty, this sustaining soup is a meal in itself.

1 medium onion, finely chopped
2 tablespoons sunflower oil
250 g large brown mushrooms, chopped
2 teaspoons fresh thyme
1 cup finely chopped fresh celery
1½ litres good beef or chicken stock
Sea salt and black pepper to taste
1 litre milk
½ cup finely chopped fresh parsley
1 cup rocket flowers

Sauté the onion in the oil until it starts to brown. Add the mushrooms, thyme and celery and stir-fry for a few minutes. Add the stock and seasoning. Simmer for about six minutes. Add the milk and simmer gently for another six minutes. Serve in big bowls with croutons, and sprinkle with parsley and rocket flowers. Add a squeeze of fresh lemon juice if desired, and place a lemon wedge on the edge of each soup bowl.

Potato and ham frittata with rocket

SERVES 6

Potato and ham has to be one of the most delicious combinations there is! Every Christmas I cook a leg of pickled pork, which my family finds more delicious than ham, and I make this light, old-fashioned dish with the leftovers.

6 large potatoes, peeled
3 tablespoons olive oil
1½ cups chopped onions
300 g thinly sliced cooked ham, cut into neat squares
½ cup milk
Salt and pepper
Small knob butter
3 eggs, beaten with 3 tablespoons chopped parsley
½ cup grated Gouda cheese
½ cup rocket flowers

Boil the potatoes in salted water until tender. Heat the oil in a frying pan and sauté the onions until lightly browned. Add the ham and stir-fry briefly. Set aside. Mash the potatoes with the milk, a little salt and pepper and a small knob of butter. Lay the onions and ham in a baking dish. Spread the potatoes on top of them and pour the egg and parsley mixture over the top, making holes in the potato layer so that the sauce can penetrate. Sprinkle with cheese and bake at 180°C for about 10 minutes or until the eggs are set. Sprinkle the rocket flowers over the frittata just before serving. Serve with a green salad.

Rocket leaves are picked before the flowering head appears. The flowers are considered a gourmet treat, as they are so rich in flavour, as are the green seeds. Ripe rocket seeds are pressed for oil and sold in the most selective delicatessens as a sublimely flavourful oil, which is so concentrated that a mere touch is required to turn an entire dish into something exquisite.

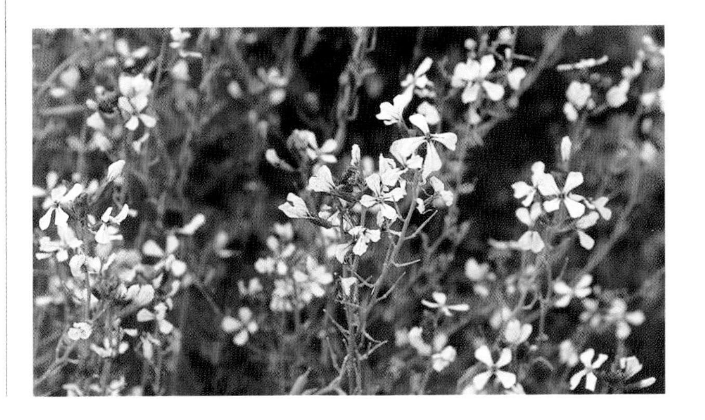

Rose-scented pelargonium

Pelargonium graveolens

The great *Pelargonium* genus originated in South Africa, and all species are wonderfully fragrant. They were introduced to England in the mid-17th century and from there spread throughout Europe. The scent of the leaves ranges from rose, peppermint, pine and spice, to nutmeg, citrus, chocolate and apple; lightly crushing a leaf will release the glorious fragrance. Today pelargoniums are widespread throughout the world and are valued as both pot and bedding plants.

CULTIVATION

Growing scented geraniums is easy. Cuttings broken off and rooted in wet sand strike remarkably easily and this can be done at any time of the year, except during the coldest months. Plant them in a sunny position with a little compost in the early stages and keep them protected until they are sturdy. They require no more than a weekly watering once established. Cut the plants back at the end of the growing season to prevent them from becoming straggly and untidy, and make a mass of cuttings for new plants with the clippings.

MEDICINAL USES

Rose-scented pelargonium is primarily a relaxant. Both the leaves and flowers retain a beautiful, calming fragrance that helps relax muscles and nerves, reduces tension and restores circulation. It is used to break down intense areas of spasm where knotty tight muscles cause pain, cramps and spasms.

The leaves and flowers are antidepressant, antiseptic, anti-inflammatory, diuretic, fungicidal and deodorising. As an antidepressant and a mild and safe diuretic, the rose-scented pelargonium has been listed in pharmacopoeias through the centuries as a valuable treatment for haemorrhoids, for excessive blood loss during menstruation and as a stimulant to the adrenal cortex.

In my earlier work as a physiotherapist, I made a wonderful massage cream for aching muscles, stiff necks and arthritic aches and pains using rose-scented pelargonium, and to this day I make sure I am never without a jar or two.

Its precious oils are used for premenstrual tension, neuralgia, acne, bruises, broken veins and oedema, poor circulation, especially to the legs, and to restore elasticity to mature skin.

The tiny, exquisitely marked flowers have the same taste and fragrance as the leaves and can be made into soothing, calming teas and drinks that help to lessen the onslaught of face-paced modern life. Rose-scented pelargonium tea can be made by pouring a cup of boiling water over ¼ cup fresh leaves and flowers. Allow the tea to steep for five minutes, then strain and sip it slowly; it will calm and relax you. This tea will soothe and ease a sore throat during a bout of tonsillitis. The tea is much loved by children!

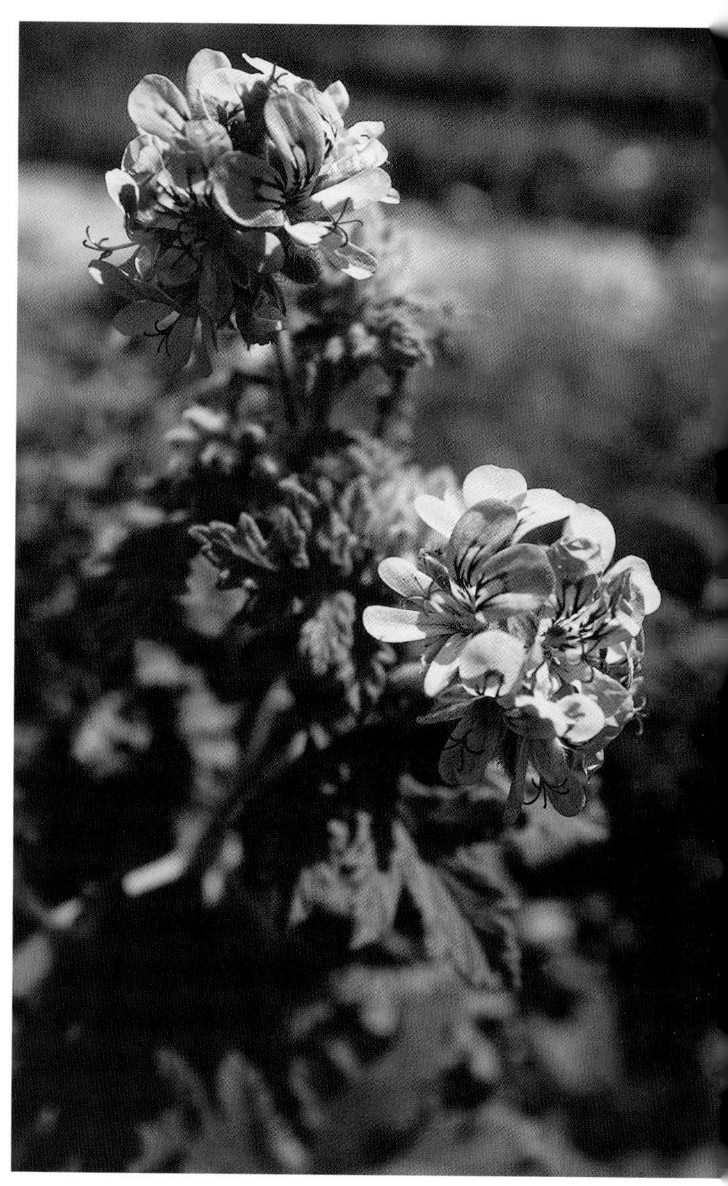

Rose-scented pelargonium massage cream

This cream for sore muscles and arthritic aches is the one I used when I worked for many years as a physiotherapist. I usually make it in spring and early summer, when the flowers are abundant.

1 cup rose-scented pelargonium leaves and flowers
1 cup boiling water
1 cinnamon stick
6 crushed cardamom pods
6 crushed cloves
2 teaspoons aniseed
1 tablespoon almond oil
1 teaspoon vitamin E oil
6 drops rose-geranium essential oil

Combine the rose-scented pelargonium leaves and flowers with the boiling water, cinnamon stick, crushed cardamom pods and cloves and the aniseed in a double boiler. Simmer for 20 minutes, stirring frequently. Allow the cream to cool for 10 minutes and then strain. Discard the flowers, leaves and spices, and add the almond oil, vitamin E oil and rose-geranium essential oil. Mix well and pour into sterilised screw-top jars. Use this cream generously and frequently.

Rose-scented pelargonium oil for aching muscles

1 cup rose-scented pelargonium flowers
1 cup rose-scented pelargonium leaves
1 cup grapeseed oil

Simmer the flowers, leaves and oil in a double boiler for 30 minutes, constantly pressing and stirring. Strain, discarding the flowers and leaves. Pour the oil into a dark glass bottle with a good screw-top lid. Use the oil warmed up to massage over aching muscles.

COSMETIC USES

To make a rose-scented pelargonium wash for oily and problem skins, tie a big handful of rose-scented pelargonium leaves and flowers in a bunch using an elastic band. Pour two litres of boiling water over it, and holding the bunch by its stems, swish it around in the water for a few minutes. Leave the bunch in the water until the water has cooled to a pleasantly warm temperature. After cleaning the face with a good cold cream, wash the face with this scented lotion as a final rinse.

CULINARY USES

Rose-scented pelargonium mousse

SERVES 6–8

This luxurious dessert is unforgettable – I make it for Christmas lunch as it goes beautifully with Christmas pudding.

2 tablespoons gelatine
6 tablespoons hot water
8 rose-scented pelargonium leaves
2 large eggs, separated
4 tablespoons castor sugar
200 ml cream cheese
200 ml plain Greek yoghurt
½ cup rose-scented pelargonium flowers
200 ml cream, whipped

Dissolve the gelatine in a little of the hot water and pour the rest of the water over the scented pelargonium leaves, and leave to cool. Whisk the egg whites until they are stiff. Whip the egg yolks with the castor sugar until light and creamy; add the gelatine and then the cream cheese. Whisk well, then add the yoghurt and the water from the soaked leaves. Fold in the scented pelargonium flowers, whipped cream and the egg whites. Pour into a glass bowl and refrigerate until set. Decorate with scented pelargonium leaves and flowers.

Rose-scented pelargonium filo baskets

SERVES 6

Use whatever fruit is in season to make this elegant dessert.

3 sheets filo pastry
1 tablespoon melted butter
1½ cups thinly sliced strawberries, raspberries or peaches, sprinkled with sugar
1 cup plain Greek yoghurt
½ cup whipped cream
1 cup rose-scented pelargonium flowers
Icing sugar

Preheat the oven to 200°C. Cut the sheets of pastry into squares measuring about 10 cm (one sheet divides into six). Brush each square with a pastry brush dipped in melted butter. Arrange a single square at a time in a patty pan, layering them in threes to form a little basket. Bake for six minutes or until they turn golden brown, then turn them out and cool very carefully as they are fragile. Once cool, mix the fruit mixture into the yoghurt and spoon into the basket. Top with whipped cream, sprinkle with scented pelargonium flowers and dust with icing sugar. Serve on glass plates.

Rose

Rosa species

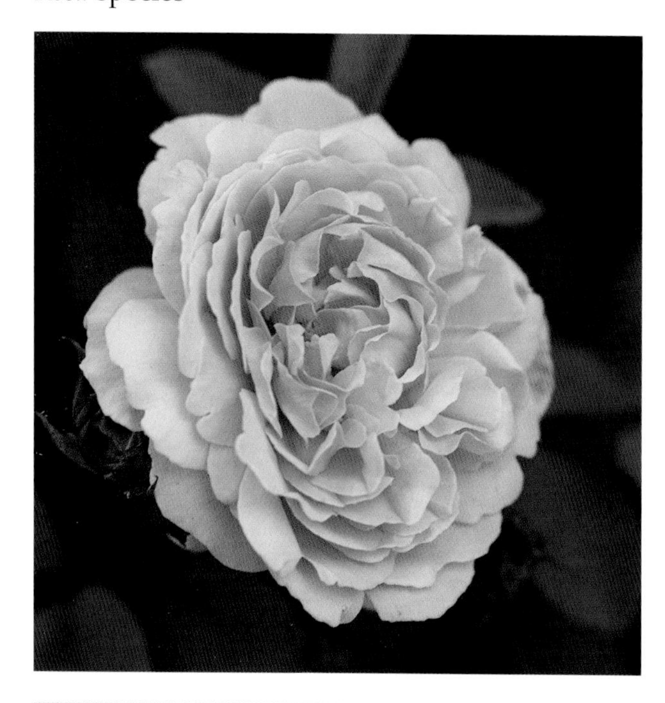

Roses date back thousands of years and are without doubt the most loved of all flowers worldwide. Through the centuries they have been revered for both their fragrance and their medicinal and cosmetic properties.

The ancient Greeks and Romans used rose petals and hips in cooking, and preserved the petals in vinegar. The Romans used roses for ceremonial purposes and built the first hot houses to ensure blooms all year round, controlling the temperature with pipes of hot water.

CULTIVATION

There is a rose for every type of garden and for every gardener's taste. However, my favourites are the old-fashioned roses, such as the exquisite, fragrant, shell-pink 'Margaret Roberts' rose (see photograph). Roses require very little; all they need is a large, deep hole in full sun, filled with compost and a sprinkling of moisture-absorbent crystals to keep the plant from drying out. They require a deep, twice-weekly watering, and must be fed with an organic fertiliser two or three times a year, and a good mulch of compost during the winter. Pruning is essential in midwinter, and deadheading will ensure masses of blooms.

MEDICINAL USES

Rose petal tea has a calming, tranquillising effect. To make the tea, pour a cup of boiling water over ¼ cup fresh, unsprayed rose petals. Leave the tea to stand for five minutes, then strain and sweeten with a touch of honey if desired.

Rosewater dates back to AD 980–1037, when the Arab physician Avicenna used it to treat skin ailments and mixed it with honey for use as a cough syrup. Rosewater may be splashed on the outside of the eyes in cases of conjunctivitis. It has an antiseptic and soothing quality and can be used even on sensitive skins.

Rosa gallica, which is native to the Middle East, was used in the Middle Ages as a treatment for depression and anxiety and to aid circulation. Modern medical research has proven these properties and nowadays the precious rose oil, known as attar of roses, is used in aromatherapy to treat these same ailments.

Rose hips form once the petals have fallen and the swollen calyxes ripen; they can be used in cough mixtures, syrups, jellies and jams. Their high vitamin C content and fruit acids, as well as beta-carotene, pectin and tannin content boost the body's immune system and make an excellent tonic that will give energy and vitality and strengthen artery walls, thus aiding circulation.

Rose petal night cap

This drink will help you unwind after a rough day.

¼ cup fresh rose petals
1 cup boiling water
Honey
2 teaspoons sweet sherry

Pour water over the rose petals. Allow to stand for five minutes. Strain it, add a little honey and the sweet sherry.

Rosewater for skin ailments

Use this lotion for dry, cracked skin, eczema, rashes, sunburn, grazes and itchy, dry areas.

6 cups rose petals
A small twist of lemon rind
4 cloves
1 litre water

Boil the rose petals, lemon rind and cloves gently in the water for 15 minutes, with the lid on. Remove from the heat, strain and pour into glass bottles with screw tops.

Use either sprayed onto the area with a spritz spray bottle, or apply it with a pad of cotton wool, wiping it onto the face after washing. It is especially effective for oily acne and spotty teenage skin. Use this rosewater twice daily, morning and evening, for quick results.

Rosehip cough treatment and winter tonic

This delicious, health-giving syrup will boost the immune system and soothe a cough. Keep it in the fridge in hot weather.

2 cups ripe rosehips, trimmed of stamens and stalks and finely chopped
2 cups brown treacle sugar
1½ cups water
1 cinnamon stick

Simmer the ingredients together in a covered pot for about 20 minutes. Pour into hot sterilised jars and seal well. Take two teaspoons at a time, chew well, and follow up with a little hot rose petal tea.

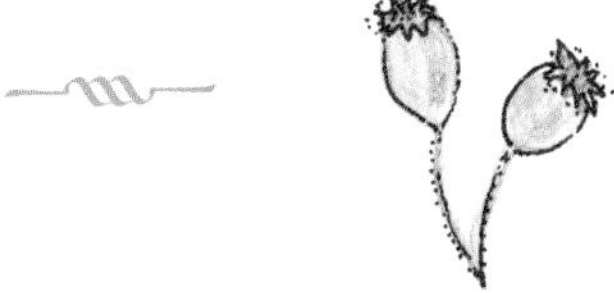

CULINARY USES

Rose petal syrup

SERVES 4–6

Serve on ice-cream, rice or sago puddings. It can also be added to drinks or served with chilled water and ice, in a 1:3 ratio.

4 cups red and pink rose petals
2½ cups water
1 cup honey
1 cinnamon stick

Simmer the petals in the water and honey with the cinnamon stick for 15 minutes. Allow the syrup to cool, then strain. To give extra sweetness, simmer with half a cup of stevia flowers.

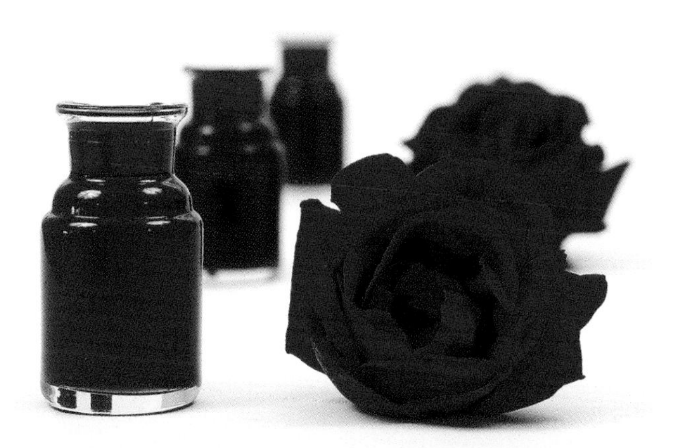

Rose petal cream jelly

SERVES 6

This is a lovely dessert for a summer party and so easy to make.

3 tablespoons gelatine
1 litre red grape juice
½ cup white sugar
1 cup red wine
2 cups fruit, e.g. strawberries, sliced peaches, youngberries or mixed fruit
1 cup mixed rose petals
1 cup cream, beaten
Icing sugar

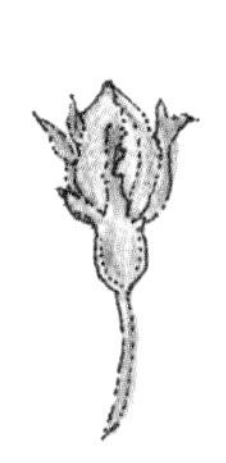

Dissolve the gelatine in a little warm water. Add it to the grape juice, sugar and red wine. Pour into a pretty glass bowl or tall individual glasses and gently lower in the fruit and rose petals. Place in the fridge until set. Just before serving, spoon the cream on top, and make a delicate pattern with more fresh rose petals. Dust liberally with icing sugar.

Rose punch

SERVES 8–10

This light and refreshing punch looks magnificent served in a glass punch bowl with whole roses set into a big block of ice or rosebuds set in individual ice cubes to keep it beautifully chilled.

2 litres white wine, chilled
4 tablespoons Kirsch
1 cup rose petal syrup (see recipe alongside)
1 litre water
Juice of 2 lemons

Mix the ingredients together gently and serve in a glass punch bowl with frozen roses (see below).

FROZEN ROSES FOR PARTY PUNCH

The day before the party, choose perfectly formed pink rosebuds that are just opening, and trim the stalks. (I find the old-fashioned 'Margaret Roberts' rose perfect here as it keeps its shape and it is tender and sweet to the taste.) Select a bowl that holds about two cups of water and fill the bowl with the rosebuds. Add the iced water and freeze overnight, keeping the bowl in the freezer until you are ready to serve the punch. Just before serving the punch, dip the bowl in hot water, then turn it upside down to release the block of ice. Slide it into the punch. Alternatively, freeze rosebuds in individual ice cubes.

Roselle

Hibiscus sabdariffa • **Rosella** • **Indian sorrel** • **Jamaican sorrel** • **Florida cranberry** • **Oseille rouge**

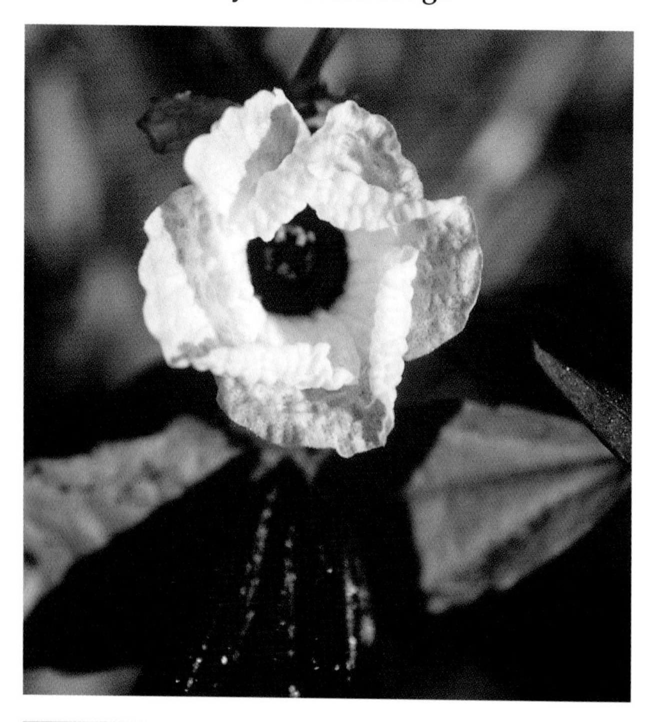

Roselle is a spectacular annual that reaches about 2 m in height, with pretty, pale cream flowers typical of hibiscus. Native to India and southeast Asia, it is said that it was taken to Africa and the West Indies by slaves. The earliest recording of the plant was by the Flemish botanist M. de l'Obel, in 1576, and the edibility of the leaves and flowers was documented in Java around 1682. It is used primarily as a food colouring and flavouring, and has been grown sporadically as a commercial crop in various parts of the world.

CULTIVATION

Roselle is a quick, prolific annual that will do well in just about any soil as long as it is well dug and richly composted; it also needs full sun and twice-weekly watering. I sow seeds in autumn and keep them protected for planting out in spring (roselle is very frost-tender), and then sow again in October for a late summer crop. Roselle is a rewarding plant to grow as all parts are edible.

MEDICINAL USES

Roselle has a high vitamin C, iron and potassium content, and contains numerous amino acids. It is good for coughs, colds and sore throats, and the seeds can be roasted to make a coffee. It is a good diuretic, it stimulates the digestive processes and is antispasmodic and antibacterial. Roselle is a good tonic, building blood and boosting the immune system. It can also be made into a gargle for sore and strained throats.

One of my favourite teas is the sour-tasting astringent, energising bright red health tea made from the brilliant calyxes of the roselle (fresh or dried calyxes can be used). The tea helps to soothe colds, clear sore throats and coughs, open the nose, and clear up mucous. It is astringent and so full of vitamin C that it helps to clear skin conditions like acne. The tea is particularly refreshing and can be used as a base for healthy cool drinks.

Roselle gargle for sore and strained throats

½ cup roselle flowers and calyxes
1 litre water
½ cup sage leaves
Juice and rind of 2 lemons

Boil the roselle flowers and calyxes in the water with the sage leaves and the lemon juice and rind. Simmer gently for 10 minutes, with the lid on. Cool and strain. Use as a gargle and also sip and swallow a little frequently. Sweeten the gargle with honey if desired.

Roselle health tea to clear colds and acne

MAKES 2 LITRES

Hibiscus sabdariffa *is the species used in commercial hibiscus tea, not the bright-flowered species commonly grown in the garden. Hot roselle tea taken with honey is also an excellent remedy for a hangover.*

1 cup fresh or dried roselle calyxes
2 litres water

Break away the five-pointed calyxes from their marble-sized seed capsules, and use only those bright red pieces in the tea. Boil the calyxes in the water for 20 minutes, then set the tea aside and let it steep. When pleasantly hot, discard the calyxes, sweeten with honey and stir with a cinnamon stick. Sip a cupful slowly. Cool the rest of the tea and let it chill. Mix in equal quantities of grape or litchi juice to make

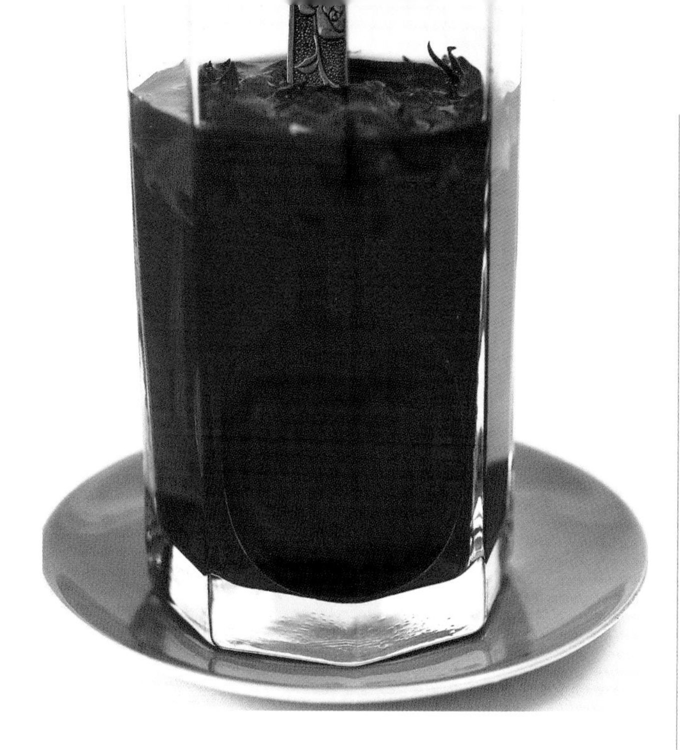

an energising cold drink. Add sliced strawberries and mint leaves and a dash of good red wine for a party punch, and as a bonus you will feel no alcohol build up!

COSMETIC USES

A strong lotion of roselle flowers and calyxes is wonderfully astringent. The lotion is excellent for cleansing oily problem skin and can be dabbed onto blemishes and inflamed spots.

Roselle scrub

½ cup roselle lotion (see below)
½ cup hot water
½ cup large flake oats

Pour the lotion and water over the oats. Allow to swell and soften for a few minutes. Use as a scrub for problem skin.

Roselle lotion

Use this lotion for problem skin, blemishes and inflamed spots. The witch hazel can be purchased at your local pharmacy.

3 cups roselle flowers and calyxes
2 litres water
10 cloves
1 stick cinnamon
3 tablespoons witch hazel

Simmer the roselle flowers and calyxes in the water with the cloves and cinnamon for 20 minutes, with the lid on. Leave to cool. Strain, and add the witch hazel. Pour into a sterilised screw-top bottle and shake well. Use on a pad of cotton wool as a cleansing lotion after washing the face, morning and evening, for oily problem skin, acne and pimples. Also drink a cup of roselle tea to keep the skin unblemished. It is an excellent cleanser.

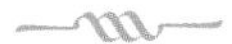

CULINARY USES

Roselle jelly

SERVES 4–6

This jelly is delicious with ice-cream, pancakes, waffles and rice puddings, or with cold meat and chicken.

1 kg fresh calyxes and flower petals broken off their seed capsules
1 litre water
2 cups honey
1 cup stevia flowers
4 tablespoons gelatine

Boil the ingredients together briskly for about 40 minutes, stirring well. Strain. Add the gelatine mixed into a little warm water and stir well. Pour into shallow bowls and allow to set in the fridge.

Roselle salad

SERVES 4–6

Roselle's high vitamin C, iron, calcium and potassium content makes this salad a superb health builder. It may be served as an accompaniment to a meal or as a substantial meal in itself, with brown bread.

4 cups watercress
1 cup roselle leaves, torn up
2 cups roselle flowers and calyxes broken off their seed capsules
2 cups finely chopped sweet peppers
2 cups chopped celery leaves and stalks
1 cup chopped button mushrooms
2 cups cooked chickpeas
½ cup finely chopped parsley
1 cup chopped onions (optional)
½ cup olive oil
Juice of 1 lemon

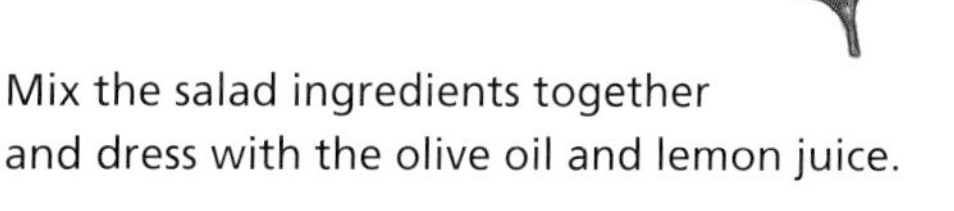

Mix the salad ingredients together and dress with the olive oil and lemon juice.

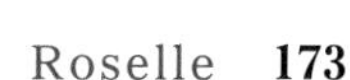

Rosemary

Rosmarinus officinalis

One of the world's best-loved herbs, rosemary gets its name from the Latin *rosmaris*, meaning 'dew of the sea'. It is native to southern Europe, particularly the Mediterranean area, and has been used by cooks and apothecaries for centuries. Rosemary is traditionally a symbol of fidelity between lovers, as well a symbol of remembrance. It is carried in bridal bouquets and used in wedding arrangements and wreaths, and given to friends to strengthen friendship and commitment.

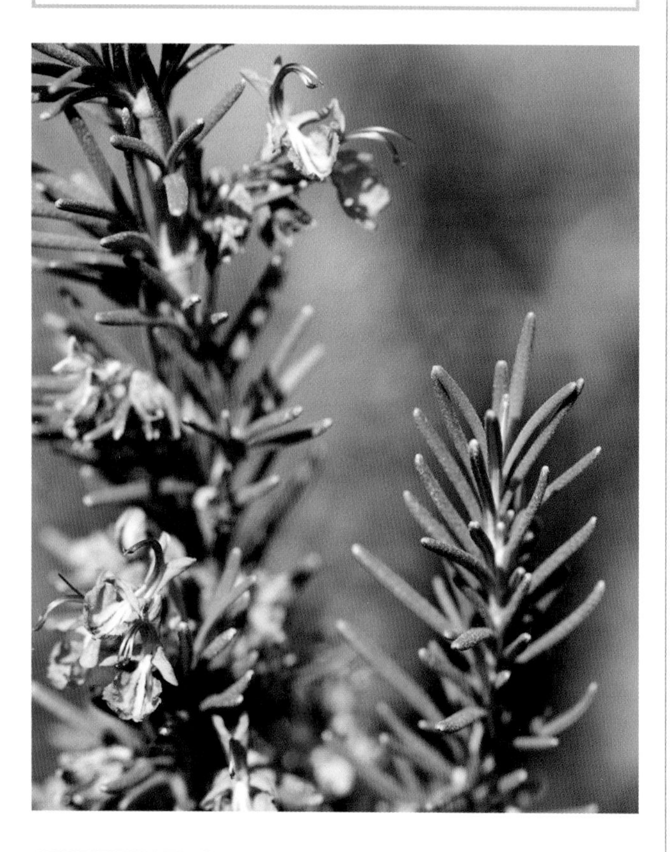

CULTIVATION

Rosemary is a dense, woody prolific shrub that reaches about 1 m in height and spread. All it requires is a well-dug, richly composted hole in full sun and a deep weekly watering. Propagation is by means of cuttings at any time of the year. Take slips about 7 cm long, strip off the lower leaves, and root the sprigs in wet sand. Once they have rooted, plant the new plants 1 m apart. Other than occasional clipping into shape, rosemary needs no attention.

MEDICINAL USES

Rosemary stimulates the circulation and eases aching rheumatic joints and stiff muscles. It is antiseptic, antispasmodic, antibacterial and a remarkable restorative herb, aiding recovery from long-term stress and chronic illness. It is also energising and uplifting, and is associated with raising low blood pressure and lowering and levelling high blood pressure. It is helpful for depression, headaches and premenstrual tension, and is also an excellent anti-inflammatory.

Rosemary tea is excellent as an antiseptic gargle and a mouthwash. It tightens the gums and clears halitosis and any mouth infections. Sipped in small amounts, rosemary tea eases flatulence, and stimulates the smooth muscles of the digestive tract and gall bladder, thus increasing the flow of bile. To make rosemary tea, steep one thumb-length sprig of fresh rosemary flowers and leaves in a cup of boiling water. Let the tea stand for five minutes, then strain and sip slowly.

COSMETIC USES

Rosemary is useful as an astringent, tonic herb and scalp treatment – one of its astonishing benefits is that it stimulates hair growth, even after chemotherapy. It can also be made into an effective lotion for acne and problem skin.

Rosemary lotion for acne

1 cup fresh flowering rosemary sprigs
1½ litres water

Boil the flowering rosemary sprigs in the water for 15 minutes, with the lid on. Cool, strain and apply on soaked cotton wool pads after washing the face.

Rosemary hair restorer

3 cups rosemary leaves and flowers
2 litres water

Boil the rosemary leaves and flowers in the water for 15–20 minutes with the lid on, giving the brew an occasional stir. Cool, strain and store in the fridge. Use as a rinse after shampooing, and massage into the scalp daily with pads of cotton wool soaked in the lotion.

CULINARY USES

Lamb chops with rosemary

SERVES 4

This is my favourite meat dish! The chops must be well browned and slightly crisp.

Sunflower oil
8 lamb loin chops
2 large onions, sliced into rings
6 large potatoes, peeled and sliced
Sea salt and black pepper to taste
Juice of 1 lemon
2 thumb-length sprigs fresh rosemary
A little water
1 tablespoon rosemary flowers

Put a little sunflower oil into a cast iron pot and brown the chops until they are almost cooked through, moving them frequently. Add the onions and potatoes, sprinkle with salt and pepper, and stir-fry until the vegetables start to brown. Add the lemon juice, rosemary sprigs and a little water to make a rich gravy. Simmer with the lid on for about 25 minutes, until the potatoes are cooked. Taste and adjust the seasoning if necessary and sprinkle with rosemary flowers. Serve in the pot, with brown rice and vegetables.

COOK'S NOTE

Rosemary is a superb herb in cooking, particularly in lamb and pork dishes as it helps to break down fats, and the flowers add a subtle taste to sweet or savoury dishes. However, rosemary has a strong flavour, and should be used sparingly.

Grilled rosemary sosaties

SERVES 4–6

The home-made rosemary skewers used in this recipe impart their delicious fragrance and flavour to the sosaties. The fruit can be varied according to what is in season.

12 rosemary branches, about 25 cm long, leaves stripped, and sharpened at one end
24 pickling onions, peeled
24 chunks aubergine
24 thick wedges green pepper
24 wedges yellow peaches, mangoes or apples
24 blocks mozzarella cheese
24 wedges tomato
24 button mushrooms

Marinade
2 cups good tomato sauce
½ cup vinegar
½ cup rosemary flowers
½ cup honey
1 tablespoon wholegrain mustard
2 tablespoons Worcestershire sauce
Sea salt and black pepper to taste

Thread each rosemary skewer with alternating chunks of vegetable, fruit and cheese. For example, start off with an onion, follow by aubergine, green pepper, peach, cheese, tomato and mushroom, then repeat until the skewer is full. Whisk the marinade ingredients well and lay the sosaties in the marinade, turning them to coat them evenly. Place the sosaties under a hot grill; turn them so that they cook evenly. Sprinkle with rosemary flowers and serve with baked potatoes.

Tiramisu with rosemary

SERVES 6

This is a delicious variation of this famous Italian dessert.

1 cup strong black filter coffee
2 tablespoons brandy
175 g sponge fingers
1 cup plain Bulgarian yoghurt
1 cup cream cheese
4 tablespoons honey
3 egg whites, well beaten
2 tablespoons rosemary flowers, pulled from their calyxes
3 tablespoons grated milk chocolate

Mix the coffee and brandy together in a flat bowl. Briefly dip half the sponge fingers into the mixture and line the bottom of a glass bowl with them. Mix the yoghurt, cream cheese and the honey and beat lightly until smooth. Fold in the beaten egg whites and rosemary flowers. Spoon this mixture over the sponge fingers. Briefly dip the remaining sponge fingers into the coffee and brandy and lay them neatly on top of the cream cheese mixture. Sprinkle with the grated chocolate and fresh rosemary flowers. Cover and chill before serving.

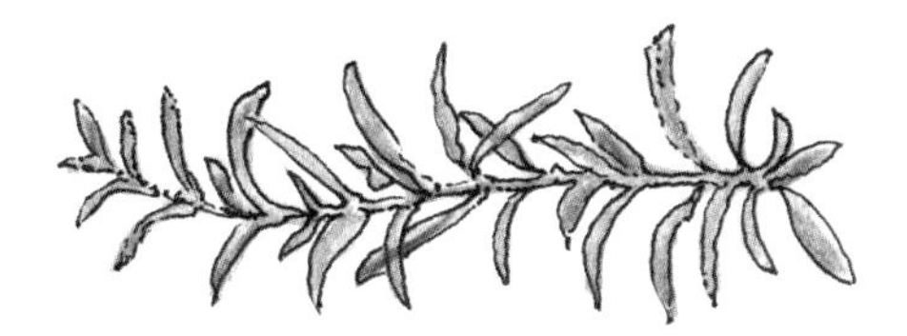

Sacred basil

Ocimum sanctum • *O. tenuiflorum* • **Tulsi**

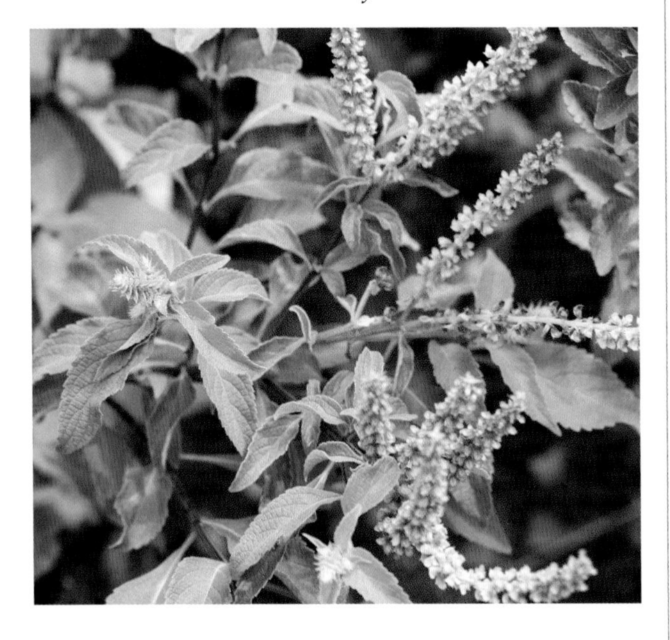

CULTIVATION

Sow the seed in trays in a mixture of sand and light compost, using just enough soil to cover the seed. Place the tray in a larger tray so that the seed tray can stand in water; the seed is very fine and easily disturbed so it is better not to water from above. The seed must never dry out. When the little seedlings have reached the four-leaf stage they are usually big enough to handle. Prick them out for planting into large compost-filled bags. Keep them shaded and protected, and move them into the sun for longer periods each day.

Plant out in full sun in richly composted soil about 1 m apart as sacred basil easily grows up to 1 m in height and width. Water plants 2–3 times a week depending on the weather. Sacred basil is frost-tender, so cover it with a frost-protective covering as soon as the weather gets cold, opening it up to the sunshine during the day and covering it at night.

The tender young flowering heads are prolific and are used in medications and foods, but always see to it that there are enough of the drying brown flowering spikes for seeds, and look out for tiny new sacred basil plants in spring. They transplant easily when they are about 6 cm high and have a long tap root so be careful to dig deep and replant immediately into big compost-filled bags or into a deep moist compost-filled hole in full sun. Keep the transplanted sacred basil well watered until it establishes.

Sacred basil is a sanctified herb in India and one of the world's precious herbs. It is native to India and parts of Asia, where it is planted around shrines, holy places, places of celebration and religious festivals, in front of homes and in courtyards. Its fragrant presence deters flies and mosquitoes, it keeps the atmosphere pure, supplies oxygen, and is said to bring peace, prosperity and health to the household.

Known as 'tulsi' in Sanskrit, the herb is listed in the ancient medical texts and pharmacopoeias as a medicine to treat coughs, colds and flu. It is an excellent expectorant and was also used as a poultice to draw infection from wounds, and as an antiseptic wash. Brazil's records dating back 5 000 years show that a lotion or tea made from sacred basil was used to treat internal organs and was also applied externally, for example on haemorrhoids.

Dried tulsi leaves, kept in oils and vinegars, found their place in many cultures for the snowbound winter months, and the apothecaries maintained a constant supply of the oils and vinegars, often prepared by medicine men in distant villages. Sacred basil seeds were sold for a good price on the marketplace, still in their papery flower husks, and were a valued item for travellers as the seeds could be shaken out of the husks and kept for planting, and a tea could be made from the dry flowers for what was then known as 'consumption' (tuberculosis). Trade in fresh flowering spikes was equally important for those going on sea voyages as it was used to treat illness on the ships.

Tulsi is a perennial plant, and is very different in growth, appearance and taste to sweet basil. It has a rich clove-like taste, makes an exceptional tea, and is very valuable medicinally.

MEDICINAL USES

Sacred basil tea is wonderfully soothing for coughs, colds, flu, bronchitis, thick nasal discharge, a blocked nose and sore blocked ears. It also eases disorders of the urinary system and rectum, repairs and strengthens the liver, and relieves congestion around the heart, restoring good, vibrant circulation to the body. It flushes out toxins, revitalising the skin and giving it a glow.

A cup of tulsi tea will ease anxiety, release tension, reduce a fever, treat colic, ease a headache, expel parasites, act as a diuretic, ease postpartum distress and encourage milk production in nursing mothers. I encourage its use as a gentle, easy-to-take tea for all who feel life is too stressful, with too much to cope with. To make the tea, pour a cup of boiling water over ¼ cup fresh tulsi flowering sprigs; let the tea stand for five minutes, strain and sip slowly. Sweeten with a touch of honey if desired.

A lotion of the cooled tea can be used for washing, dabbing or spritz-spraying onto oily problem skin as it is an excellent detoxifier and cleanser. Sacred basil is used in India both as a tea and as a wash to treat and prevent malaria, and chewing the fresh leaves is also a part of the treatment. Three cups of tulsi tea are taken daily to treat malaria. Try poultices of warmed leafy flowering sprigs over inflamed aching joints, and make sacred basil cream as a soothing massage application for stiff sore muscles, aching legs and feet.

Sacred basil massage cream for sore muscles and aching legs

1 cup good aqueous cream
1 cup fresh flowering sacred basil sprigs
1 teaspoon oil of cloves
2 teaspoons vitamin E oil
2 tablespoons almond oil

Simmer the aqueous cream and sacred basil together in a double boiler for 30 minutes, stirring frequently, mashing and pressing the plant into the oil. Cool and strain the mixture. Add the oils, whisk them in thoroughly, and store the cream in a screw-top glass jar. Use it warmed (stand the jar in hot water) as a gentle soothing massage cream on everyone in the family, including grandparents!

Sacred basil oil

I was given this very precious remedy by an Indian doctor to provide comfort when facing problems, grief, change and loss. It is rich and smooth and needs to be applied warm to the feet in slow and gentle movements. It is safe and comforting for children, the elderly, and those who are highly stressed.

1 cup tulsi flowering heads
A handful of tulsi leaves
1 cup almond oil

In a double boiler, warm the flowering heads and leaves in the almond oil for 30 minutes, crushing and pressing the flowering sprays and leaves all the time. It is traditional to say prayers into the mixture as you work. Leave it to cool for 15 minutes, strain through fine cheesecloth or muslin and pour into a dark glass bottle. Apply warm to the feet – spread a towel and ensure the 'patient' is sitting comfortably. Massage gently for 15–20 minutes.

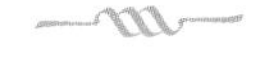

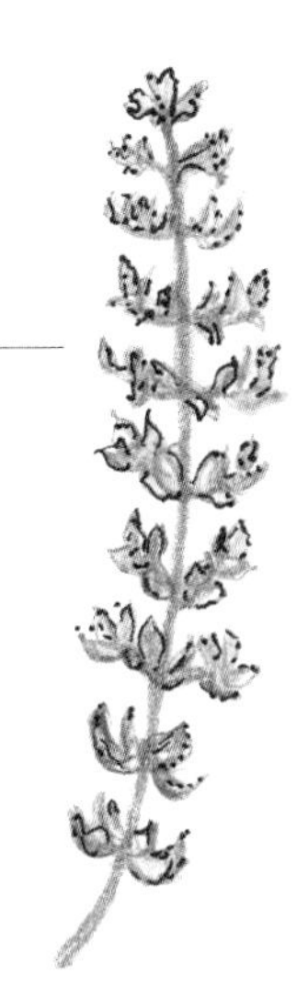

CULINARY USES

Sacred basil rub

This rub adds a fascinating bouquet of flavours to fish or chicken breasts and is easy to make.

½ cup young sacred basil flowering heads, dried and crumbled
½ cup cumin seeds, lightly crushed
½ cup crushed coriander seeds
½ cup finely grated fresh ginger
¼ cup finely grated lemon rind
1 teaspoon salt
½–1 teaspoon red pepper

Mix the sacred basil, cumin, coriander, ginger and lemon rind together well. Add the salt and red pepper (adjust the red pepper depending on how hot you like it). Mix the ingredients fresh every time, and rub into chicken or fish that has been rubbed with fresh lemon juice. Leave covered to marinade for at least three hours in the fridge. Place under the grill and turn frequently until tender and well cooked, or fry in a pan with a little olive oil, turning until it is cooked.

COOK'S NOTE

Crush dried sacred basil flowers, cumin seeds and coriander seeds together and store in a screw-top jar near the stove for quick flavouring.

Sacred basil cool drink

MAKES 2 LITRES

This healthy and deliciously clove-scented cool drink is loved by children.

1 litre boiling water
1 cup fresh sacred basil flowering sprigs
1 litre pure unsweetened fruit juice (pomegranate is particularly delicious)

Pour the boiling water over the sacred basil and allow the tea to brew for five minutes. Strain and cool. Mix with the fruit juice, and serve chilled, with ice.

Safflower

Carthamus tinctorius

Safflower is an ancient crop plant that, curiously, cannot be fully traced back in nature. It is thought to have been one of the first crops grown in ancient Syria, Turkey, Israel, Jordan and Persia, and seeds were found in Egyptian tombs from 3500 BC.

The plant was grown for its bright orange, yellow and red thistle-like flowers, rich in the pigment carthamin, and was made into the first dyes used to colour flax cloth and later cotton. A lucrative trade developed in the flowers as the colours were highly prized, and safflowers were used to dye the saffron-yellow robes of eastern monks. The bright petals of the flowers replaced the very expensive saffron styles previously used in dyeing, and to an extent, they replaced saffron in the flavouring of food and drinks too.

Safflower seed oil was cold pressed, and as it became known further afield, trade in the seed spread to India, and from there to China where it became known as *fan hong hua*, to Germany where it became known as *Fäbersaflor*, and to Spain where it became known as *cártamo*. Its valuable attributes were listed in the pharmacopoeias of different countries. Each nation developed its own treasured recipes, used in religious ceremonies and celebrations and handed down from generation to generation.

CULTIVATION

The safflower is very easy to grow. Originally I imported seed from Israel and began by sprouting it; then I planted out a few tentative rows. Virtually every seed germinated and a waist-high crop of bright flowers developed! Full sun and deeply dug, richly composted soil are required, and a slow gentle watering 2–3 times a week. Protect the furrow with a layer of dried leaves to keep seedlings cool and shaded. Safflower is a quick and easy annual and can be grown two or even three times during our long summers.

Reap the flowers when fully opened and dry on sheets of brown paper in the shade for three days (the ink print on newspaper could contaminate the soft petals). Wear good gloves as the bracts and calyxes are prickly, and pull out the tuft of flower petals and store them in a wide-mouth glass jar with a screw-top lid. To collect the seeds, allow a row or two of safflowers to mature and when the plants start to dry, cut off the

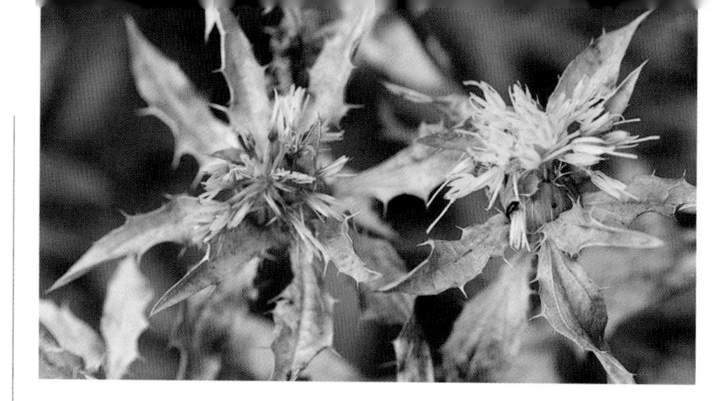

flowering heads. Spread them on a clean wooden table and crush gently with a wooden mallet to release the seeds. I use a spatula to separate the seeds from the prickly bracts, and seal the collected seeds in a glass jar with a screw-top lid for re-sowing and sprouting.

Safflowers are a good companion to mealies and beans on trellises, and under-planting with celery and coriander ensures a good crop all round.

MEDICINAL USES

Safflower has become a valuable medication: as a sprouted seed, as tender micro-seedlings, and as a tea made from the flowers. It is used for treating coronary artery disease, as a circulatory stimulant, for reducing fevers, lowering cholesterol levels, relieving pain, and for repairing and stimulating the uterus. Safflower tea is also helpful in cases of jaundice, measles, menopause and menstrual problems. To make the tea, pour a cup of boiling water over one tablespoon of fresh flowers or dried petals. Let the tea draw for 5–7 minutes, stir frequently, then strain and sip slowly. The tea can be taken twice a day.

Cold-pressed safflower oil is used in salads and cooking; it is valuable in cases of high cholesterol, and supports the heart and circulation.

Safflower is also used to colour oils and massage creams as it has pain-relieving properties. It reduces swelling and inflammation, eases and dissolves bruises, sprains and strains, and as a pain-relieving massage cream it is superb for sports injuries.

Safflower seed poultice

This is an excellent treatment for sprains and bruises.

1 cup safflower seeds
½ cup boiling water

Soak the seeds in the boiling water for 15 minutes. Drain and turn out onto a towel. Fold the edges in to keep the seeds together and apply to the affected area. Bind it in place and cover with a hot-water bottle and a blanket. Relax for 15 minutes.

WARNING: Do not use safflower in any form (not even the oil or sprouts) during pregnancy as it is a strong uterine stimulant.

Safflower massage cream

Use this cream for pain relief, and to heal wounds and scars.

1 cup good aqueous cream
1 cup safflower seeds, crushed well
½ cup fresh or dried safflower petals
½ cup almond oil
2 teaspoons vitamin E oil

Simmer the aqueous cream, safflower seeds and petals and the almond oil together in a double boiler. Keep stirring and pressing the seeds and petals and simmer for 30 minutes. Let the mixture stand, covered, to cool for 30 minutes. Strain and add the vitamin E oil. Spoon the cream into sterilised glass jars with well-fitting lids. Warm the jar in a basin of hot water for 15 minutes before using the cream to massage painful areas. The cream can also be massaged gently over scar tissue and slow-healing wounds, grazes or scratches.

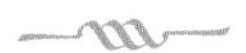

CULINARY USES

Dried safflower spicy mix

This mix makes a lovely gift for a cook. The safflower petals give a rich colour and enhance the tastes of all the other ingredients.

1 cup dried safflower petals
½ cup crushed coriander seed
½ cup cumin seed
½ cup grated ginger (dried) or 1 tablespoon ginger powder
1–2 teaspoons cayenne pepper, or 1–2 teaspoons crushed chillies
½ cup sesame seed
½ cup chopped pumpkin seeds
1 tablespoon turmeric

Shake the ingredients together vigorously in a big screw-top glass jar. Use 1–2 teaspoons of the mix in soups, stews, curries, stir-fries or as a rub over meat, chicken and fish before grilling. Use it as a delicious marinade (1 or 2 tablespoons of the spicy mix in half a cup of olive oil) before grilling thin slices of beef or chicken – it gives a gourmet taste!

NOTE: I do not add salt to the mixture, but for a marinade add 1–2 teaspoons should you like the seasoning all in one.

Safflower oil 1

This oil (and the one below) is ideal for salads and as a basting sauce over brown mushrooms, garlic, sausages, potatoes and leeks cut lengthways and roasted.

1 bottle good olive oil
2–3 tablespoons safflower seeds, lightly crushed
1 tablespoon safflower petals

Add the safflower seeds and petals to the bottle of olive oil. Stand the bottle in a large jug of hot water to warm the oil, and give it a frequent shake.

Safflower oil 2

2 cups good sunflower oil
2 tablespoons lightly crushed safflower seeds
1 tablespoon safflower petals

Pour the sunflower oil and safflower seeds and petals into a double boiler. Simmer for 30–40 minutes, stirring frequently with a stainless steel spoon. Strain, bottle and label the oil.

COOK'S NOTE

Try using safflower petals to colour cheese sauces, white sauces and liqueurs. Sprinkle in about two teaspoons of fresh and dried petals. Add more for a brighter colour.

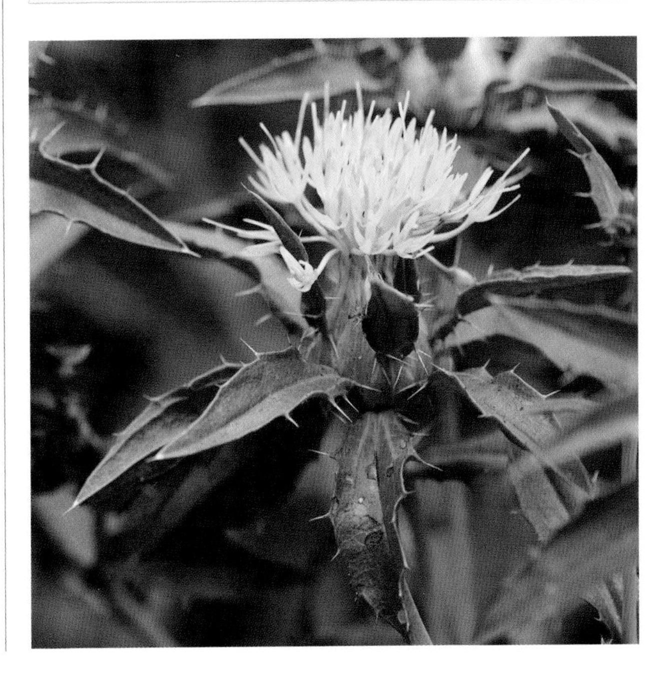

Sage

Salvia officinalis

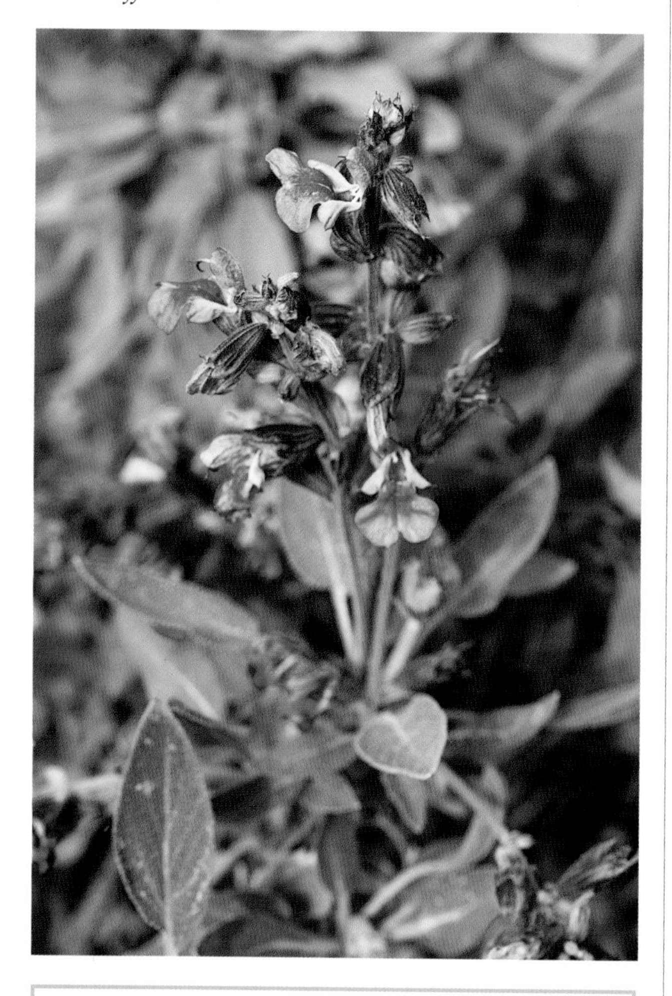

The genus name *Salvia* derives from the Latin *salvare*, meaning 'to cure'. The herb is native to the Mediterranean region and its medicinal and culinary properties have been respected for many centuries. The Romans considered sage to be a sacred herb, and gathered it with reverence and ceremony. The Chinese also valued sage highly, and Dutch merchants in the 17th century recorded that the Chinese would trade three chests of China tea for one chest of sage leaves!

CULTIVATION

Sage takes fairly easily from mature cuttings but does not like wet feet, so once your cuttings have rooted in moist sand, plant them out in individual pots in a well-drained mixture of compost and sand to strengthen. Plant them out 50 cm apart in the garden in a well-drained position in full sun. Water only once-weekly as sage will not thrive during long periods of rain or under a watering system. It needs no attention except for the odd trim of spent flowers or untidy growth. Replace the plants every three or four years. Sage does well in large pots, but make sure that these are well drained.

MEDICINAL USES

An ancient remedy for a sore throat was a gargle made from sage leaves and flowers, and sage was mixed with honey and lemon juice as a remedy for coughs and chest ailments.

Sage has been found to contain oestrogen, and as such it is used to treat irregular menstruation and the symptoms of menopause, including hot flushes and lowered oestrogen levels.

Sage also has some antibiotic properties, which is probably why it is so effective in clearing a sore throat and excess mucous from the nose, throat and chest. It was traditionally used as an asthma remedy, and with its excellent digestive and calming action, it immediately soothes spasm and anxiety. It is a nerve tonic, and its natural astringency helps to relieve diarrhoea, abdominal cramps and colic. Sage should be taken as a tea for all these ailments. To make a standard brew, pour a cup of boiling water over ¼ cup fresh flowers and leaves. Allow the tea to stand for five minutes, then strain and add a touch of honey to sweeten and a squeeze of fresh lemon juice. The usual dose during infections is one cup three times a day. As a general tonic take one cup daily, but take a break of 4–5 days every 10 days.

CAUTION: Sage is best avoided during pregnancy and should not be taken by epileptics.

Sage cough remedy

1 tablespoon fresh sage leaves
and a few flowers
1 tablespoon runny honey
1 tablespoon lemon juice
2 teaspoons fresh ginger root (optional)

Chop the fresh sage leaves and flowers very finely. Mix in the honey and lemon juice, and in the case of a runny nose, grate in two teaspoons of fresh ginger root. Mix well. Take one teaspoonful at a time frequently during the day.

Sage gargle for sore throats, mouth ulcers and bleeding gums

½ cup sage flowers and leaves
Rind of ½ a lemon
1 cup water

Simmer the flowers, leaves, lemon rind and water for 10 minutes. Leave it to stand and cool for 10 minutes. Strain. Take a mouthful, swill it in the mouth as long as possible, then spit out. Repeat at least four times daily.

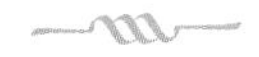

CULINARY USES

Sage flowers and bacon crisp

SERVES 4

This easy topping gives a gourmet flavour to scrambled or poached eggs. It can also be eaten on toast and in cheese sandwiches.

500 g rindless lean bacon
1 cup sage leaves and flowers
Coarsely ground black pepper
1 tablespoon parsley

Chop the bacon roughly into 2-cm pieces. In a large frying pan, fry the bacon in its own fat, turning frequently. Add the whole sage leaves and flowers. Stir-fry briskly until the bacon browns. Season with pepper, then lift the crisply fried leaves and flowers and the bacon and drain on crumpled paper towel for a few seconds. Place in a bowl. Mix with the parsley and sprinkle over scrambled or poached eggs. Decorate with fresh sage flowers.

Sage flower eggnog

SERVES 1

This refreshing 'quick fix' is excellent for all age groups, particularly students during exam time, as it energises and revitalises.

1 egg
1 glass milk
1 tablespoon honey
1 teaspoon finely grated nutmeg
1 banana
2 teaspoons sage leaves and flowers

Blend the ingredients together in a liquidiser until frothy. Pour immediately into a glass and sip slowly.

Sage and pumpkin soup

SERVES 6–8

This is real comfort food and it is a health booster too.

3 finely chopped onions
2 tablespoons olive oil
8 cups peeled and diced pumpkin
2 tablespoons grated ginger root
1 small chilli, finely chopped, or 2 teaspoons cayenne pepper
¼–½ cup chopped sage leaves and flowers
½ cup brown sugar
2½ litres chicken stock
Sea salt to taste
½ cup parsley

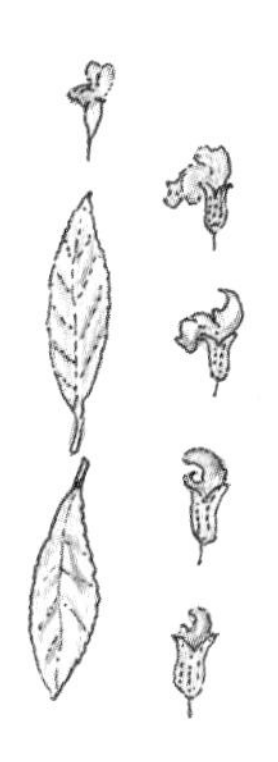

Sauté the onions in the oil until they start to brown, then add all the other ingredients except for the parsley. Simmer gently and add more water if necessary. Test if the pumpkin is tender after 20 minutes. Whirl the soup in a liquidiser until smooth. Reheat if necessary. Serve in hot bowls with crusty brown bread and sprinkle the parsley over the top. Decorate with a few sage flowers.

Sage cool drink

This recipe was used in the 1800s to counter old-age forgetfulness.

½ cup sage flowers
½ cup sage leaves
1 teaspoon aniseed
2 cups boiling water
Squeeze of lemon juice
1 or 2 teaspoons honey

Pour the boiling water over the flowers, leaves and seeds and stir for five minutes. Strain and allow to cool. Add the lemon juice, honey and an ice cube or two. Mix well and sip while chewing eight almonds.

COOK'S NOTE

Cooking with sage is a real art. As it is so pungent, it is best to use the leaves together with the flowers (which are less pungent), but remember that a little goes a long way. Sage is the herb traditionally added to poultry stuffing as it helps to break down fat and gives a fresh taste to the dish. It is excellent with eggs, cheese and vegetables. When cooking with the flowers, strip them from their calyxes and eat only the tender petals.

Snapdragon

Antirrhinum majus

The snapdragon is indigenous to Europe and has been a much-loved garden plant since before the Middle Ages, when it was considered an antidote to witchcraft. From the 15th century it was cultivated in Russia for the oil found in the seeds, which is said to be as pure and healthy as virgin olive oil. Much folklore surrounds the flowers, which open obligingly when lightly squeezed to look just like a dragon's mouth. This little mouth acts as an insect trap, which closes once the insect has entered, trapping it inside. For this reason snapdragons were once planted alongside grains and vegetables as protection for the crops.

CULTIVATION

It is best to sow the seed in autumn for a spring and early summer show. Treat the snapdragon as an annual, and sow the seed in a different area each year. Plant out the thumb-length seedlings in well-composted soil in full sun 20 cm apart and keep them moist until well established. Each flowering spike reaches 50 cm in height and mass plantings give a magnificent show. Snapdragons do not like hot weather and flower briefly in spring. However, they dry well and can be stored in a screw-top jar.

MEDICINAL USES

A cream made from snapdragon leaves and flowers will soothe hot, irritated rashes and sunburn, while snapdragon lotion is excellent at the end of a day outdoors when sunburn and windburn have taken their toll.

Snapdragon is remarkably effective for all types of inflammation, and crushed warmed snapdragon flowers mixed in a little almond oil will soothe aching sprains, strains, throbbing haemorrhoids, skin rashes and redness. Warm cotton cloths by wrapping them around a hot-water bottle, then spread the mixture on the cloths and place over an aching back or stiff shoulder or neck. Place the hot-water bottle against the area and relax for 15 minutes. This will bring quick relief and soothe away anxiety and discomfort.

In past years a gargle for mouth ulcers was made from the flowers and a few leaves, and concert and opera singers once considered snapdragon tea to be the most effective remedy for an aching, tired, strained throat. Perhaps snapdragon's mucilage, pectin, gallic

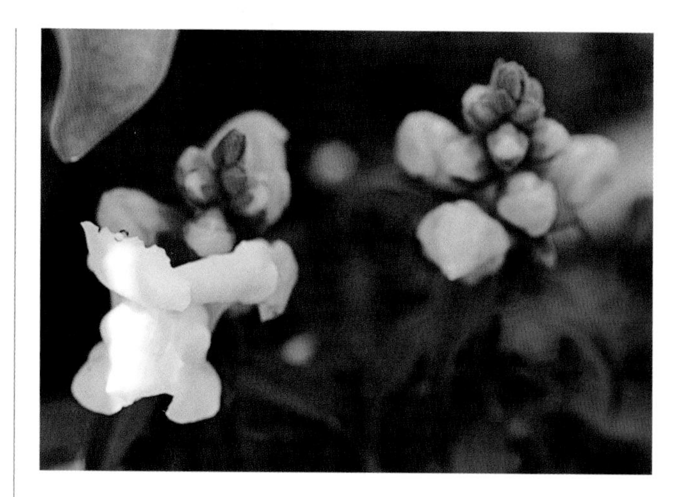

acid and resin content accounts for its soothing anti-inflammatory action. To make the tea, pour one cup of boiling water over ¼ cup fresh flowers and a few leaves, and leave to stand for 5–6 minutes. Strain, sweeten with a touch of honey, sip slowly, gargle a little, and swallow.

Snapdragon cream

Use this cream for rashes and sunburn, to soothe itching, redness and dry skin, and for cracked heels, nails and fingers.

1 cup chopped snapdragon leaves and flowers
1 cup good aqueous cream
2 teaspoons vitamin E oil

Simmer the snapdragon leaves and flowers in the aqueous cream in a double boiler for 20 minutes. Strain the mixture, stir in the vitamin E and almond oils and store in a sterilised jar. The cream will soothe hot, irritated areas and cracked heels, but it must be rubbed in well twice daily. At one time snapdragon cream was sold as a gardener's hand cream, depicting the flower on the lid. It was probably one of the first commercial hand creams.

Snapdragon lotion

This lotion is soothing for sun- and wind-burned skin, and dry, flaking skin on the nose and lips. Use it liberally. The lotion can be made using dried flowers. Dry some flowers for summer use, as it is a winter annual.

3 cups snapdragon flowers and leaves
2 litres water

Boil the snapdragon flowers and leaves in the water for 15 minutes. Strain and add the lotion to a warm bath or dab onto the area to calm the skin.

CULINARY USES

Spring pasta with snapdragons

SERVES 4

Snapdragons have a bland taste, which makes them perfect for both sweet and savoury dishes. Here they are combined with spring and early summer ingredients to make an unforgettable dish.

250 g angel hair pasta or spaghetti
3 cups mangetout peas
2 cups finely chopped onions
½ cup olive oil
2 cups thinly sliced brown mushrooms
1 cup finely chopped celery
1 cup mixed-colour snapdragon flowers, removed from their calyxes
Sea salt and black pepper to taste
2 tablespoons balsamic vinegar
¾ cup parmesan cheese
½ cup chopped parsley

Cook the pasta in boiling salted water until tender. Drop in the peas and cook for one minute. Drain. Fry the onions in the olive oil until they are transparent. Add the mushrooms, celery, snapdragon flowers and the seasoning. Stir-fry briefly until just tender. Add the stir-fry and vinegar to the drained pasta and peas. Spoon into a serving dish, sprinkle with the finely grated parmesan cheese and the chopped parsley. Decorate with a few fresh snapdragon flowers and serve hot.

Pan-fried mutton and snapdragons

SERVES 4

Hearty and appetising, this unusual dish is always a winner.

4 lean mutton loin chops, about 200 g each
3 tablespoons sunflower oil
2 onions cut into thin rings
1 tablespoon green peppercorns, soaked for about 1 hour in 1 tablespoon white grape vinegar
Sea salt and freshly ground black pepper
Juice of 1 lemon and a little grated lemon zest
6–8 early peaches, peeled and stoned
1 litre strong chicken stock
1 cup snapdragon flowers, calyxes removed

Fry the chops in the oil until brown. Add the onions and fry until they start to brown. Add the peppercorns and vinegar, sea salt, pepper, the lemon juice and zest, peaches and the stock. Gently simmer with the lid on for 10 minutes or until the meat is tender. Finally, add the snapdragon flowers and mix in well. Serve with brown rice and salad, decorated with snapdragon flowers.

Mulberry and snapdragon dessert

SERVES 4

This is a real spring dessert and can be served in attractive glass dishes as a party piece.

4 cups mulberries, stems removed
1 cup water
2 cups sugar
1 cinnamon stick
1 cup snapdragon flowers, calyxes removed
1½ cups whipped cream
½ cup chopped pecan nuts
½ cup desiccated coconut
A few mint leaves

Simmer the mulberries in the water with the sugar and cinnamon stick for exactly four minutes, no longer. Stir gently. Cool. Remove the cinnamon stick and spoon the mulberries into a glass bowl. Tuck the snapdragon flowers deeply into the syrup so that they soak it up, and dot with small spoonfuls of the whipped cream. Sprinkle the pecan nuts and coconut over the dessert and decorate with a few fresh snapdragon flowers and mint leaves. Serve chilled.

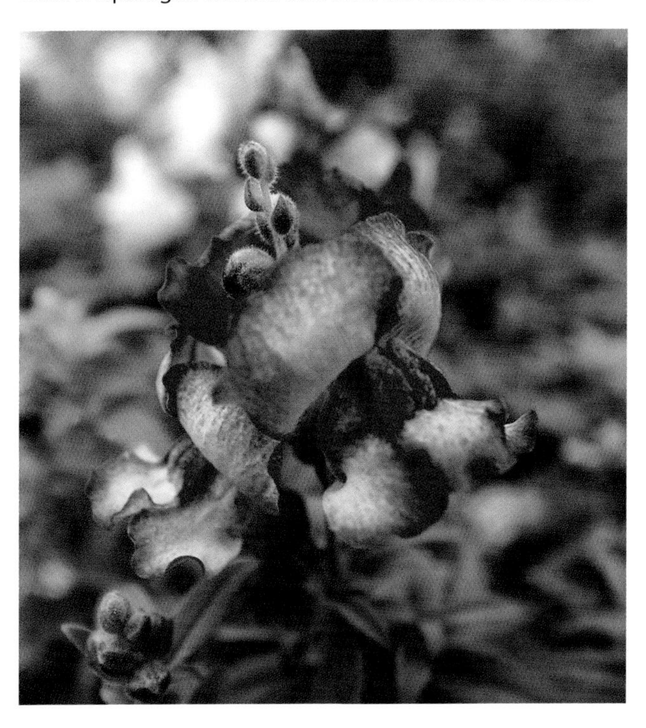

St John's wort

Hypericum perforatum

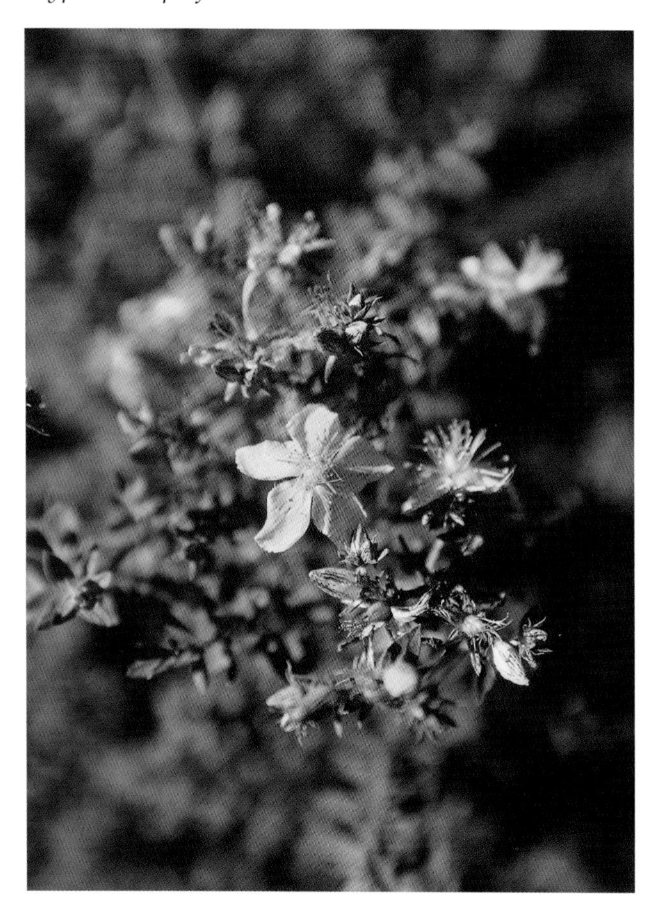

Much has been written about this ancient and revered plant, and research is still being conducted into its remarkable medicinal properties. In ancient times it was believed to have magical properties, and it was universally known as 'the Grace of God'. The crusaders took it on their journeys, along with yarrow and borage, as a pain reliever and styptic (substance that stops bleeding), and modern research has found these ancient uses to be medically sound.

CULTIVATION

Growing this unobtrusive, tiny-leafed perennial groundcover is not easy. It prefers the cool, damp meadows of its native Europe and Britain but will do fairly well even in poor sandy soil to which a little compost has been added, and with afternoon shade. Once it is established and with a twice-weekly watering, it will send up 45-cm tall heads of tiny, yellow flowers. It is these bright flowering heads that are used medicinally. Propagate St John's wort by digging off a small piece with a sharp spade and replant it immediately in a well-dug and lightly composted spot in full sun. Keep it moist for a week or two until it is well established and then water twice-weekly.

MEDICINAL USES

Hypericum perforatum is not to be confused with the other hypericums, including our own indigenous *H. revolutum*, which are unsafe to use medicinally. Dubbed 'Nature's Prozac', owing to its antidepressant properties, *H. perforatum* has also been found to be beneficial for menopause symptoms, liver and gall bladder ailments, anxiety, back pain, cold sores, chickenpox, shingles, neuralgia, stiff aching joints and muscles, lack of vitality, stress and insomnia. Its antiviral properties have been found to be so remarkable that it is being researched as a possible treatment for AIDS.

Both external and internal application of St John's wort is effective. A tea made from the flowering tops is the easiest way to take it. Pour one cup of boiling water over ¼ cup fresh flowers and buds. Leave the tea to stand for five minutes, then strain, sweeten with honey if desired, and add a squeeze of lemon juice. Use this tea for any of the ailments listed above and add one tablespoon of sage leaves and flowers for coughs, colds and menopausal symptoms.

An effective massage cream can be made to treat rashes, grazes, insect bites, cold sores, minor burns, cramp, neuralgia, aching muscles, sciatica and backache.

CAUTION: Taking St John's wort for some time may cause dermatitis in people with sensitive skin once the skin is exposed to the sun.

St John's wort massage cream

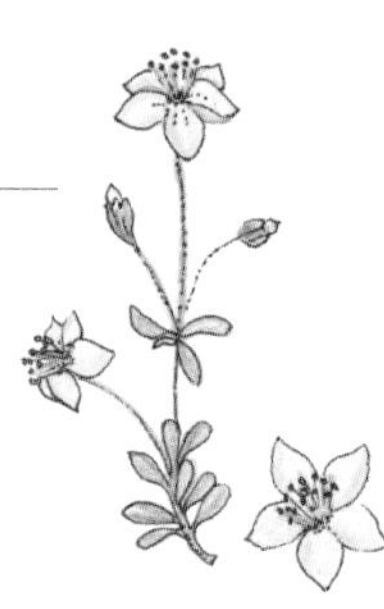

Use this cream for arthritic pains and aching muscles, as well as cold sores.

1 cup St John's wort flowering tops
1 cup aqueous cream
2 teaspoons vitamin E oil

Simmer the flowering tops and aqueous cream in a double boiler for 20 minutes, then strain. Add the vitamin E oil, mix well, and pour into sterilised jars with well-fitting lids. Store any excess cream in the fridge and rub frequently onto the affected area.

St John's wort healing oil

This oil can be dabbed on frequently for shingles, fever blisters, neuralgia, blisters and corns on the feet. This cream has many uses and is literally worth its weight in gold.

2 cups St John's wort flowering tops
1 cup grapeseed oil
1 cup olive oil

In a double boiler gently simmer the flowering tops and oils. Stir frequently. Allow to cool completely. Strain through muslin. Bottle in a dark glass bottle with a screw-top lid. In Europe, St John's wort oil is made on the midsummer solstice, 21 June. Bottles of olive oil, sunflower oil, almond oil, grapeseed oil, in which fresh St John's wort flowers are steeped, are left in the sun for four days. The oil turns ruby-red and is known as 'Turkey red oil'. Once strained, it is kept well sealed and used lavishly until the following summer solstice.

CULINARY USES

Beetroot and St John's wort health salad

SERVES 4

This is a real health-booster salad. The yellow petals brighten up the dish – and one's mood as well!

4 well-washed fresh beetroots
2 peeled apples
Juice of 1 lemon
Black pepper and coriander seeds in a pepper grinder
½ cup finely chopped parsley
½ cup St John's wort flowers

Grate the beetroots and apples. Mix well and spoon into a bowl. Pour the lemon juice over the mixture. Grind the pepper and coriander seeds over the salad and sprinkle with parsley and the St John's wort flowers.

Potato and St John's wort bake

SERVES 4

2 cloves garlic, finely chopped (optional)
8 medium potatoes, peeled and sliced very thinly
Sea salt and black pepper to taste
2–4 teaspoons freshly grated nutmeg
1 cup St John's wort flowers, petals pulled out of their calyxes
4 tablespoons butter, softened to room temperature
1 cup milk
1 cup cream

Grease a baking dish well and scatter the garlic over the base of the dish. Lay the potatoes in overlapping layers, and season with the sea salt, black pepper, nutmeg and a light sprinkling of the St John's wort petals. Dot with the soft butter. Whisk the milk and cream together and pour over the potato mixture. Bake uncovered at 180°C until the potatoes are tender and the top layer is golden and crisp, about 1½ hours.

Stuffed avocadoes with St John's wort

SERVES 4

These avocadoes make a tasty and interesting starter.

2 large avocadoes, cut in half and the stone removed
Lemon juice
1 tin sardines, drained and mashed
1 small onion, finely chopped
1 cup St John's wort flowers, calyxes removed
Sea salt and black pepper

Scoop the avocado flesh out carefully so as not to damage the skins. Mash the pulp and sprinkle with lemon juice so that it does not turn brown. Mix in the sardines, onion, St John's wort flowers and the salt and pepper. Spoon into the empty skins, sprinkle with more lemon juice and serve on a bed of lettuce. Sprinkle with St John's wort flowers.

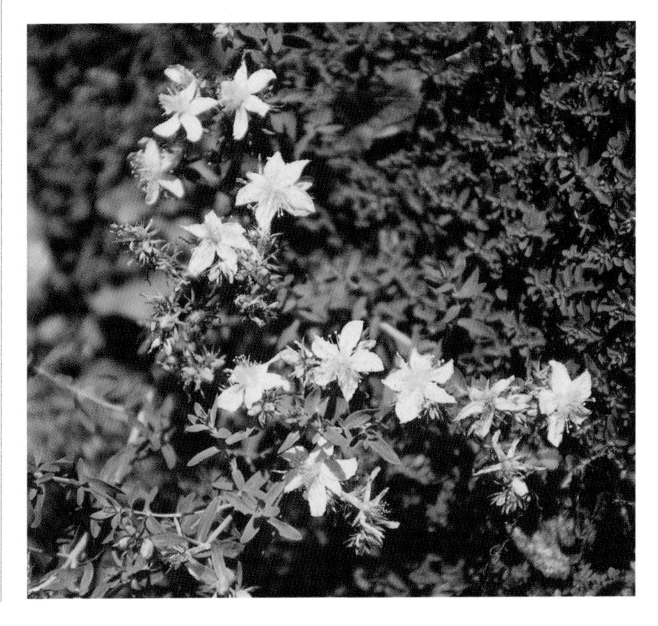

Stevia

Stevia rebaudiana

Stevia is exciting to grow – no plant offers the powerful sweetness of stevia and no plant produces a safe diabetic sugar substitute the way stevia does.

In my early trials of stevia I used only the fresh and dried leaves, but more recent experiments have shown that stevia flower syrup is nothing short of fabulous! I learned from Brazilian visitors to the Herbal Centre gardens that they preserve stevia flowers in honey as a winter medication.

Stevia's early beginnings were in Brazil and Paraguay where it is known as *caa'he* or 'sweet leaf', and ancient pharmacopoeias list it as a treatment for lowering blood sugar levels and as a contraceptive!

In 1887, stevia was recorded scientifically by two French chemists who isolated a glucoside present in the leaves, which they named 'steviocide'. The name remains in use today. They found stevia to be 300 times sweeter than sugar, and as it is a natural sweetener and safe for diabetics, tremendous interest developed in this unusual plant. By 1970 the Japanese had developed an extraction technique that removed the chlorophyll and the slight bitterness from the leaf, resulting in a fine white powder, now utilised in the food industry worldwide.

I do not use stevia powder as it is chemically processed and contains possible anticaking agents and whitening agents. I prefer to use it naturally – both the leaves (fresh and dried), and more recently the tiny white flower clusters.

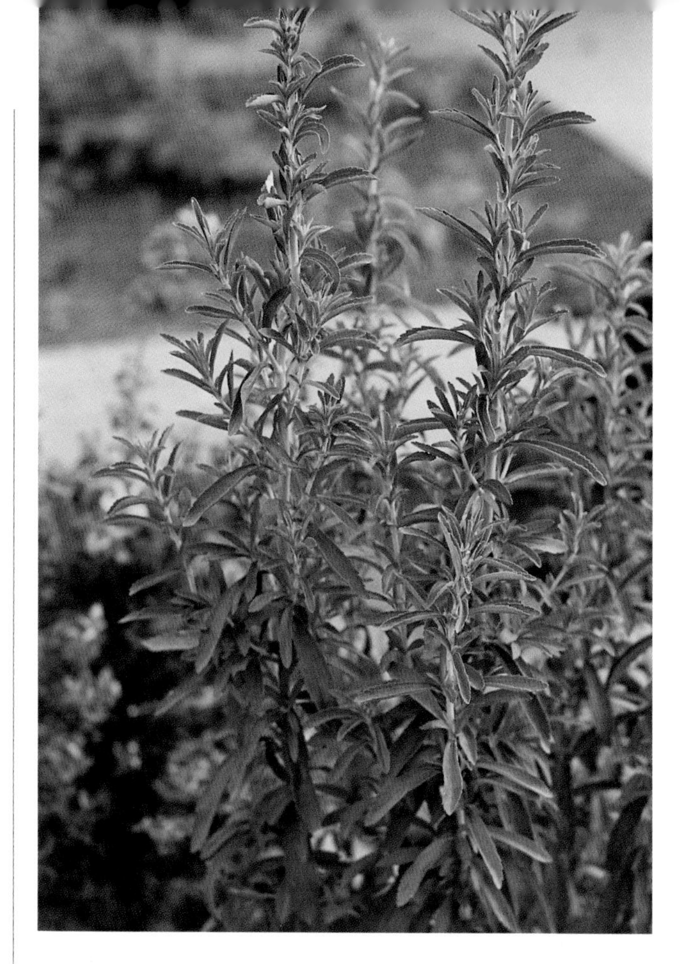

CULTIVATION

Stevia needs full sun and is a clump-forming perennial that becomes dormant in winter, sometimes dying down to almost nothing. Do not disturb it but cover it in the winter months with a protective cushion of dried leaves and prunings and some rough compost. Give it a slow once-weekly watering in winter and a good slow soak three times a week in summer.

Plant stevia in a deeply dug richly composted hole and flood with water. Space holes 1 m apart. To propagate in spring and early summer, gently dig out rooted tufts from the outside edges of the clump and immediately replant into richly composted holes. Keep it moist until it re-roots.

Sow seeds in seed trays covered lightly in moist soil (I use a sieve and sprinkle just enough soil to cover the seeds). Stand the seed tray in a big tray of water so that it is kept damp from below; in that way the fragile seed is not disturbed. It must not dry out, even for a short while.

Prick out the seedlings when they are big enough to handle and plant into composted and soil-filled bags. Keep them moist and shaded, gradually moving them out into the sun. Select their final place in the garden carefully as stevia can be quite spindly. I interplant it with other annuals in the kitchen garden and am often surprised by its self-sown seedlings, which I leave to grow wherever they are.

MEDICINAL USES

Stevia has been listed as a treatment for high blood pressure, high sugar levels and high blood cholesterol. However, discuss this with your doctor and do not exchange your present medications for stevia as it is still being fully researched.

What is known clearly is that stevia is an effective treatment for the gums and for tooth decay and plaque, and it is used in commercial toothpastes and mouthwashes.

Choose small strawberries or, if using larger fruits, cut them in quarters. Remove some of the wine and press all the additional ingredients into the bottle. Cork well and shake. Leave the mixture to stand for at least one week before opening. Strain out half a small glass of wine and sip slowly.

COSMETIC USES

Strawberry flower and fruit extracts are used in oils and creams in the cosmetic industry, and a beautiful astringent face mask can be made inexpensively at home. Strawberry tea will help to clear the skin. Use the tea as a lotion and splash onto the face after the strawberry face mask has been rinsed off in tepid water, and make an extra cup of tea to drink – it is pleasant and easily digested. The roots, buds, flowers and leaves all contain tannins (which act as toners) and, if heated with creams or oils, are exceptional for wrinkles and dry, ageing skin.

Strawberry face mask

Use this mask for blackheads, rashes, pimples, spots and dry, rough areas.

1 cup strawberry fruit and flowers

Crush the fruit and flowers together and apply them directly to the face (wash the fruit and flowers beforehand). Lie still for 15 minutes and let the fragrant pulp do its work, clearing oiliness and blackheads, healing pimples, closing and refining the pores, and soothing rashes. Wash off the mask with mild soap and rinse with water. For best results, finish by rubbing calendula cream into the skin.

Strawberry oil for ageing skin

2 cups finely chopped fresh strawberry roots, young buds and leaves
1 cup olive oil
2 teaspoons vitamin E oil

In a double boiler, simmer the roots, buds and leaves in the olive oil for 30 minutes, stirring and pressing frequently. Cool the mixture, then strain it through muslin and add the vitamin E oil. Store it in a dark glass bottle with a good screw top. Use nightly by massaging the fragrant oil deeply into the skin.

CULINARY USES

Strawberry punch

SERVES 8

Try this recipe for a party drink that is delicious and healthy.

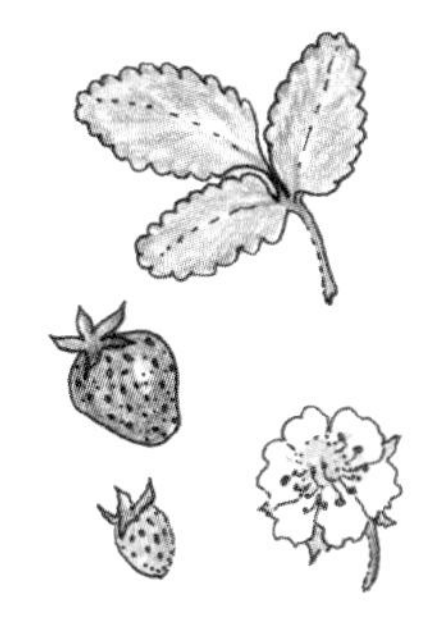

2 cups thinly sliced strawberries
1½ cups sugar
Juice of 6 lemons
2 teaspoons lemon zest, finely grated
2 tablespoons finely grated ginger
1½ litres water
1 cup strawberry flowers
1 litre rosé wine (optional)

Mash the strawberries with half the sugar and leave the mixture to stand for about two hours. Squeeze the lemons, dissolve the rest of the sugar in the juice, add the lemon zest and ginger, and set aside for about two hours. Mix everything together, pour into a jug, and float the flowers on top. As an optional extra, add one litre of rosé wine. Serve chilled.

Strawberry flower pashka

SERVES 6–8

This traditional Russian Easter cake or dessert is made in a cheese cloth-lined terracotta flower pot. The secret is the hole at the base of the pot as it allows the cottage cheese to drain beautifully.

350 g (about 1½ cups) cottage cheese
3 tablespoons runny honey
1 teaspoons rosewater or vanilla essence
1 cup plain Bulgarian yoghurt
¾ cup sultanas, soaked beforehand in hot water, then drained
1 cup fresh fruit, peeled and chopped finely – peaches, mangoes, nectarines, pears, strawberries
¾ cup strawberry flowers ('Pink Panda' is pretty but any strawberry flowers will do)

Tip the cottage cheese into a sieve and rub it through. Mix the honey and rosewater or vanilla into the yoghurt, stir until smooth, and add to the cheese. Add the sultanas and chopped fruit to the mixture. Line a new 12 cm unglazed clay flower pot with a square of fine muslin or cheese cloth. Spoon the cheese mixture into it, fold the corners of the cloth over, and put a weight on top. Stand the pot over a bowl so that it can drain. Leave overnight in the fridge, or preferably for a day and a night. Open the corners of the cloth, invert the pot on a pretty plate, decorate with the strawberry flowers, and if desired, add slices of fresh fruit. Dust with icing sugar and serve as a dessert with coffee.

Sunflower

Helianthus annuus

The stately sunflower has been a valuable crop since ancient times, and was first cultivated in South America, particularly Peru, some 3 000 years ago. It is native to South and North America and possibly Mexico, and in ancient Peru it was an emblem of the Inca sun god. In the 16th century, explorers introduced the sunflower to Spain, having brought it over from North America.

Sunflowers are a fast-maturing crop and fields of sunflowers are a breathtaking sight in summer, turning their glorious heads to face the sun as it moves from east to west. Bees love sunflowers because of their nectar and pollen and the seeds are favoured by many seed-eating birds.

CULTIVATION

Sunflowers are an easy-to-grow annual and growing them is very rewarding. In spring, dig over a patch of soil in full sun, add plenty of compost, and water it well. Press the large seeds singly into the moist soil, 20–30 cm apart and about 3 cm deep. Keep the soil moist with a light mulch of dry leaves, and do not allow it to dry out.

MEDICINAL USES

Sunflower oil is one of the most versatile of all cooking oils, and is mild, bland, and rich in linoleic, oleic and palmitic acids; it is also high in vitamins A, D and E. Like all oils rich in linoleic acid, particularly borage and evening primrose oil, it inhibits the dangerous build-up of cholesterol deposits.

The young flowering buds are highly nutritious and were a favourite food of the Incas. The buds, as well as the maturing flower petals, contain traces of zinc, beta-carotene, vitamins B_1, B_2, B_3, B_6 and E, magnesium, manganese and chromium. The seeds are a superb health food, containing the same vitamins as the buds and petals, as well as calcium, potassium, phosphorus and iron in abundance. Hulled sunflower seeds are said to be diuretic and expectorant. A handful can be eaten once or twice a day and they are delicious raw or roasted in home-made muesli.

The unhulled seeds can also be boiled and taken as a tea: Add two tablespoons of unhulled seeds to two cups of water and simmer for 20 minutes, then cool the tea and strain. Take half a cup twice a day.

Sunflower oil, seeds and young flowers are believed to help in the formation of healthy tissue, and to boost the immune system and keep the joints supple. Interestingly, all parts of the sunflower are being tested for the ability to regenerate tissue in the kidneys after infectious kidney diseases and kidney stones. The leaves are being tested in the treatment of malaria, and can be used to make a tea. Pour two cups of boiling water over half a cup of chopped fresh leaves. Leave the tea to draw for five minutes, then strain and sip it warm or cold throughout the day.

Sunflower cough remedy

This remedy is very useful for coughs, flu and bronchitis.

½ cup fresh sunflower petals
½ cup dehusked sunflower seeds
Juice of ½ lemon
2 teaspoons honey
½ cup hot water

Liquidise everything for two minutes. Spoon out into a glass jar with a well-fitting lid. Take one teaspoon at a time with a little sunflower tea. This is an excellent treatment for clearing mucous.

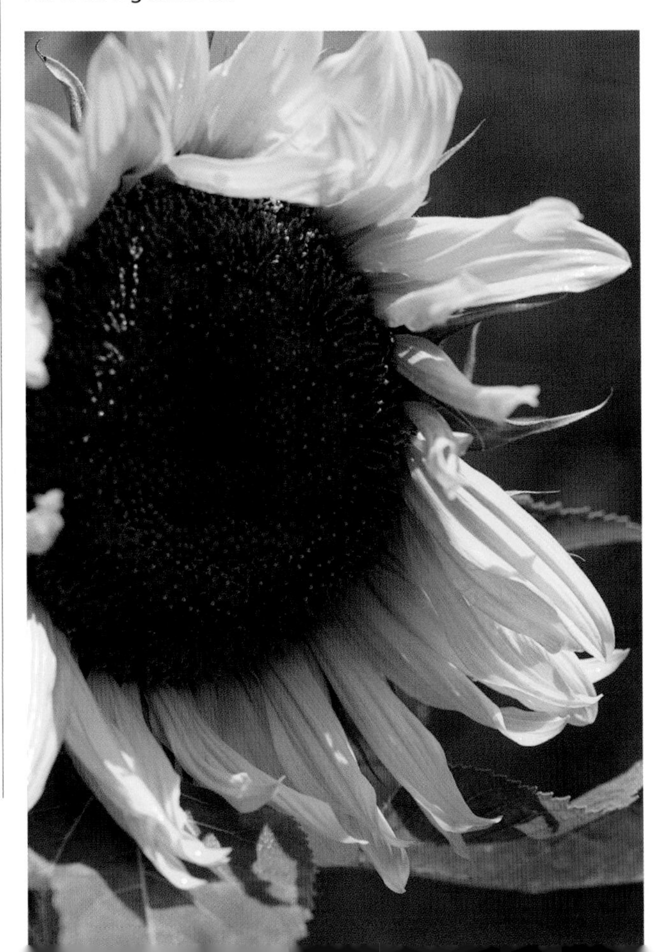

CULINARY USES

Sunflower buds with mustard sauce

SERVES 4–6

Served with a salad and cold meats, this is an unusual and delicious dish.

12–14 small flower buds, about 6 cm in diameter
2 teaspoons salt

Mustard sauce
1 tablespoon cornflour
1 teaspoon sea salt
2 teaspoons mustard powder
½ cup brown sugar
3 eggs, well beaten
½ cup brown grape vinegar
1 cup milk

Place the flower buds in a pot, cover with water, add the salt and bring to the boil. Simmer for about six minutes. Strain through a colander and repeat the process with fresh water. Boil for a further six or seven minutes or until tender. Strain, arrange in a glass dish and keep them warm while you prepare the mustard sauce.

Mix the cornflour, salt, mustard powder and sugar, and add to the beaten eggs. Whisk the mixture until creamy. Add the vinegar gradually. Warm the sauce gently on the stove on a low heat. Gradually add the milk, beating constantly, whisking while it thickens. Remove the sauce from the stove as soon as it bubbles and pour it over the cooked sunflower buds. Serve piping hot with rice.

Marinated sunflower bud parcels

SERVES 4–6

These sunflower parcels can be grilled on the coals of a fire or under the oven grill, and served directly from the foil.

10–12 sunflower buds, about 6 cm in diameter
Mild fruit chutney
Fresh lemon juice
2 medium onions, thinly sliced
Salt and pepper
Olive oil
Feta cheese, cubed

Parboil the buds for about 10 minutes in salted water. Remove from the water and rinse under a cold tap. Lay them face down in a dish and spoon the chutney over them. Leave them to marinate for about two hours, turning them over

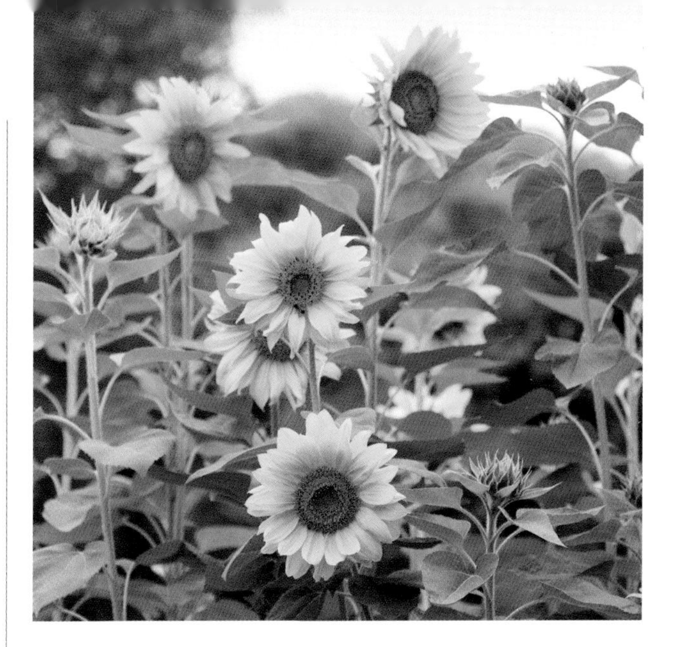

from time to time. Place each sunflower bud separately on a square of aluminium foil, squeeze some lemon juice over it, place three or four thin onion slices around it, sprinkle with salt and pepper, add a dash of olive oil and a few cubes of feta cheese, and carefully dot with the chutney marinade. Wrap the parcels neatly and place on the coals of the fire or under the oven grill for 20 minutes. Serve in the foil parcel.

Beetroot and sunflower petal salad

SERVES 6

The striking, contrasting colours in this salad give new life to an old favourite. I grow white sunflower seeds for this salad, as young, soft seeds make a delicious addition sautéed with the onions.

3 medium-sized onions, thinly sliced
3 tablespoons olive oil
12 small young beetroot, peeled and thinly sliced
1 cup water
1 tablespoon flour
2 tablespoons honey
2 tablespoons lemon juice
Sea salt and black pepper to taste
1 cup sunflower petals
Chopped parsley

Sauté the onion rings in the oil, then add the beetroot. Stir-fry briefly and add half a cup of water. Mix the flour with the honey, lemon juice, salt and pepper, and stir into the onions and beetroot. Add another half cup of water and the sunflower petals. Turn down the heat and cover the pot. Simmer gently for about 15 minutes, then remove from the heat and allow the mixture to cool. Sprinkle with a little chopped parsley. Serve as a salad with cold chicken.

Thyme

Thymus vulgaris ● *T.* × *citriodorus*

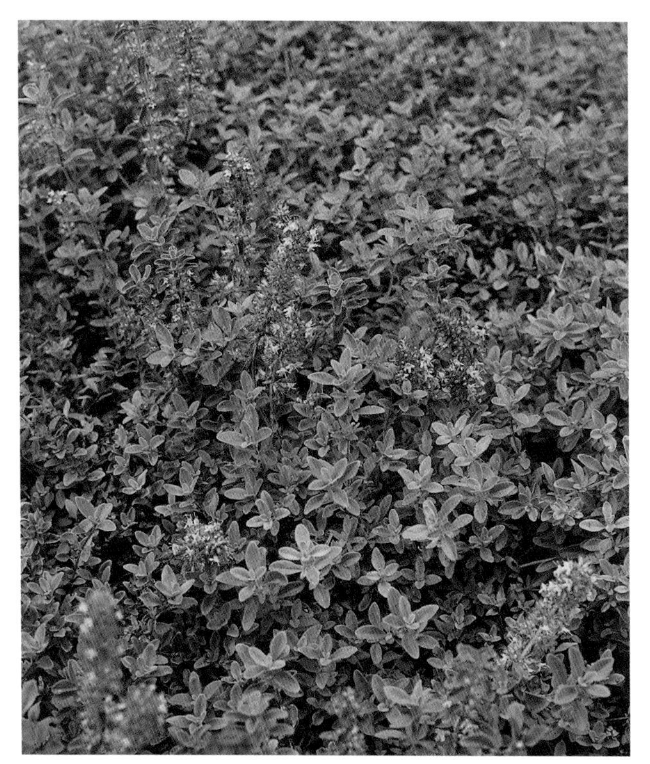

Creeping thyme

Thyme is one of the world's favourite culinary herbs and is so common that one hardly stops to think of its amazing medicinal properties. *Thymus vulgaris* is known as common thyme. The cultivated variety *T.* × *citriodorus* is called lemon thyme, and *T. serpyllum*, which is native to southern Europe, is known as mother-of-thyme. Thyme is a member of the Laminaceae family, which cross-pollinates easily, so there are literally hundreds of varieties of thyme. All seem to have similar properties and have been used medicinally by many cultures through the centuries. The Egyptians used thyme oil for embalming, and the ancient Greeks and Romans used it in their baths and as incense in their churches.

CULTIVATION

Generally, all thymes are easy to grow. They all need full sun and are not fussy about soil type, but they flourish in well-drained, sandy soil with a good bit of compost dug in. They love hot, dry conditions and demand little except a good weekly watering and occasional cutting back. Propagation is by means of small, rooted sprigs taken from the mother plant every two or three years. These should be kept protected in moist, shaded, well-composted bags until they are strong enough to take full sun, and subsequently planted out in the garden.

MEDICINAL USES

Thyme is a superb antiseptic and tonic herb, and a pleasant-tasting infusion of lemon thyme with a slice of lemon and a teaspoon of honey is a comforting treatment for a sore throat, cough and chest cold. Added to your daily food, thyme acts as a good digestive, boosts the immune system to fight colds and flu, and helps build up energy and vitality. In days gone by, savoury teas of thyme, red pepper and lemon juice were drunk to ward off colds and to keep warm and fit during the long cold winters. A few carrots, a stick of celery and chopped onions were added to make a nourishing soup to clear chest infections, backache, coughs and bronchitis, and thyme is still used in this way today.

All the thymes are superb for treating fungal infections, whooping cough, pneumonia, asthma and hay fever (especially in children), and worms in children and animals. They can be used as an expectorant to clear mucous from the body, and for soothing muscular aches and pains. A lotion of the cooled standard tea will soothe insect bites and stings, hot sore eczema areas, and will help with ringworm, athlete's foot, thrush, scabies and lice infestation. It is rich in thymol, which is a most effective antifungal, and this together with several flavonoids will relieve rheumatism and muscle spasms such as stiff neck and cramps. All the thymes taken as a tea will impart a feeling of vitality and relieve muscular and mental tiredness. The standard brew is a cup of boiling water poured over ¼ cup fresh thyme sprigs (flowering sprigs included). Allow the tea to infuse for five minutes, then strain and sip slowly.

Thyme flower lotion for aching muscles, leg cramps and rheumatism

2 cups thyme sprigs with flowers
½ cup grapeseed oil
½ cup good acqueous cream
1 teaspoon vitamin E oil
½ teaspoon rose geranium essential oil

In a double boiler, simmer the thyme, grapeseed oil and acqueous cream for 20 minutes. Strain it and add the vitamin E and rose geranium essential oils. Mix thoroughly. Spoon into a glass jar with a well-fitting lid. To use it, warm the lotion by standing the jar in hot water, then massage it into the affected area. Cover the skin with a towel and hot-water bottle and relax for 20 minutes. This wonderful lotion becomes quite a panacea.

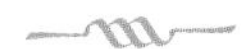

CULINARY USES

Thyme immune-boosting soup

SERVES 6–8

This is a recipe from my grandmother's day – a true comfort soup that no one ever tires of.

3 cups roughly chopped onion
A little olive oil
2 cups finely grated potato
1½ litres good chicken stock
1 cup pearl barley, soaked overnight
2 cups finely grated carrot
2 cups finely chopped celery, leaves included
1 small red chilli, finely chopped and seeds removed
  (or 1 teaspoon cayenne pepper)
Juice of 2 lemons
2 teaspoons finely grated lemon zest
½ cup fresh thyme leaves and flowers
Sea salt to taste

Fry the onions in the oil until they start to brown, add the grated potatoes and stir-fry until they start to turn golden. Add all the other ingredients and simmer with the lid on until everything is tender and the soup is tasty. Serve steaming hot with crusty brown bread.

Thyme flower savoury fish

SERVES 4

Lemon thyme is the most delicious of the thymes for this recipe.

2 beaten eggs
2 teaspoons paprika
4–6 deboned skinned fish fillets
1 cup flour seasoned with salt and black pepper
Olive oil and butter, 3 tablespoons of each
Juice of 1 lemon
2 tablespoons fresh thyme flowers and leaves,
  stripped off their stalks
Lemon wedges for serving

Whisk the eggs with the paprika until frothy. Pour into a flat dish, lay the fish in it, and spoon the remaining egg mixture over the fillets. Spread the seasoned flour in a flat dish and roll the egg-basted fish in the flour, coating the fish evenly. Meanwhile, heat the oil and butter in a large frying pan and place the fish gently in the pan. Fry until golden, using a spatula to turn the fish over carefully and fry on the other side. Drain on crumpled kitchen paper towel and place on a serving dish. Keep warm until ready to serve. Sprinkle with lemon juice and thyme flowers. Serve with mashed potato or baked potato and extra lemon wedges.

Thyme salt

A cannister of thyme salt is so useful to have at hand while cooking – it gives added zest and flavour and takes some beating!

2 cups coarse sea salt
¾ cup fresh thyme leaves and flowers
1 tablespoon coriander seeds, crushed
1 tablespoon black peppercorns, crushed
1 tablespoon mustard powder or seeds
1 tablespoon paprika

Mix the ingredients together well, and store in an airtight screw-top jar. Have a mortar and pestle next to the stove, or keep a large pepper grinder nearby. Grind the mixture before adding to food while cooking, or have it in a small grinder at the table.

> COOK'S NOTE
> **Thyme salt is perfect for all savoury dishes: meat, eggs, pastas, casseroles, soups, sauces, etc. In the case of fish and cheese dishes, replace the fresh garden thyme with lemon thyme leaves and flowers and include one tablespoon of sesame seeds and two teaspoons of lemon zest. All the other ingredients remain the same.**

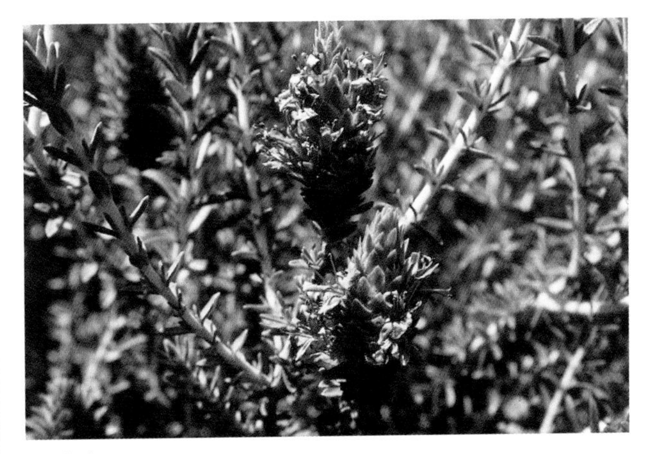

Greek thyme

Tuberose

Polianthes tuberosa

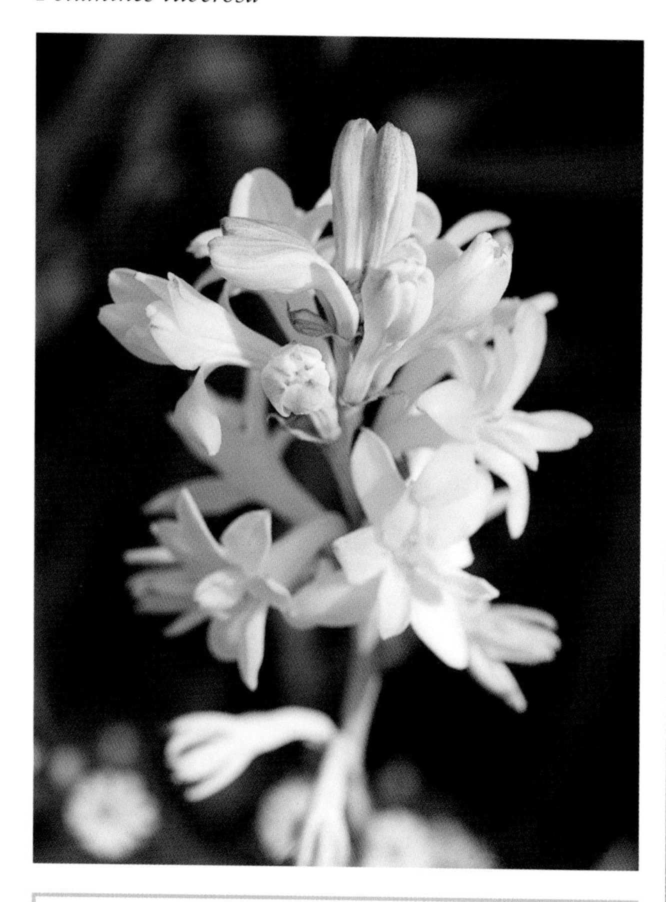

The tuberose is not commonly grown, and is an old-world bulbous plant with an exceptional fragrance. In the late 17th and early 18th centuries the first bulbs were taken from Central America to Morocco, and from there to Egypt and France, where they are still cultivated for their glorious, rich and hugely expensive oil. Pure absolute extract of tuberose is the most expensive natural flower oil in the world, worth its weight in gold. The oil is used to create exquisite perfumes, mainly in France. One flowering head of tall, creamy white, lily-like flowers will scent an entire room with its haunting fragrance for a week.

CULTIVATION

Growing tuberose is easy, as the bulb is perennial. It needs well-dug, well-composted soil in full sun and the bulbs should be spaced 20 cm apart. A single stem, 40–50 cm tall, rises through the slender tuft of pale green leaves, topped with a mass of buds and flowers. The buds are the palest shade of pink, and the flowers creamy white. Divide the clump every two years once it has flowered and replant the little corms or bulbs in new ground. The cycle usually takes two years and the bulbs can be planted in succession.

MEDICINAL USES

Centuries ago the tuberose was used in China to calm stomach disorders caused by anxiety. Around the 12th century, flower teas were introduced to soothe over-excited children, and to help relieve nausea, vomiting and fevers. A single flower added to a cup of green tea immediately imparts its rich oils and fragrance, calming and settling a wildly beating, anxious heart. Taken as an after-dinner tea, it will ease digestion and make even the most stressful day dissolve into restful calm – an ancient Chinese secret!

Recently, tuberose oil has been used with astonishing results as a treatment for stress, hypersensitivity, anger, hostility, resentment, disorientation, emotional conflict and confusion. It is becoming an important healing oil, promoting emotional stability and counteracting drug and alcohol addiction, burnout and anxiety. Research is being done into the benefits of tuberose in harmonising the emotions in terminally ill people, particularly those with AIDS and cancer.

COSMETIC USES

In Egypt, a lotion was made from the beautiful flowers to treat acne, oily skin and enlarged pores. The lotion can be made at home, as well as an easy-to-make tuberose cream for dry, brittle nails. Massage the cream into the nails and cuticles frequently – it will do wonders.

Tuberose lotion

Use this lotion for acne and problem skin, torn cuticles, split and dry, brittle nails.

2 cups boiling water
1 cup tuberose flowers and buds, finely chopped
1 teaspoon vitamin E oil

Pour the boiling water over the flowers and buds, and leave the mixture to stand until cool. Strain, add the oil and mix well. Apply the lotion with cotton wool discs, or spray it as a mist using a bottle with a spray mechanism. Alternatively, pour a little into a small bowl, dip the fingertips into it, massaging it well into the nails and torn cuticles. Do this for at least five minutes to get the benefit of the lotion.

Tuberose cream for brittle nails

1 cup chopped tuberose flowers
1 cup good aqueous cream
2 teaspoons vitamin E oil

Simmer the chopped flowers in the aqueous cream for 20 minutes, then strain and add the vitamin E oil. Mix well, store in a sterilised jar, and apply frequently, working the cream into the nails and cuticles.

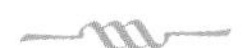

CULINARY USES

Tuberose vegetable soup

SERVES 6

This soup is adapted from an old Chinese recipe. It is light and refreshing, perfect as a starter to be followed by a rich meal.

2 cups finely chopped onions
2 tablespoons olive oil
2 cups thinly sliced mushrooms
2 cups chopped green peppers
4 cups diced celery stalks
2 litres chicken stock
1 cup cooked brown rice
2 tablespoons pure soy sauce, with no added MSG
3 tablespoons fresh lemon juice
Sea salt and black pepper to taste
1 cup tuberose flowers, lightly sliced
Nutmeg

Fry the onions in the olive oil, add the mushrooms and brown lightly. Add the green peppers and celery and stir-fry for three minutes. Add all the other ingredients and simmer gently for about 15 minutes. Serve hot in bowls with a fresh tuberose flower floating on top. Dust with nutmeg.

Tuberose and pineapple cordial

SERVES 6–8

Offer this cordial as a treat and on special occasions – it will be long remembered!

2 well-ripened pineapples, peeled and chopped
2 litres white grape juice
2 teaspoons ground ginger
½ cup runny honey
10–15 fresh tuberose flowers

Whirl the pineapples, a little of the grape juice, the ground ginger and the honey in a liquidiser until smooth. Mix in the rest of the grape juice. Toss in the flowers (the Chinese chop them up, I like them kept whole in all their beauty), and refrigerate for at least two hours before serving. Taste for sweetness, and add more honey if needed. Serve in wine glasses and tuck a tuberose flower into each glass.

Tuberose fridge cake

SERVES 6–8

Serve this fridge cake as a dessert with ice-cream or custard, or as a teatime treat. It is quick, easy, nourishing and delicious, and keeps well in the fridge.

4 tablespoons butter
1 teaspoon ground cinnamon
1 teaspoon ground pimento (allspice)
1 teaspoon ground nutmeg
3 tablespoons treacle or honey
3 tablespoons sherry
5 tablespoons sultanas, soaked for an hour in hot water
225 g digestive biscuits, coarsely crushed
4 tablespoons chopped glacé cherries
4 tablespoons candied peel
4 tablespoons chopped pecan nuts
3 tablespoons chopped tuberose flowers

Melt the butter with the spices in a double boiler. Add the treacle or honey and the sherry and mix well. Drain the sultanas and mix with the remaining ingredients. Combine with the butter, honey and sherry mixture. Stir thoroughly. Line a loaf tin with greaseproof paper. Press the mixture down firmly into the tin, cover with more greaseproof paper, and weight it down. Chill for at least two hours. Turn the fridge cake out onto a flat plate, slice thinly, and decorate with tuberose flowers.

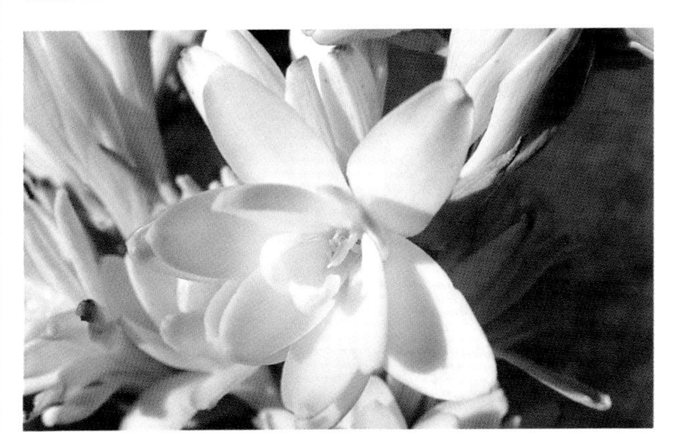

Tulip

Tulipa species

The tulip is a popular cool-weather bulb indigenous to Persia. The name derives from the Turkish word *tulipan* or *turband*, indicating its turban shape, while its Latin name is *Tulipa gesneriana*. The bulbs have been in cultivation for over 1 000 years, and have long been a symbol of perfect love. Tulips grew wild along the Bosphorus and young men supposedly gathered them to send as a symbol of love to girls in the harems beyond the palace gates, which is probably how the symbolism originated. In 1556, tulip bulbs were taken to Vienna and from there to France and finally Holland, the country with which tulips have become synonymous.

Cooking with tulips dates back to the end of the 16th century, when the unopened buds were cooked with peas or finely cut green beans. The petals were also sugared and eaten with syrup as a dessert. Owing to the increase in exotic vegetables on offer in the world's marketplaces today, this charming practice has largely died out.

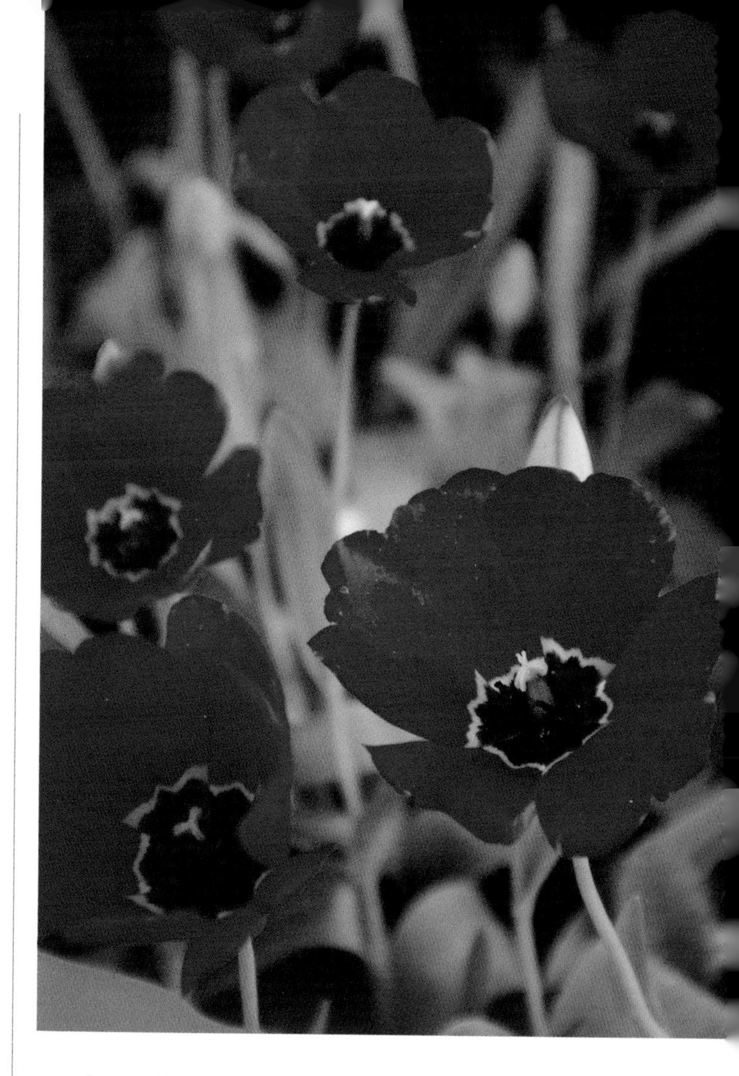

CULTIVATION

Tulips can be used to great effect in the spring garden, particularly when massed in areas of a single colour. The bulbs should be planted in late autumn when the soil has cooled down, spaced 15 cm apart in full sun, in well-dug, richly composted soil with a cooling mulch of rotted leaves. Give them a deep twice-weekly watering to ensure uniform growth. The bulbs will take about 9–10 weeks to flower. Modern bulbs are cold-treated and seldom excel after their first year of blooming, which means that new bulbs should be planted every year. Some tulip experts shade their bulbs in autumn between 11h00 and 15h00 to keep them cool. Tulips need cold to flower, so only plant them in cold areas where it freezes most nights.

MEDICINAL USES

There are only a few references to tulip poultices in the ancient herbals – perhaps the flowers were so expensive even then that they were not often crushed for medicinal purposes! However, in the case of burns, skin rashes, insect bites and bee stings, a soothing poultice of the petals was often used.

In the 17th century young girls crushed red tulip petals and rubbed them into their cheeks so that the petals would impart their colour, and the juice would help to clear up any spots. Tulip petals greatly soothe cuts, grazes, corns, callouses, scratches and infected insect bites.

Given that tulip growers in Holland still use crushed petals and the juice from the base of the flower to soothe scratches and rough skin on work-worn hands, it seems surprising that a hand and nail cream containing tulip extract has not yet been formulated by an enterprising grower.

Tulip poultice for burns and insect bites

4 tulip flowers
Hot water
Castor oil

Warm the flowers in hot water and break off the petals. While still hot, roll the petals in a warm, wet towel to soften them, then unroll and place the crushed petals over the affected area. Hold the petals in place with the hot towel for 10 minutes. Some recipes suggest smoothing a little castor oil onto the burn or insect bite before placing the petals over the area.

Tulip skin cream

Apply this cream on corns, scratches, grazes and chafed, raw skin.

1 cup good acqueous cream
½ cup olive oil
4 tulip flowers, finely chopped
2 teaspoons vitamin E oil
Few drops rose essential oil

Simmer the acqueous cream, olive oil and tulip petals together in a double boiler for 20 minutes. Strain through muslin. Add the vitamin E oil and rose essential oil and mix well. Spoon into a sterilised glass jar with a well-fitting lid.

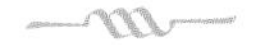

CULINARY USES

Three bean salad with tulips

SERVES 6

Perfect for a vegetarian meal, this salad keeps well in the fridge.

1 cup large white butter beans
1 cup haricot beans
2 cups green beans, finely sliced lengthways
Petals of 3 or 4 tulips

Dressing
½ cup runny honey
½ cup good olive oil
½ cup fresh lemon juice
2 tablespoons balsamic vinegar
3 teaspoons mustard powder
½ cup finely chopped onions
A little garlic (optional)
2 teaspoons sea salt
1 tablespoon crushed coriander seed
1 tablespoon crushed sesame seed

Soak the butter beans and haricot beans overnight. The next day, boil them until they are tender. Boil the green beans until tender but still fairly crisp. Allow all the beans to cool.

Shake the dressing ingredients together vigorously in a jar with a tight-fitting lid. Pour the dressing over the salad and fold in well. Place the petals of three or four tulips around the dish, filling them with a little of the bean salad, and grind black pepper over everything. Serve with crusty bread.

Tulip syrup

SERVES 6

This unusual recipe dates from the 17th century and is delicious spooned over rice or sago pudding, and custard or cream desserts. It keeps well in the fridge.

2 cups white sugar
3 cups water
6 cloves
1 cinnamon stick
Juice of 2 lemons
Petals from 8 tulips, cut into thin strips
(reds and pinks are prettiest)

Place all the ingredients except the tulip petals in a pot and simmer gently for about 12 minutes, stirring occasionally. Allow the syrup to cool for 10 minutes, remove the cinnamon stick and cloves, and stir in the tulip petal strips. Refrigerate when cool.

Tulips stuffed with chicken mayonnaise

SERVES 4–6

This is the perfect recipe for a luncheon party to celebrate the arrival of spring!

1 medium-sized cold roast chicken
2 tablespoons chopped fresh parsley
¾ cup finely chopped celery
½ cup finely chopped green pepper
½ cup finely chopped spring onion
Sea salt and black pepper to taste
1 cup good mayonnaise
12 tulips

Slice the chicken from the bone and chop finely. Mix all the ingredients together, except for the tulips. Remove the stamens and pistils from the tulips, leaving a little bit of stalk attached. Stuff the flowers with the chicken mayonnaise mixture. Arrange the flowers neatly in a circle on a bed of butter lettuce and pile any leftover chicken mayonnaise in the centre. Dust with black pepper and serve chilled.

Turmeric

Curcuma domestica

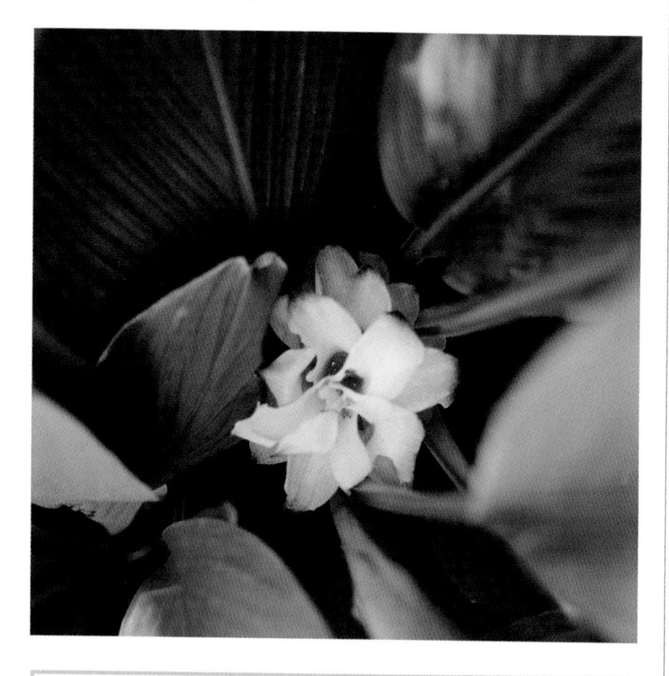

Turmeric grows in seclusion in light shade under the protection of its large smooth leaves where no one ever looks. It is a unique plant with a brilliant yellow root and exquisite flower of pale bracts that opens at ground level where you least expect it.

Over the years I have been so intrigued by this secretive plant that I set out to grow, draw and photograph it, and to share its beauty. I have also researched old herbals to ascertain its uses and found it to be one of the rare botanical treasures dating back to ancient times.

Turmeric belongs to the ginger family, Zingiberaceae, and is native to Asia. Due to its beginnings along the trade routes, it is often commonly known as 'Indian saffron'. In ancient Chinese pharmacopoeias, turmeric is listed as being a treatment for sores, bruises, ringworm, chest pains, colic, indigestion, menstrual problems and toothache. In those days the root, leaves and flowers were all included in remedies.

Today we know turmeric only as a bright yellow root, conveniently powdered for use in stews, curries and as a popular spice mixture. India, Jamaica, Haiti and Indonesia are the main producers of turmeric. Turmeric oil is still distilled in Europe and the USA, while the flower oils are made in Malaysia and Indonesia in small amounts and can very rarely be found in the market places.

CULTIVATION

Turmeric is a true exotic from the tropical parts of the world. It needs light shade or partial shade and deeply dug richly composted moist soil to flourish. Water it three times a week, but only every 10 days in winter when it becomes dormant. Cover the area with raked leaves once the long leaves of the plant have died down. Do not cut the dried leaves away; leave them to disintegrate of their own accord.

Keep the area well mulched and water with a gentle soaking spray once spring arrives. Also add a layer of good moist compost over the area. Do not dig it in or you will destroy the tender rhizomes just below the surface; set a gentle soft spray over the area for about an hour or so. By mid- to late spring tightly curled leaf tips will appear like little spears through the soft soil and will quickly unfold.

Look out for 'turmeric tubers' or rhizomes at Asian stores and plant these in moist compost-filled bags until they sprout. Do not let them dry out but also do not overwater or the tubers will rot.

MEDICINAL USES

In ancient herbal texts and pharmacopoeias, turmeric flower oil has been recorded as a massage treatment for anorexia (or emaciation as it was then recorded), for liver congestion, arthritis and sore stiff swollen joints, for poor circulation, rheumatism and muscular aches and pains and to restore a feeling of wellbeing.

Interestingly, the distilled oil from the boiled, cleaned and sundried rhizome was used as an insect repellent, as an analgesic oil for arthritic joints, as a laxative massaged over the abdomen, as an antibacterial agent over infected wounds, and as a liver stimulant over a sluggish liver.

Today the precious distilled essential oil of both the flower and the root is only sold to qualified aromatherapists or masseuses. Its actions are analgesic, diuretic, laxative, anti-arthritic, anti-inflammatory and bactericidal and it is a rubefacient and stimulant.

In Ayurvedic medicine, turmeric roots and flowers were made into a liqueur with honey and alcohol as a treatment for respiratory infections and gastric ailments. Today tender leaves and crushed flowers are still used as a warm poultice over aching joints. In India, turmeric oil is used to treat several skin ailments, and it is an ingredient in Indian cosmetics and skin cleansers.

The Sri Lankans have made turmeric into a valuable crop that is processed into medications for indigestion and for liver and stomach complaints. They also boil a little piece of flower or root in milk with honey as a tea for colds and flu.

COSMETIC USES

Turmeric flower massage oil for dry skin

1 turmeric flower and its stem, finely sliced
1 cup almond oil
20 drops vitamin E oil
10 drops rose essential oil

Watch for a flower to appear at the base of the plant. When the flower is mature and fully open, cut it off with sharp secateurs and wash it carefully. Place it on a sterilised chopping board (sterilise the board with boiling water) and slice the flower and stem finely. Place the slices in a double boiler with the almond oil. Stir gently and continuously with a stainless steel spoon (a silver spoon was used in old recipes!) for 15 minutes, submerging the bracts under the oil. Remove from the heat and let the oil stand to cool (keep it covered). When it is lukewarm pour through a strainer, discard the bracts and pour the oil into a sterilised jar with a good screw top. Add the vitamin E oil and rose essential oil. Tighten the lid, shake well, and label the jar. Use as a massage oil over dry skin areas, especially on the neck and chest and over the cheekbones, avoiding the eye area.

NOTE: Always test a little of any massage oil on the inside of the wrist before using it. Allow it to saturate the area for at least 5–10 minutes. If there is any redness, wash off immediately with warm soapy water and avoid use.

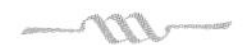

CULINARY USES

Turmeric flower stir-fry

SERVES 4–6

3 tablespoons olive oil
½ cup finely chopped onions
1 cup young fresh turmeric flowers and roots, finely chopped
1 cup lentils
1 cup rice

Heat the oil in a pan and stir-fry the onion, turmeric flowers and root. Cook the lentils and rice in separate pots, then drain and mix. Mix the stir-fry mixture into the lentils and rice. Serve with cold meats and salads or as an accompaniment to chicken stew.

Turmeric flower chicken salad

SERVES 6

This is a delicious cold salad for a hot day and is made festive by the flowers and the beautiful presentation.

1 butter lettuce
4 cups cubes of bread
Olive oil
Sea salt and pepper
2 cups chopped onions
2 cups pineapple pieces, cut into cubes
2 cups chopped green peppers
4 cups cubed, cooked chicken breasts, cooled
2 cups green rocket leaves, chopped
1 turmeric flower, chopped into bracts
1 cup fresh parsley, chopped

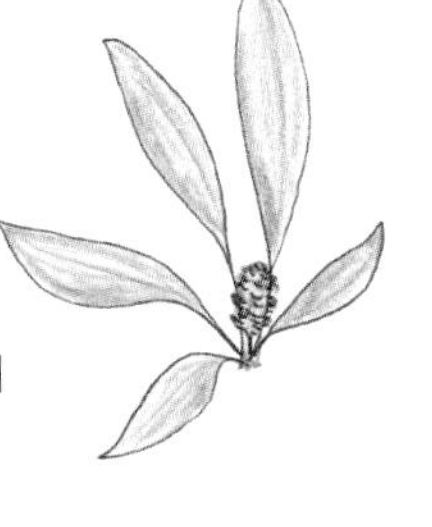

Place the lettuce leaves on a large platter. Sprinkle salt and pepper on the bread cubes and fry lightly in olive oil. Fry the chopped onions and mix with the bread cubes.

Mix the onions, bread, pineapple pieces, green pepper, chicken and rocket together and spoon into the lettuce leaves. Lightly fry the chopped turmeric flower in olive oil. Sprinkle the fried flowers and chopped parsley over the filled lettuce leaves. Pour the salad dressing over it and serve at once, decorated with other flowers, such as day lilies, gardenias and borage. Serve with naan bread.

Dressing
½ cup lemon juice
½ cup honey
1 teaspoon turmeric powder
½ cup olive oil
2 teaspoons Dijon mustard

Shake the ingredients together in a screw-top jar.

COOK'S NOTE

Peel turmeric root the way you would peel ginger, with a sharp knife on a chopping board, and remember that it will stain everything – including your hands! Once peeled, you can grate, chop, slice or grind it to a paste with other spices as an appetising addition to stews, lentil dishes, bean dishes and curries, the way you would use fresh ginger. It will add colour and flavour to the dish, and increase your gastric juices, thus making it an excellent therapeutic treatment for gastric disorders.

Violet

Viola odorata

The sweet violet is an ancient plant that has been grown and loved all over the world. It is native to Britain and widespread throughout Europe and Asia, and records of sweet violet from the first century AD in Turkey, Syria and Persia suggest that it is native to these areas as well. The violet was a favourite flower in ancient Greece and became the symbol of Athens. It was also the flower of Aphrodite, goddess of love, and the flower of her son Priapus, the god of gardens and male procreative power. Homer relates how the Greeks drank violet tea to 'temper their anger', and how they made crowns and garlands of violets to save them from drunkenness, and added the flowers to wine to give an extra bouquet.

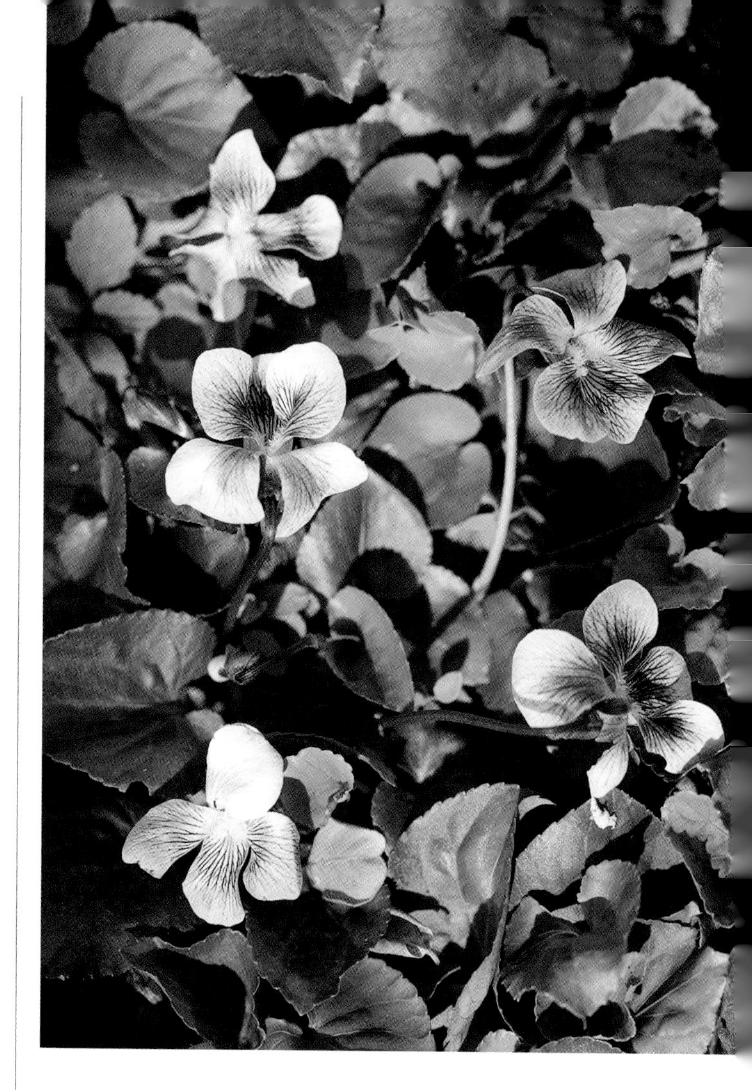

CULTIVATION

Growing violets is rewarding, as they demand little and give so much in return. They thrive in cool, partially shady positions in rich, well-composted, moist soil. The clump spreads by runners, which can be separated from the mother plant and planted elsewhere, 30 cm apart. Keep them moist and shaded until they establish. They reach a height of no more than 10 cm and so make a lovely border or groundcover. The flowers are at their best at the end of winter and early spring, and the more you pick the more they bloom. Water them deeply twice a week and give them an occasional spade of compost.

MEDICINAL USES

Violets were used medicinally by the ancient Greeks and Romans, and later in the 15th and 16th centuries violet syrup was prescribed for coughs, colds, pneumonia and bronchitis. A tea of violet flowers and leaves will soothe a headache and help one unwind after a demanding day, and it was popular as an after-dinner tea in the 18th and 19th centuries. Violets have a relaxing and calming effect on the nervous system and violet tea helps to expel mucous from the nose, chest and lungs, clear mouth and throat infections, open blocked sinuses and alleviate whooping cough and postnasal drip. To make violet tea, pour a cup of boiling water over ¼ cup flowers and leaves. Allow the tea to stand for five minutes, then strain and sweeten with honey if desired. A strong tea can also be used as a wash for eczema and rashes.

Violet flowers and leaves can be chewed to relieve a headache – chew five flowers or leaves initially and another three an hour later. Violets also have a gentle laxative effect, and bruised violet leaves make a soothing poultice for skin infections and inflammation. In Africa, violets are used as a cancer remedy, and crushed leaves are used as a poultice for skin cancer and growths. This remedy has also been used in Europe since the 12th century!

CAUTION: Do not confuse this violet with the African violet pot plant, which is poisonous.

Violet, brandy and honey cough remedy

1 cup violet flowers
1½ cups brandy
1 cup honey

Submerge the violet flowers in the brandy in a double boiler. Add the honey and simmer for 20 minutes, covered with a lid. Pour the liquid into a sterilised bottle with a well-fitting lid. Take one or two teaspoons with a cup of violet tea at least twice a day to ease coughs and clear a postnasal drip.

Violet syrup

This delightfully calming and soothing syrup is an old-fashioned remedy for winter coughs and colds. It is delicious in hot water to soothe a chill, and equally delicious in iced water to cool you down on a hot afternoon. It is also good over ice-cream and oat porridge.

4 cups violet flowers, cut off their stems
4 cups white sugar
1 cup runny honey
Juice of 4 lemons
1 tablespoon thin ginger slices
2 star anise
2 teaspoons finely grated lemon zest

Simmer the ingredients together gently in a saucepan with a tight-fitting lid for 15 minutes. Allow the mixture to cool, then strain and pour the syrup carefully into a sterilised glass bottle. Cork well and allow the syrup to stand for three or four days before using. Pour about two tablespoons into a glass of water, stir well, float a violet flower or two on top, and sip slowly. Feel the tension drain away!

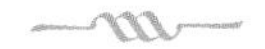

CULINARY USES

Chocolate and violet cheese cake

SERVES 6–8

Unforgettable and unusual, this dessert or tea-time treat is a no-fail favourite.

250 g ricotta cheese
250 g smooth cream cheese
6 tablespoons castor sugar
2 eggs, beaten until creamy
½ cup violet flowers, cut off their stems
2 tablespoons cocoa powder
½ teaspoon ground ginger
½ cup warm water
1 teaspoon vanilla essence

Beat the two cheeses together well. Whisk the sugar into the beaten eggs and fold into the cheese mixture with the violets. Dissolve the cocoa and ground ginger in the warm water and add to the mixture with the vanilla. Pour into an ovenproof glass dish and stand the dish in a pan of water. Bake at 180°C for 30–40 minutes or until the cheese cake is firm and lightly brown. Remove and cool. Serve covered with whipped cream and fresh and crystallised violets.

Violet liqueur

MAKES 750 ML

As a young mother I had a thriving little business making this delicious and unusual liqueur from rows of violets I grew in our farm garden. People came from far and wide to buy it and violet jam each spring. It is delicious served over ice-cream or cream cakes and it makes a wonderful gift for a special person.

750 ml good vodka
100 violet flowers, picked off their stalks
1 stick cinnamon
6 allspice berries (pimento)
250 g white sugar or 1½ cups honey
Small piece fresh ginger root

Mix the ingredients together and pour into a large, sterilised glass jar with a well-fitting lid. Shake it well and leave in a dark cupboard for two weeks, giving it a daily shake for a minute. Strain first through a muslin cloth, then through a coffee filter. Pour into an attractive glass decanter, add a few fresh violets, and serve just a little at a time in a tiny liqueur glass with a splash of thin fresh cream.

Sugared violets

MAKES 50–60 VIOLETS

This much-loved old-fashioned recipe is enjoying a resurgence of popularity. Enjoy them on their own as a delicacy or use to garnish cakes and desserts.

50–60 violets
2 egg whites
Castor sugar

Lightly whisk the egg whites. Holding each violet by its stalk, dip it into the egg whites and then into a small bowl of castor sugar, lightly sprinkling the violet with the sugar (use a small tea strainer) on every side. Lay each flower on a sheet of greaseproof paper in a warm room. Turn daily. When thoroughly dry, snip off the stem and pack the fragile sugared violets into a tin with layers of greaseproof paper.

Waterblommetjie

Aponogeton distachyos • **Cape pond weed**

The waterblommetjie, or Cape pond weed, is part of a small genus of monocotyledonous water plants and is one of South Africa's most famous edible plants. Its spectacular free-flowering, forked inflorescences in late winter through to midsummer look like masses of white blossoms scattered over the surface of the water, keeping bees and dragonflies busy. The entire plant is high in vitamins and minerals and the early Cape settlers were taught by the indigenous KhoiKhoi to use the plant both medicinally and as a nutritious food. Thanks to enterprising Boland farmers, fresh waterblommetjies are now available not only in other provinces, but all over the world. Because they are so tough and adaptable, they are hardy enough to grow in the warmer parts of Europe and the British Isles, where they are fast becoming a popular pond plant.

CULTIVATION

The tuberous rootstock settles easily into mud or a large compost-filled tub. The slender, oval leaves are about 2 cm long and often mottled with dark speckles, and the long flowering stalk with its forked cluster of succulent scales and white petals emerges from between the leaves.

Propagation is by division of the rootstock, as well as self-seeding seeds. Slice off a piece that has an eye on it and press it firmly into rich compost mixed with a little sand in a large plastic tub about 40 cm deep. Soak it well and when it has stood for an hour or two to settle, lower it slowly and gently into the pond, deep enough to cover it with about 30 cm of water. It is surprisingly tolerant, but it does need full sun and still water. It can remain there for 2–3 years, after which it needs to be lifted, the old soil and compost replaced and the waterblommetjie plants divided again. The plant easily seeds itself, and threadlike, baby seedlings can be found in the ponds, drifting, awaiting a suitable soft spot.

MEDICINAL USES

The KhoiKhoi used the high juice content of the stems to treat burns, sunburn and rashes. Children growing up in the Cape near dams filled with waterblommetjies used crushed stems and flowers and squeezed the juice onto minor cuts, grazes, insect stings, mosquito bites and itchy areas. Leaves and flowers were used as a poultice, first warmed and washed in hot water and then held in place with a crêpe bandage on sprains or strains, bruised or inflamed areas and rheumatic joints.

In cases of pimples and acne, crush the flower petals, apply to the area with a little stem juice, and leave to dry on the skin. Repeat whenever necessary.

Soothing waterblommetjie gel for burns and sunburn

Waterblommetjie stems, leaves and flowers

Crush and mash the stems, leaves and flowers to a pulp and spread this over the area to form a protective covering. Leave it on for as long as possible and repeat frequently until the pain and redness subside. The same method can be used for grazes, sores and infected bites. Often a washed arum lily leaf was cut and bound over the waterblommetjie pulp to hold it in place.

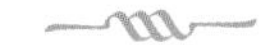

CULINARY USES

Traditional Cape waterblommetjie bredie

SERVES 6–8

A Cape farmer's wife taught me this recipe when I was 22 years old, and I have loved it ever since!

1 kg waterblommetjies
1–2 kg lamb loin chops, rib or leg trimmed of fat
¾ cup runny honey
3 large onions, chopped
2–4 tablespoons fat or cooking oil
2–3 cups water
1–2 cups fresh sorrel leaves or Cape sorrel (*Oxalis pes-caprae*)
Sea salt and black pepper to taste
4 large potatoes, peeled and diced
4 carrots, peeled and diced (optional)
1 cup chopped celery stalks (optional)
1 cup white wine

Soak the waterblommetjies in water to release any grit that may have lodged between the petals and scales of the flower. Brush the lamb with honey. Place the oil or fat in a heavy-based saucepan and brown the onions and then the lamb, turning them often. Add all the other ingredients except the wine, lower the heat, cover and simmer gently until the meat is tender. Stir every now and then, taking care not to break up the potatoes. Add more water if necessary, and add the wine last. Serve piping hot on a bed of rice.

Waterblommetjie stir-fry

SERVES 4

Quick and easy, this is an ideal supper dish.

2 cups waterblommetjies, well washed
2 cups chopped onion
½ cup extra-virgin olive oil
2 cups finely chopped lean bacon
2 cups thinly sliced brown mushrooms
2 cups grated potato
Juice of 1 lemon
½ cup parsley
Sea salt and black pepper to taste
1–3 teaspoons grated fresh ginger root
2 teaspoons fresh marjoram
Dash of balsamic vinegar

Soak the waterblommetjies to release any grit. Sauté the onions in the oil until they become transparent, then add the bacon and mushrooms. As they start to brown, add the potato, then the waterblommetjies and lemon juice. Add the parsley, seasoning, ginger, marjoram and lastly the balsamic vinegar. Serve piping hot with crusty brown bread or brown rice and a salad.

Waterblommetjie soup

SERVES 6–8

This soup varies from area to area in the Cape and all sorts of vegetables can be added.

2 large onions, finely chopped
3 tablespoons olive oil
2 cups finely chopped celery
2 cups finely grated carrots
6 cups waterblommetjies, well washed
3 cups peeled and diced tomatoes
4 potatoes, peeled and finely grated
½ cup honey
1 litre chicken stock
Juice of 1 lemon
Sea salt and black pepper to taste
1 litre milk

Sauté the onion in the oil. Add the celery and carrots and stir-fry until the onions are golden and the carrots and celery start to turn light brown. Add all the ingredients except for the milk. Simmer until tender, adding a little extra chicken stock if necessary. Stir every now and then. Add the milk just before serving and serve piping hot with crusty brown bread.

I once tasted a waterblommetjie dessert and found it simply delicious. I was told several cupfuls of boiled waterblommetjie were fried in a little butter, then laid in a dish. Mashed bananas with fresh grated ginger and grated guavas were mixed in, and it was topped with a dribble of honey and whipped cream. It is a great party dish, especially if sprinkled with grated dark chocolate and chopped pecan nuts.

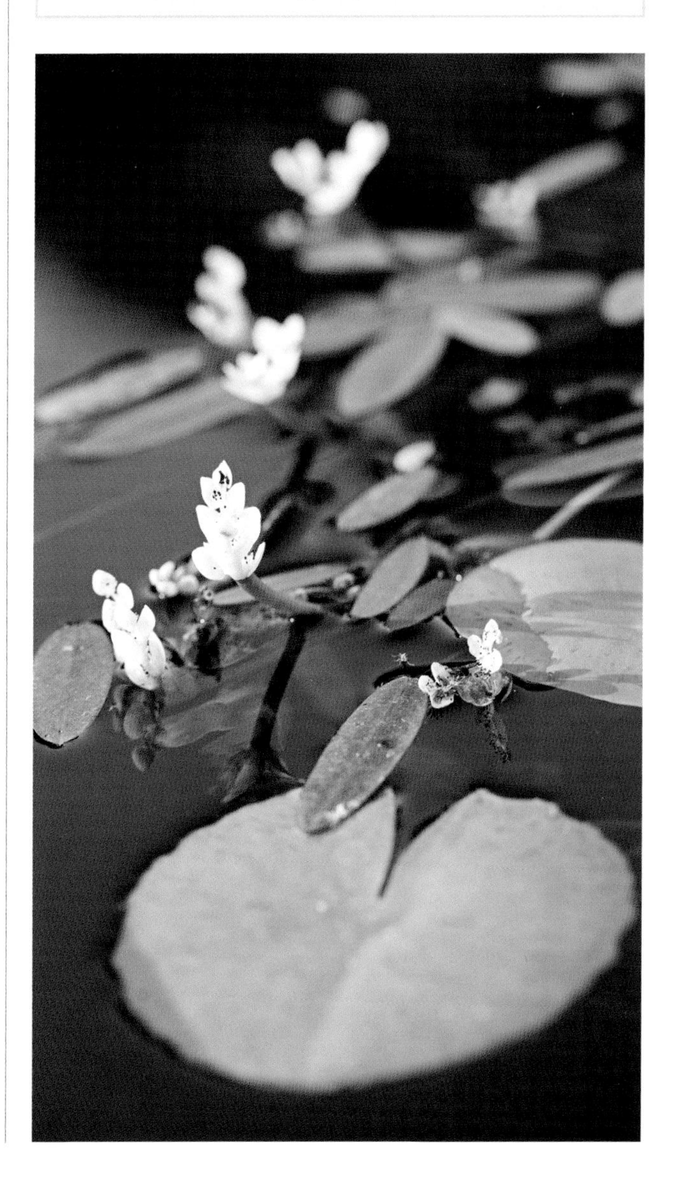

Water lily

Nymphaea alba

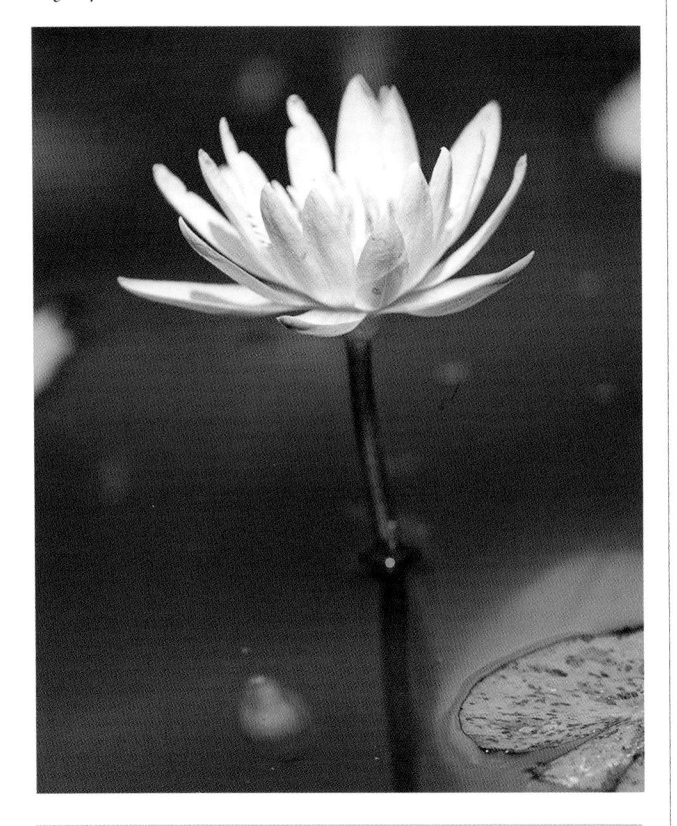

The exquisite water lily is an ancient healing plant and has often been woven into legend and fairy tales. Although most herbals describe the white water lily, *Nymphaea alba*, the other colours (red, pink, yellow and the exquisite blue *Nymphaea caerulea* from Africa) are to a large extent also used medicinally and in cooking. The scientific name *Nymphaea* is believed to have derived from the virgins in Greek mythology, with whom the water lily was associated. The plant was a symbol of purity, chastity and coldness, and in ancient Greece it was believed to have anti-aphrodisiac qualities. Modern research has actually proved the opposite to be true!

In the Middle Ages the water lily symbolised the priesthood, and young virgins had a water lily painted on their doors. The lily's manner of rising unblemished, pristine and beautiful from the mud and slime of lakes, still mountain pools and dry water courses after the first rains has symbolised regeneration since the earliest times, as well as immortality, resurrection and life after death.

CULTIVATION

Growing water lilies is very rewarding and can become an engrossing hobby. The rhizome should be planted firmly in a 30–40-cm plastic pot with a good mixture of compost and sand, covered with pebbles. Once the rhizome has been watered and soaked well, the pot can be lowered into a still-water pond in full sun. Divide the clump every three years by cutting off the new little rhizomes neatly, and replanting them in fresh soil and compost.

MEDICINAL USES

The white water lily was used medicinally by monks in Britain from the 12th century, and in the 17th century the herbalist Culpeper described it as being 'good for agues', and recorded that a 'syrup of flowers produces rest and settles the brain of frantic persons, the juice from the crushed petals and leaves takes away sunburn and freckles, from the face'. He also noted that the 'oil from the flowers cools hot tumours, eases pains and helps sores'. Interestingly, the leaves and petals have been proved to do just that!

Chemical compounds in the flower and rhizome have been found to have tranquillising properties, and the stem, juice and leaves are excellent for treating burns, sunburn, eczema and rashes and even freckles, as noted by Culpeper.

Water lily cream for rashes, sunburn and freckles

4 water lily flowers
1 small water lily stem with 4 leaves, chopped finely
1½ cups aqueous cream
2 tablespoons grapeseed oil
1 tablespoon castor oil
3 teaspoons vitamin E oil

In a double boiler, simmer all the ingredients, except the vitamin E oil, together for 30 minutes, stirring and pressing the water lily parts to extract all the juices. Strain using a fine strainer. Add the vitamin E oil and whisk in well. Pour into a sterilised jar with a well-fitting lid and label clearly. Apply lightly and gently to sunburned areas and to freckles and spots.

For freckles: Include Tissue Salt No. 5 Kali Sulph – 10 tablets dissolved in a tablespoon of water and added to the cream – and also suck two tablets three times a day to lighten freckles.

Water lily massage oil

For aches and pains in the back, shoulders, joints and feet. Exquisitely soothing, this old-fashioned remedy is still made today and remains a fabulous aromatic relaxing oil for pain and exhaustion.

4 water lilies
4 water lily leaves, finely chopped
1½ cups olive oil
½ teaspoon rose essential oil
2 teaspoons vitamin E oil
10 drops neroli essential oil

In a double boiler simmer the water lilies and leaves with the olive oil for 30 minutes. Stir frequently, pressing the petals and leaves well to release their moisture. Strain through a muslin cloth. Add the rose, vitamin E and neroli oils. Mix well and pour into a dark bottle with a screw-top lid and store in a dark cupboard. Before using the oil, warm it by standing the bottle in hot water.

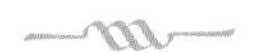

CULINARY USES

Water lily salad

SERVES 4

Multi-coloured water lily petals look festive in a salad and have a pleasant, crisp texture.

1 pineapple, thinly sliced
1 small cucumber, thinly sliced
1 apple, peeled and finely grated
1 medium-sized raw beetroot, finely grated
1 green pepper, diced
Petals from 2 or 3 water lilies,
  pulled from their calyxes
Juice of 2 oranges
2 tablespoons honey
2 tablespoons chopped pecan nuts
2 teaspoons crushed coriander seed
Sea salt and paprika to taste

Arrange the sliced pineapple and cucumber in a flat glass dish. Mix the grated apple and beetroot together and pile in the centre. Sprinkle with the diced green pepper. Arrange the water lily petals around the beetroot and apple to create a flower-like circle. Mix the orange juice with the honey and pour over the salad. Sprinkle with the pecan nuts, coriander, salt and paprika. Serve chilled.

> COOK'S NOTE
> **In the 16th and 17th centuries the French used the rootstock of both the white and yellow water lily for beer-making. Today the rhizomes are still eaten for their starch content in many parts of the world, and the flowers grace many a salad in gourmet cuisine the world over.**

Water lily and apple dessert

SERVES 4

6 apples peeled, cored and diced
1 cup water lily petals, pulled off their calyxes
¾ cup sugar
1½–2 cups water
½ cup sultanas
1 teaspoon ground cinnamon
½ teaspoon crushed cardamom seeds, removed from their pods
1 cup whipped cream
½ cup chopped pecan nuts

Quickly cook the apples and water lily petals with the sugar and water, sultanas, cinnamon and crushed cardamom. Mash well or put through a blender. Spoon into individual bowls, pile a mound of cream on top and sprinkle with the chopped pecan nuts. Spike with five or six fresh-water lily petals and dust with more cinnamon. Serve either warm or chilled.

Watermelon balls with ricotta and water lily

SERVES 6

This is such a pretty starter for a Christmas dinner that your guests cannot fail to be impressed! Choose three or four different-coloured water lilies and strip the petals off their calyxes.

Half a watermelon
250 g ricotta cheese
4 tablespoons finely chopped fresh mint
1½ cups fresh multi-coloured water lily petals
1½ cups litchi juice
2 teaspoons ground ginger or 2 tablespoons grated fresh ginger

Scoop out neat balls from the watermelon half and arrange them in individual glass dishes. Using a teaspoon, scoop out small amounts of ricotta cheese and drop them over the watermelon balls. Sprinkle with chopped mint. Tuck the water lily petals all around the edges, drizzle with a little litchi juice and finally sprinkle with ginger. Serve chilled.

Wild garlic

Tulbaghia violacea

Who would have thought that South Africa's wild garlic, a member of the *Tulbaghia* genus, would become so popular overseas? Today it is planted out in some of the most fascinating gardens in the world. It is known there as 'society garlic' and the leaves, stems and flowers are used to flavour and decorate dishes in expensive restaurants and hotels. It fetches high prices as a culinary herb in market places and as a plant in garden centres in the USA, Britain and Australia.

Wild garlic has been around forever in South African gardens, with the plants arranged close together in banks and borders to discourage snakes, as they dislike the smell of it. In South Africa it has been used for centuries as a food flavouring, and as a medication that lowers fevers and has antiseptic and expectorant properties. The leaves have also been used for centuries in the treatment of throat cancer.

A larger species, known as *T. simmleri*, has a larger, taller flowering head and is loved by landscapers. It is planted as a road island feature and along embankments where it flowers continuously, needing little attention.

Another rare favourite is the browny orange-flowered *T. alliacea*, which was a respected fever herb in the Cape and a long-recorded medication for fits, paralysis and joint aches. It was also used as a purgative. Decades ago a Zulu farmworker showed me how to make a delicious and traditional Zulu relish to keep all sorts of health problems at bay (see recipe on facing page).

In 2009, quite by chance, I came across a new cultivated variety, *T. simmleri* 'Alba'. It has pure white flowers, and its upright compact appearance lends itself to path borders, parterre plantings, and mandala designs with white stones.

The genus *Tulbaghia* is named after Ryk Tulbagh (1699–1771), who was Governor of the Cape of Good Hope. In his home town, Tulbagh, the plantings of tulbaghia were breathtaking when I was a child, lining streets, walkways and garden paths.

CULTIVATION

Few plants are as undemanding and rewarding to grow as wild garlic! Small clumps of juicy stems can be levered off the side of the main clump, and should be planted in well-composted soil, 30 cm apart in full sun. This species will survive in heat, drought and bitter cold.

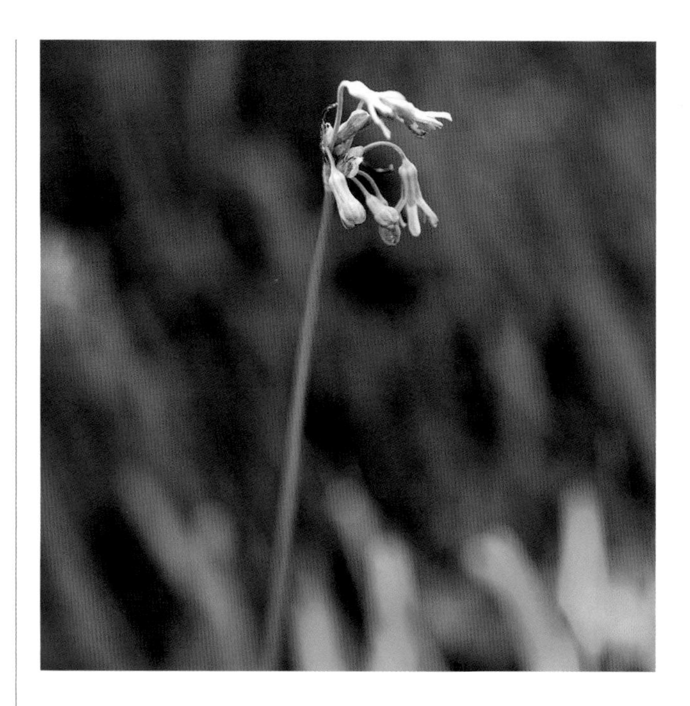

MEDICINAL USES

Wild garlic leaves, flowers and bulblets are all used fresh, either raw in salads or made into a tea with lemon juice. Known as *isihaqa* in Zulu, wild garlic is taken traditionally as a crushed pulp, or boiled in water with salt and taken as a gruel or thin soup three times a day for fever, colds, coughs, sore throats, asthma and tuberculosis. In cases of asthma and tuberculosis, chopped leaves and bulblets can also be eaten with every meal, and wild garlic tea can be taken between meals to ease chest tightness and coughing. To make the tea, pour a cup of boiling water over ¼ cup fresh chopped leaves, stems and flowers. Let the tea stand for five minutes, strain, add a squeeze of lemon juice and sip slowly. This tea is also given for fits, with a little sipped every hour.

Poultices of crushed wild garlic leaves and flowering stems are still used in country districts to treat rheumatism, paralysis and joint aches, and some tribes use the fresh bulblets boiled in water as an enema. Wild garlic is rich in antiseptic properties and it is thought to have antifungal and antibacterial properties like real garlic.

Bathing with wild garlic extract is an age-old treatment for aching rheumatism – simply soaking in a bath of wild garlic extract is said to be good for all the above ailments! The garlic smell is not as pungent as real garlic, I am told, and it quickly disappears.

Wild garlic leaves have long been used to treat cancer of the oesophagus, which makes me wonder whether its sulphur-containing substance, alliin, could be even more valuable than we know.

NOTE: Another non-edible wild garlic is available in mauve and rare white, known as 'Winter Bride'. It is lily-scented, not garlic-scented, and flowers in winter. These flowers are not edible!

Wild garlic bath infusion

Use this for rheumatic aches, stiff joints, aching back and muscle spasm.

Wild garlic flowers and leaves
Water to cover

Fill a big pot with wild garlic, cover with water, and simmer for 20 minutes. Allow the mixture to cool, strain and add to the bathwater.

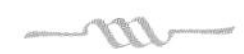

CULINARY USES

Zulu wild garlic relish

SERVES 4–6

½ cup olive oil
2 cups chopped onions
2 cups chopped wild garlic bulblets, well cleaned
Crushed coarse sea salt
2 cups chopped fresh wild garlic leaves
1 cup wild garlic flowers
¾ cup mild chopped chillies
Juice of 1 lemon, or ½ cup vinegar
1 cup sultanas, soaked in warm water until plump
1 tablespoon crushed coriander seeds (optional)
2 teaspoons crushed cardamom pods (optional)
1 tablespoon finely grated ginger (optional)
2 tablespoons honey (optional)

Heat the oil in a heavy-bottomed pot and fry the onions, then gradually add the chopped wild garlic bulblets. Stir-fry until lightly browned, adding a little more oil if needed, and a light sprinkling of crushed coarse sea salt. Add the garlic leaves and flowers (and finely chopped stems of the flowers too if desired), and stir-fry. Once the mixture starts to brown, add about ¾ cup mild chopped chillies (for those who like it hot, a few finely chopped hot chillies can also go in). Add the lemon juice or vinegar, stir-frying all the time. This was how the Zulu recipe ended.

Add the soaked sultanas and stir-fry. Check for taste, add a little water if needed, and add the coriander, cardamom, ginger and honey. Mix everything together and serve with fish or sausages or spread on croissants with cheese.

COOK'S NOTE

'Zulu relish' has become so popular over the years that visiting chefs and hotel schools have started to grow rows of wild garlic for its taste and rarity.

Wild garlic salad

SERVES 4–6

This salad can become a masterpiece! Add whatever is in season and be adventurous.

1 butter lettuce, broken up into separate leaves
1½ cups chopped celery stalks and leaves
1 cup chopped green pepper
1 cup chopped wild garlic bulblets and leaves
1–2 cups cubed peeled cucumber pieces
2 cups cubed avocado, with a squeeze of fresh lemon juice over it
2 cups cubed pineapple pieces
½ cup chopped parsley
2 cups fresh rocket leaves
½ cup wild garlic flowers

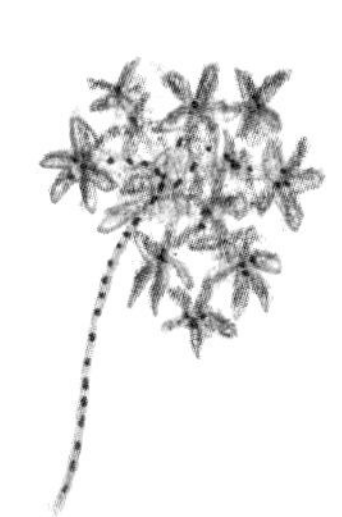

Dressing
½ cup olive oil
½ cup honey
½ cup lemon juice
1 teaspoon mustard powder

Build up the salad layer by layer so as not to crush anything. Mix the dressing ingredients in a glass jar. As you go, add a squeeze of fresh lemon juice and a drizzle of the dressing between each layer. Decorate with wild garlic flowers. Serve with cold chicken and crusty home-baked bread.

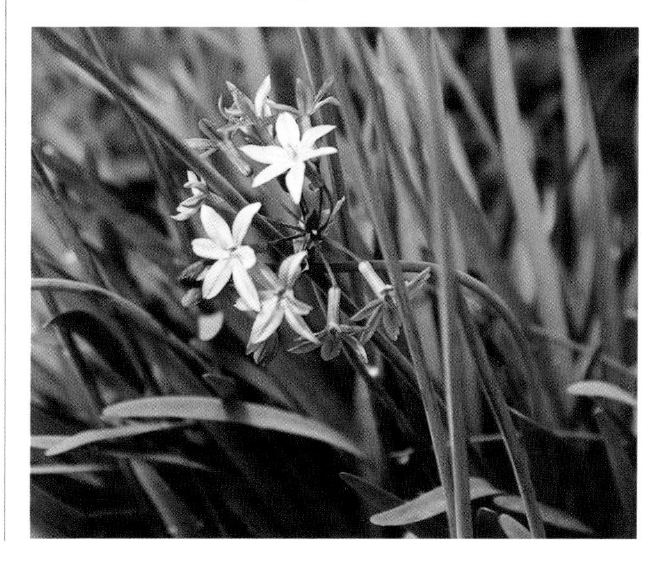

Winter savory

Satureja montana

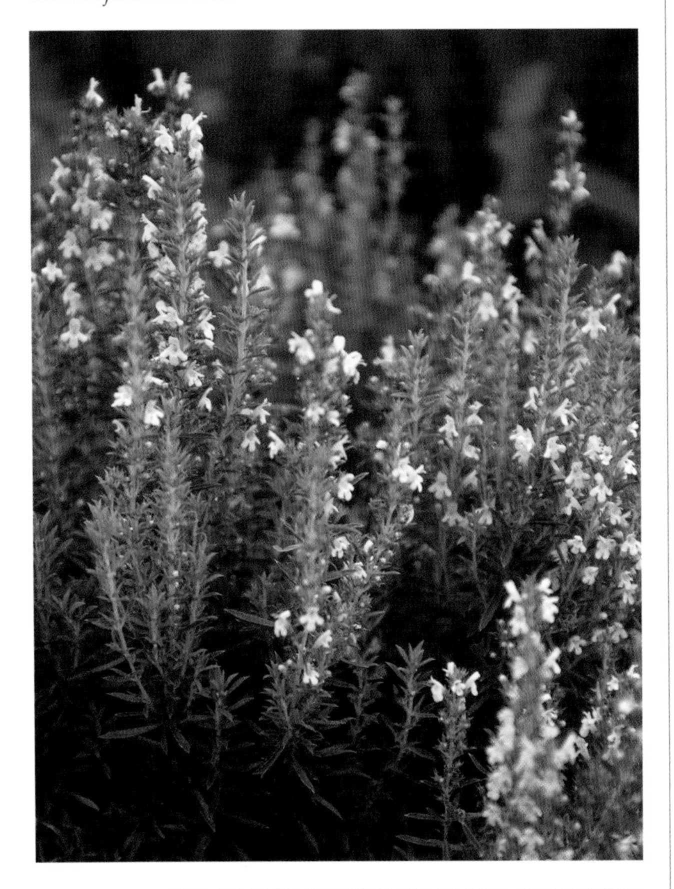

Winter savory is an exceptionally pretty herb, forming a bright green, perennial groundcover about 14 cm in height, with a charming cushion-like spread. It makes an ideal path edging, container plant and focal point for hanging baskets. In spring and early summer it is covered with sprays of tiny white flowers that set bees humming and send butterflies into a frenzy of delight. The warm sun releases the plant's strong oils; should you step on it, you will be instantly refreshed by the scent of the pungent oils containing precious components like thymol and linalool.

CULTIVATION

Plant rooted cuttings 50 cm apart in full sun in well-composted, well-dug soil. Winter savory is a most successful companion plant to tomatoes and keeps aphids and whitefly at bay.

MEDICINAL USES

Native to southern Europe and North Africa, winter savory has been used since ancient times to aid and stimulate digestion and to ease colic, flatulence and a feeling of fullness. Herbals from the Middle Ages through to the 18th century show that the monks used it with honey to make a strong syrup for digestive problems as well as for coughs, colds and chest ailments, and kept it at hand as a powerful remedy for these ailments. Modern science has proved those medieval herbalists to be correct and in recent years doctors at Montpellier Hospital in France ran a series of tests using winter savory and lucerne (alfalfa) as a treatment for coughs, bronchitis, pneumonia, chest infections, asthmatic wheezing and persistent sore throats, and found winter savory to be a superb antiseptic for clearing infection, as well as a powerful antibacterial agent.

Modern research has also found that the essential oil extracted from winter savory is beneficial in treating *Candida* overgrowth, the fungus that causes thrush, as well as other fungal infections. A standard tea of winter savory drunk twice daily (not during pregnancy) also greatly relieves the condition. To make the tea, pour a cup of boiling water over half a cup of fresh flowering tops. Leave the tea to stand for five minutes, then strain, sweeten with honey, and sip slowly.

Interestingly, the classical Greek physicians Galen and Dioscorides used winter savory with thyme and classified them as heating and drying medicines, prescribing them for clearing mucous from the chest and sinuses. They also considered winter savory to have aphrodisiac qualities, following on from the ancient Egyptians who used winter savory in love potions.

Winter savory tea for respiratory ailments

This powerful tea will help to loosen a cough and clear the nose and chest naturally.

½ cup winter savory fresh flowering tops
¼ cup fresh lucerne leaves and flowers
Honey
Lemon juice

Pour a cup of boiling water over the winter savory and lucerne. Allow the tea to infuse for five minutes, then sweeten with honey to taste, and add a squeeze of lemon juice. Take a cup three times a day during a cold or bronchitis.

CULINARY USES

Butter beans and winter savory

SERVES 6

This is the best bean dish I make – it is tasty, rich in protein and fibre, and keeps well in the fridge. The winter savoury greatly reduces indigestion and flatulence from the beans.

400 g large white butter beans
2 sprigs winter savory
2 cups chopped onions
½ cup good olive oil
2 cups chopped celery
1 cup honey
½ cup winter savory flowering sprigs, stripped off their stalks
Sea salt and black pepper to taste
Juice of 2 lemons
½ cup balsamic vinegar
1 cup tomato paste
Parsley

Soak the beans and winter savory in warm water overnight. The next morning discard the water and rinse the beans. Bring to the boil (use enough cold water to cover them) and tuck in two or three winter savory sprigs. When the beans are tender, drain, discard the sprigs and return the beans to the pot to keep warm. In a large pan, fry the onions in the olive oil until golden brown, add the celery and then stir-fry all the remaining ingredients, including the beans. Add a little water to prevent burning, stir frequently, and simmer for 10 minutes. Serve piping hot sprinkled with parsley and a few winter savory flowers pulled from their calyxes. This is a sustaining meal when served with brown bread and a green salad.

Winter savory and cabbage mealie soup

SERVES 6–8

Use fresh mealies in season and 'samp' in winter to make this hearty, warming and delicious soup.

½ cup olive oil
4 finely chopped onions
2 cups chopped brown mushrooms
2 cups finely chopped celery
4 cups green outer cabbage leaves, finely shredded
2 tablespoons winter savory flowering sprigs
2 cups 'samp' or 'stampmielies', soaked for at least 3 hours in warm water or 4 cups green mealies cooked and cut off their cobs
Juice of 2 lemons
2 teaspoons crushed coriander seed
2 tablespoons chopped parsley
2 litres good strong chicken stock
Sea salt and black pepper to taste

Pour the oil into a large heavy pot and fry the onions until golden brown. Add the mushrooms and fry until golden, then add the celery and finally the cabbage and winter savory sprigs. Stir-fry well. Add all the other ingredients and simmer gently for about 40 minutes. Serve the soup in individual bowls and sprinkle a little chopped parsley and lots of little winter savory flowers pulled from their calyxes over the top. Serve with brown bread rolls.

Winter savory sauce for pasta

SERVES 4–6

This simple cheese sauce is easy to make and can be served on top of toast, pasta, cauliflower and cabbage.

1 litre milk
3 tablespoons flour, whisked into 2 eggs
Sea salt, black pepper and paprika to taste
3 teaspoons mustard powder
1 tablespoon winter savory flowers and a few tiny leaves
2 cups finely grated cheddar cheese
1 cup ricotta or smooth cream cheese

Simmer the milk in a heavy saucepan, then add the flour and egg mixture, whisking all the time. Add the sea salt, black pepper, paprika and mustard powder and the winter savory. As the sauce starts to thicken, turn down the heat and briskly stir in the cheddar cheese and the ricotta or cream cheese. If it gets too thick, add a little milk and stir to a smooth paste-like consistency. Pour immediately over the hot pasta and dust with more paprika or serve over hot buttered toast.

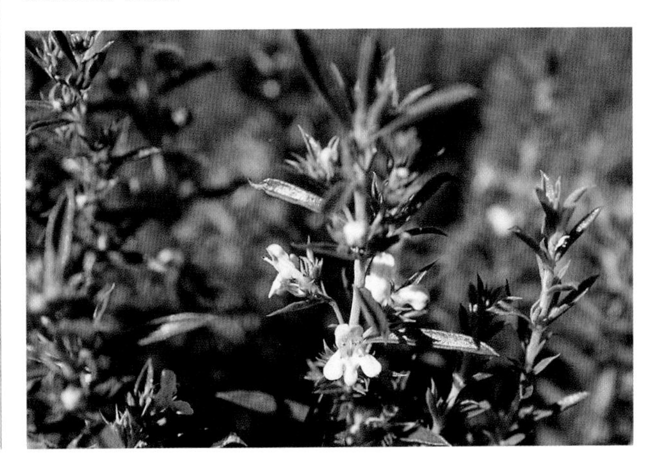

Wisteria

Wisteria sinensis

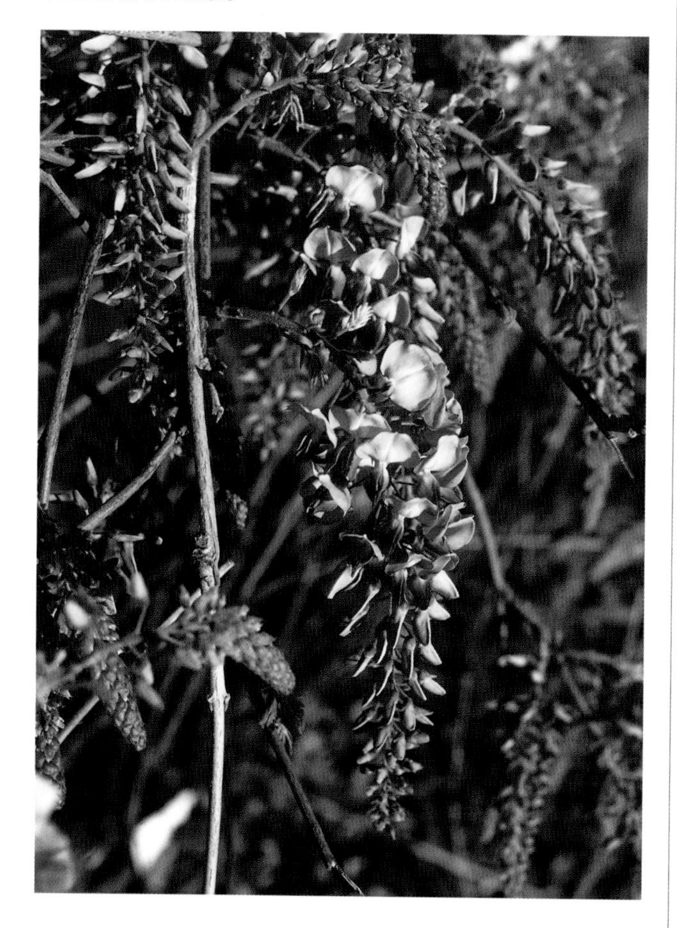

This elegant vine with its beautiful pendulous, fragrant flowers in spring has been a popular garden subject in western countries for a few hundred years. It originated in China, but in 1818 it was named after an American physician and philosopher, Casper Wistar, professor of anatomy at the University of Pennsylvania. It had been cultivated in Britain and then in Switzerland for about 100 years before that. In America it was commonly known as the 'Carolina kidney bean'. *Wisteria floribunda* is a smaller, less showy wisteria from Japan, which is also edible, but it is *W. sinensis* that is commonly found in gardens today.

To the Japanese and Chinese, wisteria is a symbol of friendship and unity within the family, and most Japanese homes have at least one plant in the garden, even in tiny gardens. In the past, Japanese emperors and their retinues took flowering wisteria bonsais on their travels to give to their hosts as a sign of goodwill and friendship.

CULTIVATION

Wisteria is a vigorous deciduous climber, and the sprawling, twisting vine may be trained into a standard, espaliered across a wall, or allowed to sprawl with glorious abandon over trellises, pergolas and down banks. It does need some restraining, however, as it becomes large and powerful as it ages, but its ability to adapt to temperature extremes and its vigorous speed of growth has made it a favourite the world over.

To grow wisteria it is important to obtain a grafted specimen from a nursery, as roots and cuttings could result in pale or small flowers. The plant requires a large, deep, richly composted hole and a position in full sun. Train the tendrils onto supports or twist them around sticks that can be removed once the stems are thick and mature. The buds form in midwinter on the attractive bare, grey branches. Give the vine a good bucket or two of rich compost and a deep weekly watering, which will ensure a mass of blooms. The flowers are followed by compound leaves, which provide deep, dense shade all through the summer.

MEDICINAL USES

Wisteria flowers contain a sweet, heady nectar, and bees make an extraordinary honey from wisteria that was used in Europe in the 16th and 17th centuries to alleviate coughs and dry, sore throats. The honey mixed with crushed wisteria blossoms in spring was considered to be an energising, resistance-building tonic. The spring flowers were also used medicinally in a poultice to relieve bruises and throbbing varicose veins, and bottles of fresh flowers and buds were topped up with wine vinegar, corked and stored in a dark place for use when fresh flowers were not available. Cloths soaked in this mixture were applied to ease several conditions, including pimples and infected spots.

Wisteria and apple cider vinegar for acne, pimples and infected skin spots

1 bottle apple cider vinegar
12 wisteria flowering sprays

Almost fill a glass bottle with apple cider vinegar. Push six flowering sprays into the bottle and top up with vinegar until the bottle is full. Cork the bottle firmly and place in the sun, turning and shaking it daily. After 10 days, strain, discarding the flowers. Return the vinegar to the bottle and press in the remaining flowers. Leave it in the sun for 10 days, turning and shaking it daily. Finally, strain and return the vinegar to the bottle, and label. Use the vinegar as a rinse after washing the face – simply add a dash to the rinsing water. It can also be dabbed directly onto spots using a cotton wool pad.

CULINARY USES

Wisteria fritters

SERVES 4–6

These fritters have an oriental touch and are particularly beautiful served under a bower of wisteria for a spring luncheon.

8 flowering wisteria sprays

Batter
2 eggs
¾ cup sugar
1½ cups flour
2–3 cups water
Few drops vanilla essence
1 cup sunflower oil

Whisk the eggs and sugar together. Add the flour and water alternately, and the vanilla essence. Beat to a thin batter, adding more water if necessary. Heat the oil in a large pan. Hold the flowering sprays by their stalks and dip them one by one gently into the batter. Lower them into the hot oil, being careful not to splash, and fry for about two minutes or until golden. Drain on crumpled kitchen paper towel, snip off the stems and serve warm with whipped cream and a dusting of icing sugar.

Wisteria and watercress spring salad

SERVES 4

Fresh salads are very appealing in spring, and this one especially so. The tonic effects of the fresh watercress make this an excellent health salad too.

4 cups watercress sprigs
2 cups thinly sliced cucumber
2 large, sweet oranges
2 cups nasturtium flowers and a few leaves
1 cup diced feta cheese
½ cup chopped parsley
½ cup chopped celery leaves
1 cup wisteria flowers, pulled off their stems

Dressing
½ cup balsamic vinegar
2 teaspoons ground coriander
2 tablespoons honey
1 teaspoon mustard powder

Arrange the watercress and cucumber in a salad bowl. Peel each orange segment and place on top of the watercress and cucumber, along with the nasturtiums, feta, parsley and celery. Sprinkle with wisteria flowers. Put the dressing ingredients into a jar, seal and shake. Pour the dressing over the salad just before serving.

Wisteria country borscht

SERVES 6

This rich red, refreshing beetroot soup is perfect for a warm spring luncheon and the sweetness of the wisteria makes it special. You can serve it hot without the yoghurt and with a spoon of sour cream instead, but borscht is traditionally served chilled.

1 large onion, finely chopped
1 large leek, thinly sliced
A little olive oil
1 large carrot, finely grated
2 sticks celery, finely chopped
6 medium-sized raw beetroot, peeled and grated
2 litres good stock
Sea salt and coarsely ground black pepper
Juice of 2 lemons
½ cup good red wine
1 tablespoon honey
1 cup wisteria flowers, stems removed
250 ml plain Bulgarian yoghurt
½ cup finely chopped parsley

Sauté the onion and leek in the oil. Add the carrot and celery and stir-fry until they start to brown lightly. Add all the other ingredients except the wisteria flowers, yoghurt and parsley. Simmer for about 40 minutes with the lid on until all the vegetables are tender. At this point you can strain and discard the vegetables and serve a clear soup, or put it through a liquidiser. Chill the soup if desired and serve with a spoonful or two of yoghurt in each bowl, a grinding of black pepper and a sprinkling of parsley and wisteria flowers.

Yarrow

Achillea millefolium

Often known as 'soldier's wound wort', yarrow is a remarkable ancient herb commonly found in waste areas. It originated in Europe, and as its common name implies, it has traditionally been used to staunch bleeding. The ancient Greeks used it to heal wounds, and during the Trojan War Achilles is said to have healed the wounds of his warriors by applying crushed yarrow leaves, hence the genus name *Achillea*. The crusaders took two herbs with them on their crusades: borage to give them courage and yarrow to heal wounds.

Yarrow has always been associated with magic. Yarrow stalks stripped of their leaves and small branches have been used since the time of the druids in the centuries before Christ to foretell the future and divine the weather.

CULTIVATION

Growing yarrow is easy and it is often grown in the garden for its showy sprays of tiny pink and white flowers, which are long-lasting in the vase. Clumps should be planted 50 cm apart in a sunny spot and will thrive in any type of soil. With compost and a twice-weekly watering, the flowering heads will reach 50 cm in height from the perennial clump of fine feathery leaves. Yarrow is an excellent plant doctor, and planted next to rare or ailing plants, it will give them a health boost and keep aphids away. Just a handful of leaves will speed the decomposition of a barrow-load of undecayed compost.

MEDICINAL USES

Many hybrids of yarrow are grown for their showiness in the garden, but these are neither edible nor do they have medicinal properties. Only *Achillea millefolium* is edible, but it should not be taken for long periods as the build-up can cause skin irritation and headaches. It should not be taken by pregnant women.

Through the centuries yarrow has been used in cosmetics as it is an exceptional astringent. Yarrow and chamomile are the only two herbs that contain the rare and exquisite azulene, an organic compound that is used for its blue colour and healing properties. Yarrow has a tonic action; it brings down fever, promotes sweating, relaxes the peripheral blood vessels, and eases premenstrual tension and bloated painful menstruation, restoring it to normal. It is a good anti-inflammatory, antispasmodic and anti-allergenic.

In 1597 the herbalist John Gerard noted that chewing the fresh green leaves was a good remedy for toothache, and modern medical science continues to prove these ancient remedies substantially correct and effective. A crushed leaf will stop a nose bleed (place the leaf in the affected nostril), and a poultice of leaves will stop a cut or wound from bleeding.

Yarrow flower and borage healing cream

Apply this cream to burns, scratches, grazes, bruises and stiff, sore muscles.

1 cup yarrow flowers and buds
1 cup borage flowers and buds
½ cup calendula petals
2 cups aqueous cream
1 tablespoon of almond oil
2 teaspoons vitamin E oil

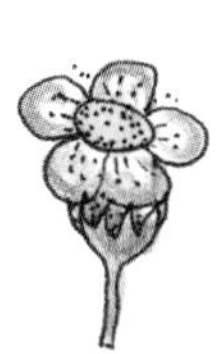

In a double boiler, simmer the flower parts, aqueous cream and almond oil for 30 minutes, pressing and mixing everything thoroughly. Strain, add the vitamin E oil and mix well. Spoon into sterilised glass jars with well-fitting lids and label. Use lavishly.

CULINARY USES

Yarrow kedgeree

SERVES 4–6

Tasty and unusual, this dish will become a family favourite.

2 cups cooked brown rice
675 g hake fillets
Sea salt and black pepper
A few lemon slices
1 bay leaf
2 onions, thinly sliced
2 tablespoons butter
3–4 teaspoons young yarrow flowers and buds, stripped off their stems
2 teaspoons mild curry powder
2 teaspoons turmeric
1½ cups good strong vegetable stock
½ cup sultanas soaked in hot water for 2 hours

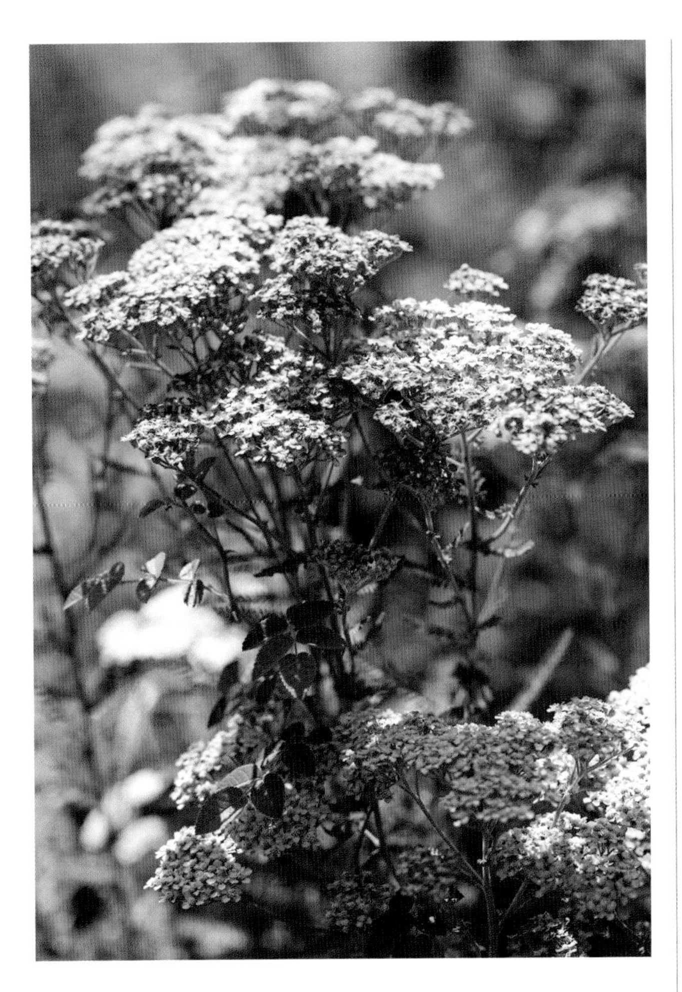

Juice of 1 lemon
½ cup chopped almonds
Finely chopped parsley

Boil the brown rice for about 40 minutes until cooked. Poach the fish in water with salt and pepper, the lemon slices and bay leaf for about 10–15 minutes or until cooked. Drain well and flake the fish. Fry the onions in the butter until they start to brown, add the yarrow flowers, and stir-fry. Add the curry powder, then the turmeric, cooked rice, stock, sultanas and lemon juice. Add the flaked fish and fork lightly until it is well mixed. Taste for seasoning. Turn into a serving dish and sprinkle with the chopped almonds and finely chopped parsley. Serve hot.

COOK'S NOTE

Yarrow has long been used by the Chinese and Europeans for culinary purposes. Very young yarrow flowers, buds and leaves have a pungent taste that is particularly good with curries and stir-fries.

Yarrow stir-fry

SERVES 4

This is a quick-and-easy supper dish.

Olive oil
2½ cups very thinly sliced lean beef
2 onions, peeled and chopped
2 potatoes, peeled and coarsely grated
½ cup young yarrow flowers and buds, stripped off their stems
1 green pepper, chopped
2 large tomatoes, peeled and sliced
2 tablespoons honey
Sea salt and coarsely ground black pepper
Juice of 1 lemon
1 teaspoon good curry powder

Heat the olive oil in a large wok or pan and lightly brown the thin strips of meat. Add the onions and stir-fry until golden. Add the potatoes and stir-fry until cooked and browned. Toss in the flowers and stir-fry for a few seconds before adding the remaining ingredients. Serve piping hot with a salad.

Yarrow and pumpkin bredie

SERVES 6

This old-fashioned, hearty pumpkin stew needs a long cooking time for the flavours to combine.

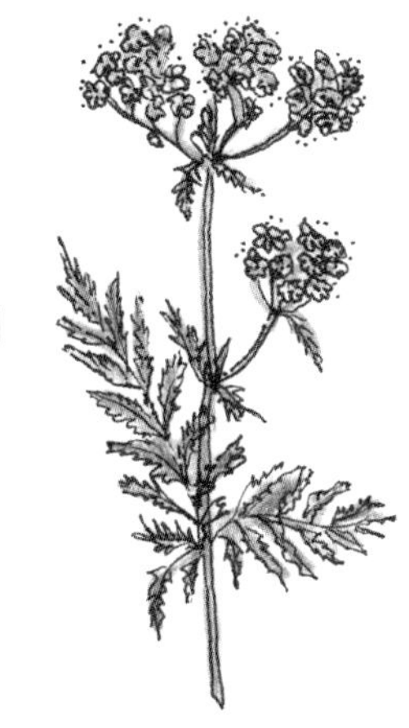

1 kg lean stewing lamb
2–3 tablespoons sunflower oil
2 large onions, sliced
2 teaspoons curry powder
2 tablespoons grated fresh ginger
2–3 tablespoons young yarrow flowers and buds stripped off their stems
3 cups good vegetable stock or water
500 g potatoes, peeled and sliced
1½ kg pumpkin, peeled and diced
2 teaspoons nutmeg
Sea salt and black pepper to taste
Juice of 1 lemon

Brown the lamb in a little oil in a heavy-based cast iron pot. Add the onions and sauté until golden. Add the curry, ginger and yarrow flowers and stir-fry until golden. Add all the remaining ingredients and cover the pot. Simmer gently for about 1½ hours or until very tender and full of flavour. Add more stock or water if necessary during the cooking time, and give the bredie a good stir every now and then to prevent sticking and burning. Serve with rice or couscous.

Yucca

Yucca gloriosa

The strange yet appealing yucca is native to the USA, Mexico and the West Indies and is part of the Agavaceae family, many species of which have tough, sword-like leaves. The leaves of the yucca are spiky, stiff and often razor-sharp, rising from the ground or from short woody trunks. In midsummer, huge panicles of exquisite lily-like, white flowers appear, in complete contrast to the leaves, often up to a metre long. These are so long-lasting and spectacular in appearance, rich and creamy in texture, and heady in fragrance, that yuccas have long been cultivated in gardens and parks around the world as a feature plant.

The yuccas have a remarkable method of pollination. About an hour after dark on a summer evening, they emit a beautiful fragrance that attracts the yucca moth. As the moth darts from flower to flower seeking the fragrance, it burrows against the crown of elongated stamens in the heart of the flower and so pollinates the flowers, which then produce juicy round seeds.

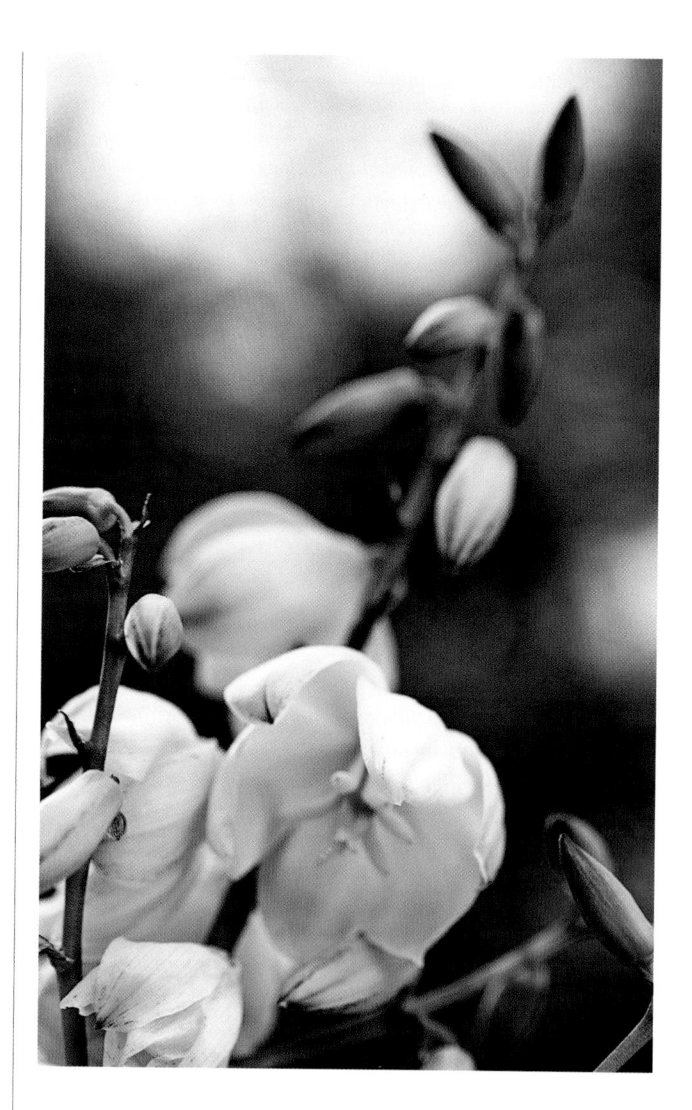

CULTIVATION

Yuccas make bold garden sculptures and are perfect for landscaping, not only because of their unusual appearance, but because they are so resilient to extremes of weather, including long periods of drought. Several yucca species are used in landscaping. Some are smaller in size, but all are edible. *Yucca filamentosa*, or Adam's needle, is virtually stemless, with long, curly threads along the edges of the spiky leaves. The species most often planted is *Y. gloriosa*, or Spanish dagger.

Plant yuccas in full sun, with two or three bucketfuls of compost. They adapt quickly to any conditions and withstand even poor soil, but with compost and a deep weekly watering they will produce several towering flowering heads during summer.

MEDICINAL USES

The seeds, trunk and roots of the yucca contain saponins, and have been used by American Indians for centuries to make a wound wash and lotion for rashes, scrapes and burns. The roots and fruits were also used for washing hair, treating scalp problems such as hair loss, and soothing insect bites and itchy, raw, sore skin. Crushed and pounded flower petals have been used to heal sore fingers and cracked skin in harsh, dry climates, and the petals provide relief when packed around cracked heels and over grazes and bruises. Stems and roots boiled in water make a good soapy brew, which was used to wash clothes.

Soothing yucca wound wash

Use this for rashes, scrapes and burns, as well as acne, problem skin and sunburn.

2 cups yucca flowers or mature seeds
3 litres water

Gently boil the flowers or seeds in the water for 20 minutes, with the lid on. Allow the mixture to cool. Strain out the flowers or seeds and wash or dab the lotion over affected areas. The liquid can also be poured into a spritz spray bottle and sprayed frequently on the affected area.

CULINARY USES

Yucca flower soup

SERVES 4

Serve as a soup dusted with paprika, or pour over a bowl of rice and eat as a main course like the Mexicans do, with garlic and chillies added.

1 cup split peas
½ cup olive oil
2 cups chopped onions
3 cups yucca petals
1 cup chopped green pepper
4–6 large tomatoes, skinned and chopped
3 tablespoons brown sugar
Sea salt and black pepper to taste
Juice of 1 lemon
Paprika to taste
2 litres good stock

Soak the split peas in boiling water for an hour. Pour the olive oil into a heavy-bottomed pot and fry the onions until golden. Add the yucca petals and green pepper and stir-fry until they start to brown. Add all the remaining ingredients, including the split peas, and simmer gently for about five minutes.

Stuffed yucca flowers

SERVES 6

Fish or chicken can be used instead of the mince in this exotic and decorative party dish.

4 cups cooked rice
2 cups chopped onions
½ cup olive oil
500 g lean topside mince
1 cup grated carrots
2 cups skinned, chopped tomatoes
2 teaspoons spicy curry powder
Sea salt and black pepper to taste
Juice of 1 lemon
1 teaspoon red hot chilli (optional)
1 teaspoon chopped garlic (optional)
24 fully open yucca flowers
1 tablespoon brown sugar
½ cup good fruit chutney

Cook the rice. Sauté the onions in the olive oil until golden. Add the minced meat and fry until brown. Add the carrots, one cup of tomatoes, curry powder, salt, pepper and lemon juice, and the chilli and garlic if desired. Add a little water and cook until full of flavour and well done. Drain the meat mixture over a pot and catch all the juices. Spoon the meat into the yucca flowers and place them on a bed of cooked rice in a serving dish. Add the extra cup of tomatoes to the meat juices in the pan, add the brown sugar and chutney, and cook for about five minutes, stirring constantly. Adjust the seasoning and pour the piping hot sauce over the stuffed flowers. Serve hot with a salad.

> COOK'S NOTE
> **The yucca is extremely easy to grow and offers such beauty and abundance in its flowering spike that we should learn from the West Indians and cook it as they do. It is superb chopped into stir-fries, casseroles, soups and pickles.**

Yucca and apple crumble

SERVES 6

4–6 apples, peeled, cored and sliced
½ cup sultanas
2 cups yucca petals, broken off the centre
1 cup brown sugar
1 cup water
½ cup butter
1 cup oats
½ cup sesame seeds
1 teaspoon cinnamon
½ cup honey

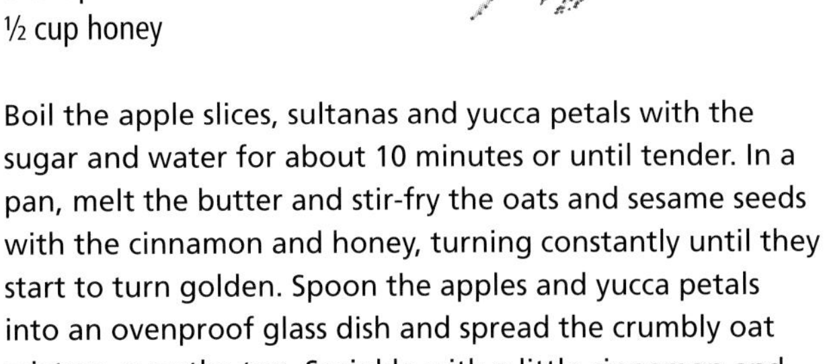

Boil the apple slices, sultanas and yucca petals with the sugar and water for about 10 minutes or until tender. In a pan, melt the butter and stir-fry the oats and sesame seeds with the cinnamon and honey, turning constantly until they start to turn golden. Spoon the apples and yucca petals into an ovenproof glass dish and spread the crumbly oat mixture over the top. Sprinkle with a little cinnamon and keep the dish hot until you are ready to serve. Serve with a generous helping of whipped cream, and top with a fresh yucca flower.

> COOK'S NOTE
> **Steep dried yucca flowers in sunflower oil, enough to cover the flowers, in a glass jar. Use it as an ingredient in stir-fries or served on home-baked bread the way the Mexicans did centuries ago – they claimed it gave strength and fleetness of foot!**

Therapeutic quick reference

The following is a list of ailments and the most effective healing flowers for each condition. Refer to the individual flower entry for information on the method of application and possible side-effects.

Always consult your medical practitioner before treating yourself or your family with home remedies.

A

abscess burdock, crab apple blossom, echinacea, hollyhock, pumpkin flowers
aching joints ajuga, anise, bergamot, chicory, coriander, cornflower, dandelion, day lily, fruit sage, sacred basil, St John's wort, turmeric, wild garlic
acidity anise, caraway, chamomile, fennel, hollyhock, mint, orange blossom
acne burdock, calendula, Cape sorrel, coriander, crab apple blossom, daisy, dandelion, echinacea, fennel, myrtle, roselle, rosemary, tuberose, waterblommetjie
aids echinacea, St John's wort
allergic rhinitis echinacea, elder flowers, hollyhock, mullein, sage
anaemia dandelion, Judas tree, lucerne
analgesic anise, Californian poppy, day lily, rosemary, St John's wort, turmeric, water lily
angina bulrush, chamomile, hawthorn
anorexia angelica, Korean mint, lucerne, turmeric
anti-allergenic chamomile, echinacea, yarrow
antibacterial calendula, lavender, mint, roselle, rosemary, sage, strawberry, thyme, turmeric, wild garlic, winter savory
antibiotic burdock, chives, echinacea, myrtle, nasturtium, sage, St John's wort
anti-cancer burdock, clover, lucerne, strawberry, violet, water lily
anticoagulant evening primrose, mullein
antifungal burdock, calendula, echinacea, Judas tree, sage, thyme, winter savory
anti-inflammatory calendula, chamomile, echinacea, fennel, goldenrod, hyssop, mint, rosemary, rose-scented pelargonium, turmeric, yarrow
anti-oxidant burdock, calendula, chamomile, goldenrod, hawthorn, mint, mullein, mustard, myrtle, nasturtium, rosemary, rose-scented pelargonium, thyme, winter savory
antispasmodic anise, Californian poppy, caraway, chamomile, coriander, evening primrose, fennel, hawthorn, honeysuckle, hyssop, mint, mustard, orange blossom, roselle, rosemary, St John's wort, yarrow
antiviral calendula, echinacea, hyssop, Korean mint, sage, St John's wort, strawberry
anxiety anise, borage, calendula, Californian poppy, carnation, catmint, chamomile, coriander, evening primrose, gardenia, granadilla, jasmine, lucerne, orange blossom, rose, sage, snapdragon, St John's wort, tuberose
aphrodisiac water lily, winter savory
appetite stimulant caraway, chives
arteriosclerosis buckwheat, hawthorn
arthritis ajuga, buckwheat, burdock, clover, elder flowers, goldenrod, mustard, rose-scented pelargonium, turmeric
asthma anise, chamomile, echinacea, evening primrose, gardenia, honeysuckle, hyssop, sage, wild garlic, winter savory
astringent calendula, myrtle, orange blossom, prickly pear, red hibiscus, roselle, rosemary, sage, St John's wort, strawberry, yarrow
athlete's foot sage, thyme

B

backache lucerne, St John's wort, thyme, wild garlic
bad breath almond blossom, anise, caraway, coriander, fennel, mint, plum blossom, rosemary
bedwetting Californian poppy, catmint, rose-scented pelargonium
bladder ailments carnation, carpet geranium, chives, cornflower, echinacea, fig, Judas tree, nasturtium
bladder tonic dandelion, garland chrysanthemum, pumpkin flowers, strawberry
bleeding calendula, daisy, gardenia, yarrow
blisters banana flower, fruit sage, fuchsia, gladiolus
bloating anise, artichoke, bergamot, caraway, carpet geranium, chamomile, coriander, fennel, garland chrysanthemum, hawthorn, Korean mint, mint, pea, yarrow
blocked nose calamint, mint, orange blossom, pineapple sage, roselle, sacred basil, sage, winter savory
blood pressure evening primrose, hawthorn, moringa
blood pressure, high ajuga, broccoli, chives, gardenia, hawthorn, pansy and viola, rosemary, stevia
blood pressure, low rosemary
blood sugar levels, regulate artichoke, burdock, rosemary
blood tonic borage, chives, dandelion, evening primrose, garland chrysanthemum, Judas tree, moringa, nasturtium, orange blossom, peach blossom, roselle
boils burdock, Cape sorrel, coriander, crab apple blossom, dandelion, echinacea, hollyhock, linseed, pumpkin flowers
bronchitis ajuga, angelica, anise, bergamot, borage, cauliflower, clover, echinacea, elder flowers, mullein, mustard, nasturtium, sacred basil, sage, thyme, violet, winter savory
bruises ajuga, buckwheat, calamint, daisy, day lily, delicious monster, evening primrose, fruit sage, gardenia, hollyhock, myrtle, peach blossom, rocket, safflower, waterblommetjie, wisteria
bunions dahlia
burns banana flower, Cape sorrel, feijoa, plumbago, prickly pear, St John's wort, tulip, water lily, waterblommetjie, yucca

C

callouses banana flower, fuchsia
calming borage, Californian poppy, chamomile, coriander, fruit sage, jasmine, Korean mint, lavender, rose-scented pelargonium, sage, tuberose, violet
catarrh angelica, chamomile, elder flowers, goldenrod, hollyhock, hyssop, mullein, orange blossom

chest pains anise, chamomile
chicken pox St John's wort, chamomile
chilblains buckwheat, calendula, echinacea, hawthorn, linseed
chills anise, Korean mint, linseed
cholesterol artichoke, buckwheat, chives, evening primrose, linseed, milk thistle, safflower, stevia, sunflower
chronic fatigue angelica, buckwheat, mint, rosemary
circulation, aid to burdock, elder flowers, hawthorn, hyssop, Korean mint, lucerne, rose, rosemary, sacred basil, safflower
circulatory ailments ajuga, angelica, buckwheat, bulrush, calendula, hawthorn, linseed, fennel, mustard, orange blossom, rose, turmeric
cold sores echinacea, elder flowers, St John's wort
colds ajuga, anise, bergamot, borage, broccoli, calamint, catmint, cauliflower, chives, crab apple blossom, daisy, echinacea, elder flowers, evening primrose, gladiolus, hollyhock, hyssop, lucerne, mullein, mustard, nasturtium, pansy and viola, pineapple sage, roselle, sacred basil, sage, St John's wort, thyme, turmeric, violet, wild garlic, winter savory
colic angelica, anise, bergamot, calamint, caraway, carpet geranium, catmint, chamomile, coriander, fennel, fruit sage, hollyhock, marigold, mint, prickly pear, sacred basil, sage, winter savory
colitis calendula, honeysuckle, prickly pear
conjunctivitis clover, linseed, rose
constipation broccoli, carnation, chicory, dandelion, fig, hyssop, linseed, mustard, orange blossom, plum blossom, turmeric, violet
corns banana flower, dahlia, dandelion, fuchsia
coughs ajuga, angelica, anise, bergamot, borage, calamint, caraway, catmint, cauliflower, chives, clover, cornflower, crab apple blossom, daisy, echinacea, elder flowers, evening primrose, gladiolus, hollyhock, honeysuckle, linseed, mullein, nasturtium, pansy and viola, pineapple sage, rose, roselle, sacred basil, sage, St John's wort, thyme, violet, wild garlic, winter savory, wisteria
cracked heels elder flowers, lavender, rose-scented pelargonium, yucca
Crohn's disease chamomile, mint
cuts and grazes banana flower, bulrush, calendula, Cape sorrel, dahlia, daisy, fuchsia, gardenia, gladiolus, linseed, peach blossom, prickly pear, pumpkin flowers, safflower, St John's wort, tulip, waterblommetjie, yucca
cystitis angelica, carpet geranium, chicory, gardenia, garland chrysanthemum, goldenrod, hollyhock, red hibiscus, strawberry

D

dandruff carpet geranium, sage
deodorant artichoke, fruit sage, garland chrysanthemum, lavender, rosemary, rose-scented pelargonium
depression buckwheat, jasmine, lavender, milk thistle, orange blossom, rose, rosemary, rose-scented pelargonium, St John's wort
detoxifying artichoke, burdock, calamint, calendula, chicory, dandelion, echinacea, fennel, fruit sage, garland chrysanthemum, Korean mint, lucerne, peach blossom, thyme
diabetes artichoke, strawberry
diarrhoea bulrush, carpet geranium, catmint, crab apple blossom, daisy, feijoa, gladiolus, goldenrod, hawthorn, hollyhock, moringa, prickly pear, sage, strawberry
digestive aid angelica, anise, artichoke, bergamot, caraway, chives, fennel, fruit sage, marigold, mint, mustard, pea, red hibiscus, roselle, rosemary, sage, thyme, tuberose, winter savory
digestive ailments anise, bergamot, calamint, chamomile, calendula, coriander, cornflower, evening primrose, fennel, fig, gladiolus, goldenrod, hollyhock, hyssop, Korean mint, linseed, mint, pea, prickly pear, sage, strawberry, tuberose, winter savory
disinfectant day lily, sage, thyme
diuretic anise, burdock, caraway, dandelion, fennel, garland chrysanthemum, goldenrod, hawthorn, Judas tree, marigold, moringa, mustard, roselle, rose-scented pelargonium, sacred basil, sunflower, turmeric
diverticulitis hollyhock, mint
dizziness lavender, mint, rosemary
dry skin almond blossom, bergamot, bulrush, calendula, carnation, carpet geranium, dahlia, delicious monster, elder flowers, fruit sage, honeysuckle, lavender, mint, sage, tulip, yucca
dysentery crab apple blossom, feijoa, gladiolus, mint, moringa

E

earache echinacea, elder flowers, mullein
eczema borage, burdock, calendula, carnation, chamomile, clover, elder flowers, evening primrose, honeysuckle, mullein, pansy and viola, peach blossom, thyme, violet, water lily
energising almond blossom, lucerne, rosemary, St John's wort, thyme
expectorant angelica, anise, calamint, caraway, fennel, honeysuckle, hyssop, mullein, sunflower, thyme
eye ailments calendula, chamomile, clover, cornflower, daisy

F

fainting lavender, rosemary, yarrow
fear borage, evening primrose, gardenia, granadilla, Korean mint, lavender, orange blossom, tuberose
fever angelica, bergamot, borage, calendula, dandelion, elder flowers, gardenia, hawthorn, Korean mint, moringa, mullein, red hibiscus, sacred basil, safflower, wild garlic, yarrow
fever blisters echinacea, elder flowers, stevia
flatulence anise, artichoke, bergamot, caraway, carpet geranium, catmint, coriander, fennel, fruit sage, marigold, mint, prickly pear, rosemary, winter savory
flu ajuga, angelica, borage, broccoli, calamint, catmint, chives, cornflower, echinacea, elder flowers, gardenia, Korean mint, lucerne, mustard, nasturtium, sacred basil, thyme, turmeric, winter savory
freckles elder flowers, fuchsia, water lily
fungicidal echinacea, rosemary, rose-scented pelargonium, Korean mint, sage, thyme

G

gall bladder ailments artichoke, calendula, chicory, crab apple

H

I

K

L

M

N

O

P

postnasal drip chamomile, elder flowers, violet
postnatal depression buckwheat, lucerne, mint
post-viral fatigue syndrome (ME) Californian poppy, echinacea, St John's wort
premenstrual tension borage, evening primrose, hawthorn, orange blossom, rosemary, yarrow
prostate problems dandelion, pumpkin flowers, prickly pear
psoriasis borage, burdock, calendula, carpet geranium, clover, elder flowers

R

rashes banana flower, borage, burdock, calendula, chamomile, clover, coriander, dahlia, daisy, feijoa, fruit sage, fuchsia, hollyhock, honeysuckle, Judas tree, linseed, mint, myrtle, pansy and viola, peach blossom, plumbago, poppy, prickly pear, snapdragon, St John's wort, strawberry, tulip, violet, water lily, waterblommetjie, yucca
respiratory ailments bergamot, borage, burdock, calamint, chives, cornflower, evening primrose, honeysuckle, Judas tree, moringa, mullein, sage, thyme, turmeric, winter savory
restlessness anise, chamomile, lavender
rheumatism ajuga, angelica, chicory, coriander, cornflower, dandelion, day lily, honeysuckle, lavender, linseed, marigold, moringa, mullein, mustard, pansy and viola, rosemary, thyme, turmeric, waterblommetjie, wild garlic
ringworm Korean mint, thyme

S

scabies elder flowers, thyme
scalp problems banana flower, carpet geranium, rosemary, yucca
sciatica St John's wort
scurvy Cape sorrel, nasturtium
sedative bergamot, Californian poppy, catmint, chamomile, hawthorn, jasmine, orange blossom, rose, St John's wort
shingles chamomile, St John's wort
shock anise, Korean mint, mint
sinus problems bergamot, calamint, elder flowers, goldenrod, linseed, mullein, violet, winter savory
skin ailments almond blossom, banana flower, borage, burdock, calendula, carnation, chicory, dahlia, daisy, delicious monster, echinacea, elder flowers, evening primrose, feijoa, fennel, fuchsia, hollyhock, honeysuckle, Judas tree, Korean mint, lavender, mint, moringa, mullein, myrtle, pansy and viola, plumbago, poppy, prickly pear, snapdragon, rocket, rose, roselle, rosemary, violet, wisteria, yucca
sore nipples calendula, chamomile
sore throat ajuga, bergamot, calamint, daisy, echinacea, elder flowers, fuchsia, Korean mint, lavender, moringa, nasturtium, plum blossom, roselle, sage, stevia, thyme, wild garlic, winter savory, wisteria
sprains and strains ajuga, burdock, calamint, day lily, delicious monster, fruit sage, myrtle, rocket, safflower, snapdragon, St John's wort, waterblommetjie
stiffness burdock, cornflower, jasmine, pansy and viola, rosemary, rose-scented pelargonium
stimulating Korean mint, lucerne, mint, rosemary
strained throat anise, chamomile, sage, snapdragon
stress anise, borage, catmint, chamomile, gardenia, hawthorn, jasmine, Judas tree, lucerne, orange blossom, sacred basil, St John's wort, tuberose
sunburn almond blossom, banana flower, bergamot, borage, calendula, delicious monster, feijoa, fuchsia, honeysuckle, linseed, mint, pineapple sage, plumbago, red hibiscus, snapdragon, water lily, waterblommetjie

T

tension anise, catmint, hawthorn, jasmine, Korean mint, lavender, lucerne, sacred basil
thrush calendula, goldenrod, sage, thyme, winter savory
tight chest angelica, anise, bergamot, borage, calamint, honeysuckle, Judas tree
tired feet banana flower, dahlia, fruit sage, gladiolus, lavender, linseed, mint
tonic almond blossom, borage, buckwheat, cornflower, mustard, pea, sage, St John's wort, thyme, wisteria, yarrow
tonsillitis echinacea, fuchsia, sage
tooth decay anise, moringa, sage, stevia
toothache anise, Californian poppy, day lily, echinacea, Judas tree, yarrow
tranquillising lavender, rose-scented pelargonium, water lily
tremors cornflower

U

urinary tract ailments angelica, chicory, chives, fennel, goldenrod, hyssop, linseed, mustard, myrtle, peach blossom, sacred basil, strawberry

V

vaginal itching buckwheat, clover, elder flowers
varicose veins buckwheat, daisy, mullein, wisteria
verrucas dandelion
vertigo cornflower, lavender, mint, rosemary
vomiting bergamot, caraway, fennel, Korean mint, tuberose

W

warts dandelion, fig, poppy
weak nails Judas tree, pineapple sage, tuberose
weight loss evening primrose, fennel
whooping cough anise, borage, caraway, clover, mint, thyme, violet
worms pumpkin seeds, thyme
wounds banana flower, bergamot, bulrush, calendula, crab apple blossom, daisy, evening primrose, mullein, prickly pear, pumpkin flowers, safflower, turmeric, yarrow, yucca

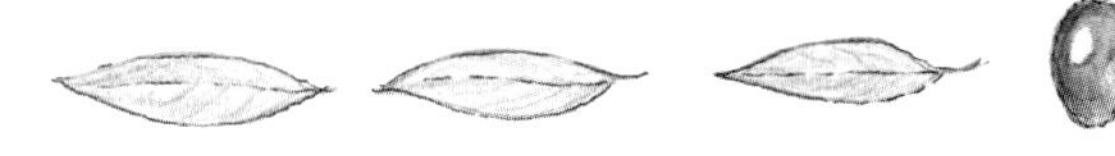
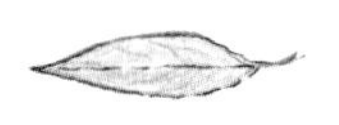
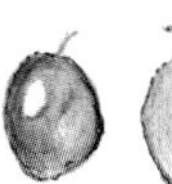
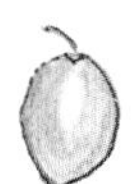
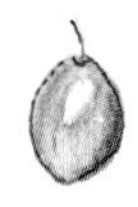
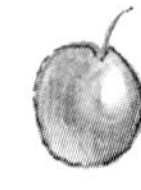
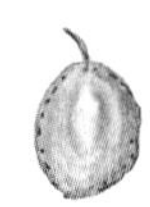

Flower index

Recipe index

Breakfast dishes:

Cakes and biscuits:

Cheese dishes:

Condiments and preserves:

Desserts:

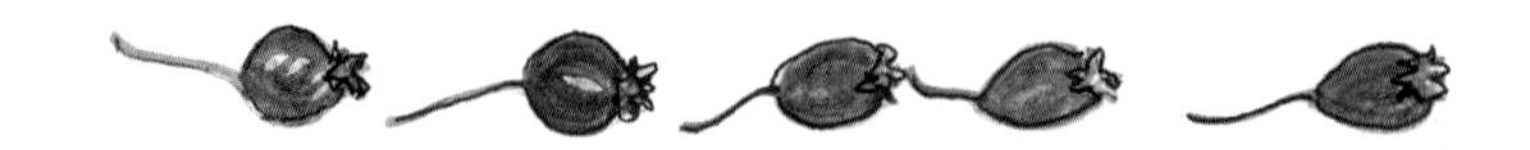